PRAISE FOR

YOGA AND THE QUEST FOR THE TRUE SELF

"This book provides a comprehensive—and blessedly comprehensible—introduction to yoga metaphysics. . . . In a market that's fairly glutted with books about the 'how' of hatha yoga, Cope provides valuable insight into the profound 'why' of this ancient science—along with a totally great read."

—*Los Angeles Times*

"Few other accessible books provide as good an overview of the spirituality of yoga. As a result, this will be in demand wherever yoga is popular."

—*Library Journal*

"Cope . . . lights up a notoriously arcane subject for Western readers."

—*Publishers Weekly*

"Amid the torrent of how-to-do-asanas titles flooding the market, *Yoga and the Quest for the True Self* is a patch of high ground where one can dry out and achieve a little perspective. [Cope is] a crisp writer and gifted storyteller. . . . [*Yoga and the Quest for the True Self*] is an authoritative yet heartfelt volume, refreshingly free of jargon, pleasing to read, full of sage advice and encouragement."

—*Yoga Journal*

"Cope shares his experiences, observations, and revelations in a highly readable blend of personal anecdotes, classic Hindu and yogic teaching stories, and in-depth considerations of the physiological and psychological benefits associated with the regular practice of asanas, yoga postures, and pranayama, the control of the breath."

—*Booklist*

"Beyond the feel-good hype—and authentic benefits—that have driven contemporary interest in this ancient art, there lies another reality that has far deeper roots in yoga's history. Cope . . . explores the psychological and spiritual dimensions of this path to liberation while insightfully bringing its practice down to earth."

—*NAPRA ReView*

"Intellectually precise, profoundly moving, and gratifyingly accessible . . . Stephen Cope has written a book that offers hope that the fruits of spiritual practice and the attainment of wisdom are not for some more enlightened person, but for you and me."

—Donna Farhi, international yoga teacher
and author of *The Breathing Book*

"With rare clarity and wit, Stephen Cope shows us how yoga can guide us through the maze of our psyche—and home to our own soul."

—Anne Cushman, former senior editor, *Yoga Journal*,
and co-author of *From Here to Nirvana*

"*Yoga and the Quest for the True Self* is a splendid bridge between traditional yoga and the concerns and needs of contemporary Western seekers. Stephen Cope takes you straight to the heart of yoga."

—Georg Feuerstein, Ph.D., founder-president of the Yoga Research
and Education Center; author of *The Yoga Tradition* and
The Shambhala Encyclopedia of Yoga

"Stephen Cope's wonderful new book captures the essential magic of yoga—brilliantly helping us to connect muscle, bone, and sinew with spirit, soul, and consciousness. An inspiring guide for anyone interested in the deepest possibilities of human existence."

—John Welwood, author of *Journey of the Heart*

"Stephen Cope dances on the spiritual path with practical feet and enticing insight."

—Marion Woodman, author of *Coming Home to Myself*

"A superb account of what it means to make yoga a part of one's life . . . accessible, engaging, and refreshingly free of pretentiousness and jargon."

—Michael Washburn, author of *The Ego and the Dynamic Ground*
and *Transpersonal Psychology in Psychoanalytic Perspective*

by Stephen Cope

The Great Work of Your Life
The Wisdom of Yoga
Yoga and the Quest for the True Self

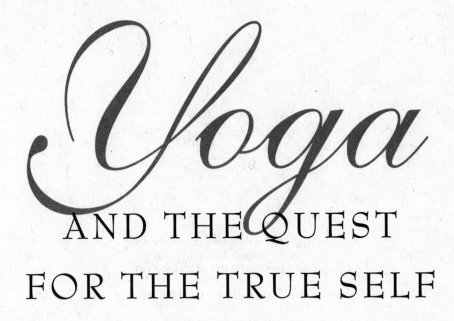

Yoga

AND THE QUEST
FOR THE TRUE SELF

STEPHEN COPE

Bantam Books

NEW YORK   TORONTO   LONDON   SYDNEY   AUCKLAND

YOGA AND THE QUEST FOR THE TRUE SELF

PUBLISHING HISTORY
Bantam hardcover edition published October 1999
Bantam trade paperback edition / September 2000

ISBN 978-0-553-37835-1

Published simultaneously in the United States and Canada

Bantam Books are published by Bantam Books, a division of
Random House, Inc. Its trademark, consisting of the words
"Bantam Books" and the portrayal of a rooster, is Registered in
U.S. Patent and Trademark Office and in other countries. Marca
Registrada. Bantam Books, New York, New York.

PRINTED IN THE UNITED STATES OF AMERICA

BVG 20 19 18 17 16 15

For my first teachers:

Robert Samuel Cope, Barbara Crothers Cope,

Oliver Frisbie Crothers, and Armeda Van Demark Crothers

CONTENTS

INTRODUCTION

Recent surveys reveal that more than eleven million Americans currently do yoga on a regular basis—in YMCAs, health clubs, private studios, senior centers, living room floors, and retreat centers around the country.[1] The Miami Dolphins and the Chicago Bulls are doing it. The Royal Canadian Mounted Police are doing it. Sting, Madonna, Kareem Abdul-Jabbar, Raquel Welch, Woody Harrelson, Jane Fonda, and Ali McGraw are doing it. With almost alarming rapidity, practices whose secrets have been handed down for thousands of years exclusively through the tradition of "whispered wisdom," from adept to student, have landed on Main Street U.S.A.

There are many obvious reasons for this rapprochement. Yoga is probably the world's most perfect form of exercise. It cultivates cardiovascular health, and musculoskeletal strength and flexibility, without the painful and damaging side effects of high-impact aerobics. It tunes up every organ system—respiratory, digestive, reproductive, endocrine, lymphatic, and nervous. It cultivates the body's capacity to relax and dramatically reduces the negative effects of stress. With regular yoga practice, we breathe better. We sleep better. We digest our food better. We feel better. We may even begin to recover from chronic illness. And, for many Americans, the best part is that none of these amazing outcomes requires long years of training and apprenticeship. The benefits of practice are immediate. We are, by and large, a very practical people. And yoga is a very practical endeavor.

Yet the immediate physical benefits of yoga—widely reported in medical journals and the mainstream press—may be only the tip of the iceberg. Regular practitioners of yoga describe a whole host of subtle transformations in their lives, changes that seem more mysterious, more difficult to quantify and even to describe. Many experience moments of sharply increased mental focus and clarity, and heightened perceptual and intuitive powers. Some describe a dramatic increase in energy and stamina, emotional evenness and equanimity. Others report a heightened feeling of connection to an inner self, ecstatic states of bliss, and profound well-being. And there are the not-infrequent stories of truly miraculous healings—physical, emotional, spiritual.

I first discovered yoga thirteen years ago. I had been practicing Buddhist meditation for some fifteen years, and had heard that yoga was a wonderful preparation for meditation. "It calms the body," said my friend Paula. "It prepares the mind for meditation. Try it." I tried it. My meditation practice deepened noticeably. But I discovered in yoga much more than just a preparation for meditation. I soon began to experience its more remarkable benefits. Intrigued, I began to look more deeply into this practice. And what I found excited me both as a suffering human being and as a psychotherapist wrestling daily with the suffering of others. Here was a methodical approach to the restoration of the full potential of the human being, a systematic path to what ancient seekers called *jivan mukti,* the "soul awake in this lifetime."

Yoga speaks in a startlingly fresh way to the concerns we Western seekers bring to our psychological and spiritual journeys. Americans suffer inordinately with what therapists call problems of the self—an inability to self-soothe; an inability to sustain a satisfying and cohesive sense of self over time; an inability to warmly love the self; an inability to maintain an ongoing sense of belonging and a deep sense of meaning and purpose in life.

"Self-estrangement" is the curious new word we've devised to describe this particular brand of suffering. We live deeply ensconced in the cult of the individual. We live what we like to think of as "our lives," often disconnected from and independent of the world of nature, as well as from the dark and mysterious world of the soul. We live cut off from a sense of our true deep mutual belonging and interdependence, and we suffer from a painful sense of separation—a separation from the life of the body; a separation from the hidden depths of life, its mystery and interiority; a separation from the source of our own guidance, wisdom, and compassion; and a separation from the life-giving roots of human community.

What a surprise to find that the psychology and practice of yoga speak directly to the problems of self-estrangement. Indeed, alienation from the self is the entire focus of yoga philosophy. Here is a language that, unlike our current psychological language, is deeply concerned with the relationship between the soul and the self, the body and the soul, the divine and the human. Here is a systematic exploration of the unconscious that predates Freud by thousands of years. Here is a psychology that described the collective unconscious and the transpersonal self several millennia before Carl Jung. Here is a philosophy that understood life as an archetypal pilgrimage to the center long before the New Age. Here is a psychological language not yet rendered impotent by cliché or commercialism, and, even more refreshingly, one that is uncomplicated by Calvinism and Puritanism and is free of the Western obsession with guilt and shame.

Nonetheless, yoga's deepest secrets are not easily accessible. Those of us who lift the lid to peer more deeply into its mysteries may find ourselves bewildered. Initially, we bump up against an incomprehensible stew of every conceivable philosophy, psychology, and metaphysic ever brewed up on the spiritually fecund subcontinent of India. Veda, Vedanta, Samkhya, Tantra; ancient and modern, esoteric and practical, magical and scientific. As novelist Arundhati Roy says of her native land, "India is a land that lives in many centuries at once." In the world of yoga, primitive and archaic religious forms lie side by side with the most sublime and sophisticated spirituality known to humankind. How are we to find our way in this strange new world?

When I first began inquiring more deeply into yoga, I lamented the fact that there were so few books about the real experience of the transformation wrought by this practice. There were plenty of how-to books to help me learn the basics about yoga postures and breathing. There were mountains of hyperbolic accounts of the lives of Indian saints and yogis—fascinating stories about time travel, bilocation, knowledge of former births, understanding the languages of animals and birds. There was a flood tide of nearly incomprehensible Hindu metaphysics, filled with high-flown descriptions of ecstatic states—the union with the One, the Absolute, cosmic consciousness, and transcendence of the phenomenal world. But where were the descriptions of neurotic Western seekers like myself? Where was my story?

For ten years now I have lived and taught at the largest residential yoga center in the world—Kripalu Center for Yoga and Health, in

Lenox, Massachusetts. Day in and day out it is my privilege to hear the stories of contemporary seekers, many of them quite a bit like myself, asking the same questions I asked. They come here to practice yoga—seventeen thousand of them a year—as I did, hoping it will help. And most often it does, in ways they hadn't imagined. But how? And why? What is all this about *kundalini* and *chakras*? Is it real? Where do these practices lead? If I persevere am I going to end up wearing *mala* beads, saffron robes, and living on a mountaintop? Whom can I trust to guide me through this fascinating new world?

In this book, I have attempted to write the Baedeker I needed as I began my own exploration—an account of the interaction of real Western human beings with the psychology, philosophy, and practice of yoga; an account that attempts to build a bridge between a sometimes complicated and esoteric theory and an essentially very straightforward and down-to-earth practice.

I begin with a classic yogic parable of transformation, "Viveka's Tale," which lays the groundwork for the entire journey that follows. In Part One, "The Discovery of the Royal Secret," I use aspects of my own story, and those of friends, colleagues, and psychotherapy patients, to describe contemporary versions of Viveka's experience of exile, hearing the call of the true self, and setting out on the royal road home.

Part Two, "The Self in Exile," takes us more deeply into the yogic view of the human dilemma and describes the fundamental components of yoga's psychology of the self. This section is supported by the appendix, "Yoga Metaphysics with a Light Touch," which offers a more detailed outline of classic yoga philosophy.

Part Three, "Encounters with the Mother and the Seer," describes the birth of witness consciousness, which is both the path and the goal of all yogic practice. This section focuses on the twin pillars of witness consciousness—awareness and equanimity—their psychological and emotional origins, and their final transmutation into the most mature forms of human consciousness.

Part Four, "The Spontaneous Wisdom of the Body," tells the story of three contemporary yogis and their very different and fascinating transformations through the regular practice of yoga postures and *pranayama* (yogic breathing). This section describes the interplay of consciousness and energy in the practice of *hatha* yoga (the form most familiar to Americans), and their relationship to the final goals of yoga.

Part Five, "The Royal Road Home," describes—through both classical and contemporary stories—some of the surprising components of mature practice in the yoga traditions.

The most interesting story in the world of yoga right now lies at the point of intersection between the ancient forms of yoga and the reality of twentieth-century lives and culture. I approach the story wearing the motley array of hats I've collected during my adult life. The first hat, of course, is that of a suffering and confused human being. But a close second and third are those of the psychotherapist, trained in psychoanalytic psychotherapy, and the yoga teacher, trained in Kripalu yoga. There are other voices, too, that make an occasional appearance—the theologian, trained at Episcopal Divinity School in my midtwenties; the anthropologist, trained as an undergraduate at Amherst College; the dancer, trained as a member of the Minnesota Dance Theater in Minneapolis.

The point of intersection that I describe is fascinating not only because of the capacity the ancient science of yoga has to change our lives, but also because of the capacity we have to change yoga. Through its intersection with the West, yoga is undergoing a time of enormous evolution. It is being feminized, democratized, and brought into relationship with contemporary medicine, Western psychology, and with Buddhism, Christianity, and Judaism.

America's love affair with yoga is just beginning. And as with all love affairs there will be highs and lows, light and shadow. As one prominent character in this book repeatedly declares, "The valleys are as low as the mountains are high." In following the story, I have tried not to shy away from the lows: the unrealistic idealization of gurus and the creation of yogic cults; the unbalanced pursuit of supernormal powers instead of liberation; the commercialization of a spiritual path; the attempts to transcend the painful realities of intimacy, identity, work.

As author Jon Kabat-Zinn has said, "Wherever we go, there we are," and yet it is my experience that for many of us, after exposure to the practice of yoga there is simply, and at times astonishingly, a great deal more of us there. More consciousness, more energy, more awareness, more equanimity, more life in the body, more connection with the mysteries of the soul. And there is that wonderful, haunting voice of the true self that calls to us, that keeps us company as we stride deeper and deeper into the world, determined to save the only soul we really can save.

A NOTE TO READERS

It is impossible to understand the living truth of yoga without getting close to the experiences of real practitioners. But in writing an "experience near" account of yoga, I have had to face a difficult challenge: How to tell the stories of my friends on the path, my colleagues, patients and students, without invading their privacy? I have chosen in almost every case to create composites—sticking as closely as I am able to the truth of real experiences with yoga, while creating essentially fictional characters. Many of us will see aspects of ourselves in these characters, but, aside from a handful (whom I have given their real names) the characters in this book do not, and are not meant to, represent any actual persons.

This book is not in any way meant to be a study of the history, sociology, or psychology of the Kripalu community. Where I have used aspects of Kripalu's story, I have done so as a doorway into more universal issues regarding yoga and psychospiritual transformation. Hundreds of students and guests who have lived through various eras in Kripalu's complicated twenty-five-year history will have had considerably different experiences than I have. I represent here only my own story.

Viveka's Tale

The voice hesitant,
and her hand trembling
in the dark for yours.

She touches your face
and says your name
in the same instant.

The one you refuse to say
over and over again.
The one you refuse to say.

—David Whyte,
"The Soul Lives Contented"

We are not who we think we are.

"Viveka's Tale," an archetypal parable of the Indian religious imagination, reveals the single most pervasive theme in yogic scriptures and folktales: Our true self remains deeply hidden, incognito, submerged beneath a web of mistaken identities.

Once upon a time, in a small kingdom in northern India, a beautiful young queen named Atma gave birth to a son, whom she called Viveka. Auspicious signs accompanied the birth. There was a rainbow. Flocks of white doves were sighted, and a lush rainfall sweetened the ripening fields of the kingdom. Little Viveka was loved by all. Around him, however, a silent contagion festered. In the absence of the king, who was away fighting infidels on the northern border, an internecine struggle broke out in the royal household. Finally, as a result of the sinister backroom plotting of several courtiers driven by greed for the throne, the young prince, the sole heir to the throne, was stolen from the nursery and abandoned to the elements—sent floating down the river in a basket to his certain doom.

As fate would have it, however, the young child was rescued by a group of very poor peasants and social outcastes who lived in a remote area of the kingdom near the mouth of the river. They reared Viveka as one of their own, sharing with him all they had to give, in a life of grinding poverty and deprivation. The peasants did not reveal to Viveka the mystery surrounding his true origins, and Viveka grew up identifying himself as an outcaste, immersed in the life of poverty and hopelessness that he had learned.

But something else lived inside Viveka. He had a recurring dream of palaces and lush green fields and a mother's love. Viveka had an enduring and secret fantasy that he had another home, another family. Inside him remained subtle traces of the paradise he had lost. Meanwhile, back at the court, others, too, were dreaming of him, dreaming and praying that he still lived. On the morning of his sixteenth birthday, Viveka's mother appeared to him in a dream. She called him by his true name, which he recognized at once. In the early hours of the morning, Viveka awakened in a cold sweat. His mother had called him home and had sent him a vision of the landmarks he should seek in his pilgrimage back to his true family.

Just before dawn that morning, Viveka set out on a quest for his true home and family, with nothing but the clothes on his back and several days' rations of food. For seven years, Viveka searched, looking for the landmarks his mother had given to him in the dream. Along the way, he encountered every conceivable obstacle—wild animals, thieves, sorcerers, bands of outlaws, hunger, fear, hallucinations. But as he roamed the mountains and plains of northern India, he also encountered naked ash-smeared yogis, seers, ascetics in caves, countless holy men and women who shared with him all their yogic wisdom and assisted him in his quest.

Among these wandering *sadhus*, Viveka discovered Rudra, his first important mentor, whom he met as he huddled in a cave during a wild thunderstorm on a mountaintop, and with whom he lived and studied for a year and a quarter. With Rudra, Viveka studied the secret practices of yoga and meditation. Through the "whispered wisdom" he learned from this great sage, Viveka eventually trained himself to enter deep states of concentration, in which his awareness could penetrate the unmanifest realms. In the last days of his apprenticeship, Viveka learned to merge his consciousness with the one transcendent ground of being, *brahman*. He mastered the art of transcending time and space, and could send his body anywhere he wished. Eventually, he used his supernormal powers of bilocation to visit his mother and to reassure her that he was coming home.

Viveka now saw clearly where he had to go. In order to arrive home, he had to cross a final obstacle—a dangerous forest, filled with tigers, vipers, and evil spirits of every sort. Just at the end of his perilous journey through the forest, at the far edge of the darkest section, Viveka was seriously wounded in an encounter with a tiger-spirit. His battered body was dragged from the forest by a wise woman who lived in a small hut in the marketplace of the village, just at the forest's edge. The wise woman was known in the village simply as Mother, and she was to be Viveka's next important mentor. She brought Viveka to her hut, where she tended him. Over the course of the year and a quarter he spent with Mother, Viveka learned the next stage of yoga. Mother taught him to see God in all beings, and to see the soul in the phenomenal world, even in the tiger who attacked him. Viveka learned to open his heart to himself and to all of life, practicing reverence for the many beings and dedicating himself to the awakening of all beings.

Viveka's final lesson in yoga still awaited him, however. Having taught him many of the secrets of life and of his true nature, the wise woman told him that he must now finish his pilgrimage. He must reach home in his physical body, to embrace his real mother, the queen, and to take up his *dharma*, his rightful place in the order of things. When Viveka finally entered the doors of the palace, he was greeted with great celebrations; he was told that his father had died during his long war in the north and that Viveka himself was now the king. At first, he could not comprehend what this meant, and he shrank from his duty. He could not find "king" anywhere inside himself. Under the patient tutelage of his final teacher, a renowned seer who lived near the palace, and over a period of many months, Viveka was eventually able to see through the final remnants of his mistaken identity. He discovered his true royal nature inside. He knew, beyond a shadow of a doubt, that he was a king. Finally, Viveka assumed the throne, where he ruled wisely and well for many years.

Stories of "hidden realities," such as "Viveka's Tale," are central to the yogic view of the human dilemma.[1] Though the details of these parables vary greatly, their moral is always the same: We live in alienation from our true nature. Like Viveka, we are a magnificent possibility in disguise. Like him, we intuit these possibilities. We dream about them. We long for them.

Viveka is the archetypal yogi (literally, "one who practices yoga"), and his story is meant to dramatize the fundamental yogic view that our lives only make sense when understood as a sacred quest for the true self. The practices of yoga, which Viveka encountered on his pilgrimage home, are organized around the belief that all human beings have the innate capacity and longing to mature to full aliveness, that all human beings are born with the seed of awake, conscious mind. Yogis believe that this inborn seed of consciousness will trouble us, as it did Viveka, will call to us, and, finally, will compel us on our own pilgrimage to awakening. Like Viveka, when we finally commit to the quest for the true self, we will discover that we are not alone on our journey. One day, to our astonishment, we will find that the true self for which we are searching is also searching for us.

Part One

THE DISCOVERY
OF THE ROYAL SECRET

1

WAKING UP IS

HARD TO DO

You see, I want a lot.
Perhaps I want everything
the darkness that comes with every infinite fall
and the shivering blaze of every step up.

So many live on and want nothing
and are raised to the rank of prince
by the slippery ease of their light judgments.

But what you love to see are faces
that do work and feel thirst.
You love most of all those who need you
as they need a crowbar or a hoe.
You have not grown old, and it is not too late
to dive into your increasing depths
where life calmly gives out its own secret.

—Rainer Maria Rilke,
Das Stundenbuch

I leaned against a doorframe and quietly surveyed the party swirling
around me. Laughing revelers spilled through the doors of Mark's big
living room onto the bluestone terrace and down the sweep of lawn. It
was just dusk, and a warm May breeze brought the scent of lilac. Mark
throws parties like his theatrical productions, I thought: lavish and well

attended. I wondered anxiously if Sean would show up with his new lover.

I took a deep breath and sighed, turning back into the big kitchen at the rear of the house. The antique harvest table in the center of the room was abundant with the kind of food we eat when we're supposed to be having fun—casseroles stuffed with ricotta; desserts made with whipped cream; salads sprinkled with pine nuts and feta cheese. The odor of warming lasagna, my contribution to the party menu, wafted from the oven. It was a relief to be alone for a moment. My eye caught the pile of dirty dishes near the sink, and I filled the dishpan with soapy water and began to wash a pot. The warm water felt good on my hands.

"Want some help with that?" came a voice from the door. I hadn't heard her come in. Paula stood in the doorway looking particularly elegant in a slim black sheath, her brown hair cropped in a perky new style I hadn't seen before.

"Did you get tired of the party, too?" she asked as she picked up a stray dishtowel.

"Just not in much of a party mood." I attacked the burned edge of a cake pan with my Brillo pad. "But Mark swore he couldn't have a party unless I made my vegetable lasagna. He only loves me for my casseroles."

Paula's smile lit up her fine features. She was beautiful in the way only a forty-five-year-old woman can be, and I was glad for her quiet company. Paula picked up the pot I'd just washed and began drying. I pulled the lasagna out of the oven and set it down on a hot plate on the sideboard. We worked together in silence for a moment, then she asked me if I was OK. I felt relief admitting I was not, that I was depressed.

"You sure do a good job of covering it up," she said, referring to the little riff I'd done at the piano that broke everybody up. She told me how well she thought I was handling the situation.

"It's still hard being at parties by myself . . . without Sean. I'm not used to it yet."

Paula put her hand on my shoulder. As usual, her instinct was just right.

"How're things with you and ol' Geoff?" I asked, pulling back from the moment of closeness.

Paula was silent for a moment. "Have I told you that I've been on Prozac for the last year?" I was surprised. Paula and I studied with the same yoga teacher in Cambridge, and we saw each other once or twice a week in class. I'd always thought of Geoff and Paula as the together "power couple." Geoff was a well-known lawyer, currently experiencing his fifteen minutes of fame in a notorious political case in Washington, D.C. Paula was a successful marketing executive for a large mutual fund in Boston.

"Let's talk," I said, scooping out two small plates of lasagna. She poured two glasses of wine, and we cleared a place at the table.

In the last two months, Paula and I had grown closer. Her seventeen-year-old gay nephew, Matt, of whom she was particularly fond, had made a suicide attempt, and I'd sat up most of one night with Paula and her sister in a hospital waiting room. We'd had coffee or a phone chat weekly since then, talking mostly about Matt.

"Prozac? How come you never told me?"

She said she'd been embarrassed, covering it over, minimizing, doing what I'd just done with her. She reached out a hand and touched my arm. "You're a really good friend, Steve. I don't want to have to put on a face with you."

"I don't either. But you know, I'm the ultimate Lone Ranger. All those years of heavy-duty WASP training—'never complain and never explain.' But you first. I want to know how you're doing."

Slowly, Paula began to reveal another side of herself. Under the surface of her successful corporate career, she felt a sense of desperation. Her job had always been a pressure cooker, she said, but now she seemed less able to tolerate it. For the past year, she'd regularly had panic attacks on Sunday nights as she contemplated going back to work after the weekend. Work nights, she would often go to bed early, hoping for a refreshing night's sleep, only to sit bolt upright at two AM with her mind racing: deadlines, pressure to perform, competition with a rival rising star who was, as Paula put it, "younger and hungrier than I am."

"You know, I truly don't remember why I'm doing this work," she lamented. "I don't really care about it anymore. If I'm going to pour out my energy the way I do in that job, I want to be doing something that matters." I was aware that it was Sunday night and Paula was facing a new workweek.

"I don't know if my work life feels empty because I'm depressed, or if I'm depressed because it feels empty." Paula went on to describe how she'd begun to feel melancholy and confused a year earlier, when both children had been out of the house for the first time. Katy, nineteen, was now in college in California, and Marc, twenty-four, was in New York, struggling with a nascent career in music.

"But it's not just that I miss them. It's like I'm lonely for myself. I feel like I'm missing life. And I'm sad about that."

It was a relief to be talking to somebody else whose life was falling apart. "I've been feeling like that for the last eight months, since Sean left. It's like, Humpty-Dumpty had a great fall, and I can't seem to put the pieces back together again."

"Tell me about that," she said.

"He was in the middle of some kind of midlife lunacy, I guess." I told her the worst part—that he was having an affair with a guy in his twenties, whom everyone said looked exactly as I had at that age. "He actually took him to our goddamned summer place when I wasn't there. It just walloped me, experiencing betrayal like that after fifteen years together." I had been living in a state of shock, uncomprehending. How could he leave all that we had?

"It's unbelievable. You just watch as the whole infrastructure of your life collapses—friends, extended family, rituals, holidays, the cat and dog, neighbors. I mean, Sean is my niece's godfather. I adore his family. And we had so many friends who looked up to us as a stable gay couple." I wasn't feeling self-pity so much as bewilderment, like standing on a dock in a storm, watching helplessly as the boat that contains your most precious possessions comes off its mooring and drifts slowly out to sea.

I wondered secretly if I would be ruined beyond repair by this loss. I felt sure that I would never have the treasure of a relationship lasting long into old age the way my parents and grandparents had had. And I'd always assumed I would have this. I took another sip of wine and looked into the middle distance. What had I done wrong? Was there a great big *L* for loser plastered on my back that nobody had told me about?

"Here's the thing that's really got me, Paula. Forgiving betrayal like this seems to require some huge grown-upness, a maturity I don't seem to have. It's the hardest thing I've had to face in my life."

"Forgiveness, yes," she murmured, dragging a fork across her empty plate. I wondered, then, whom she had yet to forgive. After a moment, I smiled. "Help!" Paula pantomimed a big, hysterical scream. We both laughed, and I reached for one of Mark's nasty death-by-chocolate brownies, gulping it down as though it was the only thing that could give me comfort.

I told her how I'd spent the last few months trying to rebuild my life—purchasing a new house that I'd been renovating, seeing thirty-five patients a week, running myself ragged schlepping around town to meetings, volunteering for the AIDS action committee, receiving and giving clinical supervision, feverishly working out at the gym five days a week. And making an effort to appear marginally social.

"I'm exhausted," I said with a sigh. Paula placed the back of her hand against her forehead, in such a perfect expression of the neurasthenic housewife that we both cracked up. Like a good therapist, she'd picked up the not-so-subtle strain of hysteria in my personality and reflected it back to me.

"You know what my fantasy is?" she asked, shifting in her chair and pulling her knees up to her chin. "Have you ever read that little book about the guy who spent a year alone in that house on the beach at Truro?"

"*The Outermost House*! I can't believe that's your fantasy, too." As we continued to talk, we discovered that we shared a fascination with other solitary beings—Thoreau, Annie Dillard, Thomas Merton.

"I have this huge need right now to get quiet," she said, brightening as she told me about her early morning walk with the dog, her quiet weekends away on the Cape, her long bath after work, and especially her Sunday mornings spent at Quaker meeting. Sometimes in the midst of this quiet, she said, she would begin to sense a voice inside that she barely knew, but for which she longed.

"My real life is right there, you know. But just out of reach. It's buried beneath the mountain of things to do, people to take care of. My worst fear is that I'll die and not have lived fully. Not have found myself. What's that bumper sticker say, 'Don't die curious'? I keep asking myself, what was I made to do? What is my real calling?

"I have to make some decisions," she went on. "But I'm too confused. I'm afraid of hurting my family. I feel trapped. And I can't tell you how guilty and selfish I feel for even thinking any of this."

As Paula spoke, I found myself feeling safe. It was a relief to hear her describe a landscape of conflicts, hopes, and fears that were so similar to my own. Somehow, it made me feel much less alone on the planet.

"I know just what you mean," I said. "My heart's just not in all this trying so hard, either. I've got this huge life whirling around me, but

somehow it's just not right. It's my old life. It's like my breakup with
Sean ushered me through some hidden doorway into a new dimension.
The reality I'm facing is calling up a whole new person. But I seem to
keep trying to build my new life on the pattern of the old, and it's just
not working. I don't want to rebuild. I want a whole new design."

Paula brightened. "Ironic, isn't it? Captives of our own lives. So how
do we break free, Steve?"

Midway through life, Paula and I were each facing a serious crisis of
meaning—mine triggered by a devastating disappointment in love, hers
by a bewildering disappointment in a career in which she was outwardly quite successful. Our crises were, of course, not at all unusual.
But they were serious. We were both suffering painful symptoms—
anxiety, depression, and a difficult sense of internal disorganization and
fragmentation. But as we would come to understand much later, our
crises each contained the seed of a magnificent gift. We were both
forced, by pain, to look under the surface of things. To investigate
deeper into the nature of our human-beingness—its impermanence, its
lack of continuity, its disappointment, its suffering.

Over the coming months, Paula and I forged an important friendship
out of our shared experience of breakdown. We shared our confusion
and our grief. We occasionally acted like lunatic adolescents together.
We talked about the Big Questions. And in the midst of our angst, our
yoga practice took on a new urgency.

Three or four times a week we found ourselves stretched out on big
blue mats, surrounded by fifteen or twenty other students. Gina, the
instructor, always began the class with the same soothing words: "Just
let go of all the rest of the day, now. Let all of your worries roll off your
shoulders; let's just enjoy being home in the body for the next hour and
a half."

What a relief those words were. Just breathing. Just stretching. The
faint smell of sweat. Nothing to do but explore the inner world of
sensation and breath. I discovered it was impossible to obsess or worry
when I was breathing deeply or when I was focused on the details of
my body's alignment in a posture. Through those months, my yoga mat
became a dear friend, a kind of home base. As soon as I unrolled it, my
stress level ratcheted down. During this period I felt too restless and
upset to meditate. But yoga became, for me, a kind of meditation-in-

motion. It seemed to produce some of the same effects as my previous daily hour on my meditation cushion.

Gina talked about how the breathing "balanced the hemispheres of the brain" and "slowed down the brain wave frequencies," how the postures both stimulated and calmed the nervous system, creating clarity in the mind. I didn't really understand the theory, but I knew I felt calm and centered after class. My practice took the edge off anxiety and depression. And after a workout I never felt compulsive. I didn't want to overeat. I didn't want to zone out in front of the TV. I felt alive.

I began experiencing something else, as well, something a tad more mysterious, something that felt vaguely spiritual. In the midst of my focused workout, I routinely had insights, moments of clear seeing into my dilemmas, and occasional epiphanies. I felt connected with some hidden source of wisdom inside. Out of the blue would come an answer, a perspective, a sense of knowing the right thing to do. On the mat I often felt as though I was digesting my life, my experience, my traumas.

Paula and I sat one evening after class in the coffee shop beneath the yoga studio, discussing our lives. We discovered we both secretly felt our breakdowns were a kind of spiritual crisis. And we shared the sense that the disappointments of our lives had launched us on a holy quest of some kind. As we identified, together, the aspects of this search that we shared, I scribbled them down on the paper place mat in front of me with a big red crayon:

~ A search for "the quiet" in which the small inner voice could be heard
~ A longing for the authentic and the real
~ A visceral need for self-expression
~ A sense of rebellion against the "captivity" of our old lives
~ An inchoate sense of something unimaginable about to be born out of the disorganization of our lives

As we left the shop that night, I folded up the place mat and stuck it in the back of my journal, where I found it as I began to write this book.

WAKING UP

In my midthirties, I'd noticed a remarkable number of clients coming to consult me with some version of the story Paula and I were living out. These were adults with a reasonably functional sense of self, who'd managed to establish themselves at least tolerably well in life, finding satisfying work and developing stable relationships. They often showed up at my office because they had symptoms of depression or anxiety, sometimes psychosomatic symptoms, or what appeared at first glance to be unresolved identity issues.

But while the story changed, the core problem was often remarkably similar. Some disappointment in work or in love, some illness, or some breakdown in the familiar structures of their life, or perhaps something more positive, like a love affair or a serious promotion at work, had awakened them from the trance of their daily life. A crisis had forced them to look under the surface of things. In the process of falling apart, these clients had been forced to discover a richness of inner resources they had not known existed. And in the process, they found a hidden depth to themselves and the world around them.

Dennis's fifty-million-dollar company went bankrupt just as he reached his fifty-fifth birthday. As he worked through this devastating loss over the course of two years in therapy, he discovered that in many ways it was a blessing in disguise. He was, for the first time in his adult life, free to pursue his deepest inner passion—painting. By the end of our therapy, he wondered aloud whether he might have unconsciously engineered the business failure so his soul could find its expression in art.

When Dennis came to see me, he was not sick. He simply needed support in his search for the self he had not, at first, realized he had lost. The internal structures of meaning around which he'd built a complicated and seemingly full life during his first twenty-five years of adulthood no longer served his deepest internal needs and longings. Through the apparently disastrous drama of the bankruptcy, he was actually being initiated into a new but hidden aspect of his humanness.

Emily, a thirty-six-year-old physician who worked as a top administrator in a large oncology center, spent a year and a half undergoing treatment for breast cancer. Though the treatment was successful, the experience turned her life inside out, and through the course of her therapy she reevaluated her values and decisions about work. She and her family made the decision to move to their farm an hour from the city, where she set up a smaller practice, specializing in women's medicine, and began developing the property into a working farm.

By the time he reached his thirty-fifth birthday, many of my friend Jim's career goals had been met. He had developed his own software business, and had sold the business to an eager buyer for almost ten million dollars. Jim spent the next two years feeling anxious, depressed, and restless, moving from one business pipe dream to another until, in the process of therapy, he realized that the second half of his life would look extremely different from the first half. He could not use the familiar pattern of his early adulthood to find the prototype for the second half of life. He would have to look deeper. Through a courageous inquiry, Jim discovered that his heart's desire was to live simply in San Francisco, to teach yoga, to learn the violin, and to write the coming-of-age novel he had had in his head for many years.

As I looked more carefully at the dilemmas of friends like Paula and Jim, of clients like Dennis and Emily, and at my own dilemmas at midlife, I discovered that for many of us, the developmental tasks of the second half of life are primarily spiritual. Carl Jung had come to the same conclusion fifty years before:

> Among my patients in the second half of life—that is to say, over thirty-five—there has not been one whose problem in the last resort was not that of finding a spiritual outlook on life. It is safe to say that every one of them fell ill because he had lost what the living religions of every age have given to their followers, and none of them has been really healed who did not regain his spiritual outlook.[1]

Jung believed that at midlife, most of us have refined our external selves, what he called the *persona,* the mask we wear to assure some stable, ongoing sense of identity. In his view, the persona represents only one limited aspect of the personality, and by midlife, most of us are outgrowing it. At some point during the middle years, Jung said, "the glowing coals of consciousness buried deep within the personality begin to break into flames." When this occurs, the hitherto repressed and hidden aspects of the self may seem to overwhelm the conscious self, initiating a difficult period of disorganization of the personality.

The developmental demands of this newly awakening self are enormous, but they are mostly overlooked in our culture. While the awakenings of early adulthood, which are mostly about identity, are culturally supported with rituals and celebrations—weddings, graduations, ordinations, baptisms—the more subtle spiritual awakenings of the middle years are culturally invisible. Jung was outraged by this.

> Are there not colleges for forty-year-olds which prepare them for their coming life and its demands as the ordinary colleges introduce our young people to a knowledge of the world? No, thoroughly unprepared we take the step into the afternoon of life; worse still, we take this step with the false assumption that our truths and ideals will serve us as hitherto. But we cannot live the afternoon of life according to the programme of life's morning; for what was great in the morning will be little at evening, and what in the morning was true will at evening have become a lie.[2]

Somewhere in the middle years of life, Dennis, Emily, Jim, Paula and I were ready for a deep new pilgrimage to the center to find what Jung called "the whole self." And for each of us in our own way, the return to the center of the self was inextricably linked with the return to God. Jung believed that the symbols for the self are indistinguishable from the symbols for God, and that the journey to the center of the self and the journey to God are one and the same. But in order to find this center it was necessary for each of us, in our own way, to deliberately enter the darkness of the unconscious, to begin what Jung called the "night sea journey." This entry into the unknown began, for each of us, a period of disorganization and metamorphosis that would eventually allow us to accomplish the goals of the second half of life— the integration of opposites, bringing into awareness all the banished aspects of the self.

Many of us found that it was in the quiet moments of life that we picked up the thread of an altogether new sense of realness: Dennis found it in front of his canvas, Emily in quiet moments with animals and family members on her farm, Jim in his writing, Paula at Quaker meeting, and I found it in yoga. All of us discovered that when the sensory overload was tuned way down, the connection with that elusive center seemed remarkably automatic. Insight arose, along with happiness and a kind of sweetness, even in the midst of pain. Many of us had brief glimpses of living in the flow of life, reconnected to the sources of our energy. We wanted more. Perhaps, in the words of Rilke's poem, we wanted everything.

THE WANDERER EMERGES

Several months after the party at Mark's, I called Paula early one morning to ask if she could meet me for coffee. "I've had a remarkable dream," I said on the phone. "I really want to know what you think." Paula had been a student of dreams for many years, and I had come to rely on her insights.

When we met later in the morning, I recounted the dream in detail. "I'm on a trip to my family's summer house, a gray Victorian cottage on the shores of Lake Ontario. I'm wandering along the rich green landscape surrounding the lake. I smell the familiar scent of lake, and I know the house is about a day's journey away. But as I move toward it, I find floodwaters are rising around me, threatening to overwhelm me on the sandy spit of road on which I'm walking.

"I can see the house in the distance, rising above the whitecaps of the bay. I am told at an inn that I have just a day to get there and back, or I may be flooded in and stranded. I determine to push ahead. When I arrive at the house, it's just as it was when I was a child—calm, warm, and serene inside. In the center of the living room is a small altar, glowing with light. On the altar are precious pieces of French china, which I recognize as pieces that used to belong to my grandmother. The whole altar is pulsing with light and energy. I feel completely at home. I feel OK. I look up and see myself. This other version of me is childlike, and glowing with an intense warm light. I am looking calmly and lovingly at myself. We recognize each other in a profound way—really see each other. I know who the child is. He knows who I am. I begin to sob and to hold him. And then I wake up."

Paula stirred her coffee and thought for a moment. "It's the Wanderer archetype," she said, staring into the middle distance.

"And?" I said.

"I think it was a classic dream about the quest for the true self," Paula continued excitedly, now seeming more sure of her analysis. She reminded me of the house in our *Outermost House* fantasy. "It's obvious. You're setting off through the waters of unconsciousness to find home. The house is a symbol of the self. I think it means it's time for you to go on a pilgrimage."

I looked at her and could feel a big smile spread across my face. It was wonderful to have a friend who knew me so well. And one who had read Carl Jung and Joseph Campbell cover to cover.

Both Freud and Jung believed that much of our mental and physical life is hidden from our awareness, playing itself out in the unconscious mind. Jung believed that water was the most frequent symbol of the unconscious found in dream images, and that its presence often indicated the flooding of the conscious mind by the unconscious. This entry into the flood could be what Freud called a "regression in service of the ego." Jung called it a "night sea journey," in which the light of consciousness intentionally descends into the dark, watery world of the unconscious, where no road maps suffice. After a period of intentional disorganization, the self emerges reorganized, with new energy, new life, and a new experience of wholeness.

Viveka's quest is the yogic version of the night sea journey. The hero of this journey, as Joseph Campbell taught us, appears to be a universal archetype. He or she inevitably has a wonderful, divine birth. Through a variety of circumstances her divinity becomes hidden, she hears a mystic call, journeys forth, and undergoes great testing in order to reach the goal. The best of these heroes purposefully expose themselves to the dark waters and to the demons living in the forest.

Psychologist and author Carol Pearson calls this archetype "the Wanderer." The Wanderer intentionally sets out to confront the unknown, taking a journey that, as she says, "marks the beginning of life lived at a new level. During their travels Wanderers find a treasure that symbolically represents the gift of their true selves."[3] And to find this gift, the Wanderer will suffer a deep reorganization of life. The Wanderer sets off, always alone, on the "road of trials," which is the initiation into heroism.

As Paula and I talked that morning, we acknowledged that we had both had many dreams and fantasies about travels and quests. We found ourselves haunted by the literature of pilgrimage, both interior and exterior: Thomas Merton's *The Seven Storey Mountain*, St. Teresa's *The Interior Castle*, Peter Matthiessen's *The Snow Leopard*, Isak Dinesen's *Out of Africa*, Henry David Thoreau's *Walden*. Since my breakup with Sean, I had been full of plans. I was going to set off across Europe on my bicycle. I was going to go, like Thoreau, to the woods, "to live intentionally." I was going to go back to South America, where I had lived and traveled extensively.

The Wanderer, like Viveka, is visited by an intense but unsettlingly vague sense of homesickness. She is not sure where home is, but she knows that she will recognize it when she sees it. And she knows she must pursue it at all costs. In my dream, my unconscious was speaking to me of my own homesickness. I knew that it was time to make the quest real. I found that my *Outermost House* fantasy was most persistent. I dreamed of a quiet year of reading, meditating, doing lots of yoga, getting close to nature again, working harder at the piano, and writing. I was ready for a break from the intensity of doing psychotherapy. I knew that because I was not currently in a relationship, I was free to let the Wanderer emerge. If not now, when?

THE WANDERER DEPARTS

"So, what are your great thoughts on the eve of your departure, Swami?" asked Geoff as he got up to pour Paula and himself a cup of coffee. We were seated around my big dining room table, with Mark and my good friends Tom and Nina, the night before I was to begin a yearlong sabbatical. The first four months were to be spent at Kripalu Center for Yoga and Health in the Berkshire Hills, where Paula had taken me several times on yoga retreats. I would be doing lots of yoga and meditation, and would have time for writing and practicing the piano, and for walking in the beautiful mountains. My luggage was stacked by the door.

I swallowed another forkful of Mark's brownies. "I feel like I'm heading off for summer camp. All I need are those little name tags Mom used to sew into my underwear."

"Is it true they get up at 4:30 in the morning so you can do yoga for two hours?" asked Mark. "This is not like the summer camp I went to."

"In yogic tradition, the earliest hours of the morning are the most auspicious for spiritual practice. But, you don't have to get up then if you don't want to. There's another practice period at the end of the day, before dinner. But I'll get up. This is my chance to really go for it. Haven't you ever wanted to connect with your inner spiritual warrior, you couch potato?"

"What do you think is going to happen?" Nina asked. "Are you going to discover some deeply buried karma at the core of your neurotic structure?"

"Whatever you do," Mark said, "you better take plenty of notes. This will make great material." Mark was a playwright, and the adventures of life for him were always "material."

"You better be careful," Tom, one of my psychotherapy partners, said. "Can't you have some kind of weird *kundalini* experience? You could just vaporize yourself. Then what would we do with all that office furniture you just bought?"

"Go ahead and enjoy my new chair, Tom. I'll think of you stuck there, swilling two cups of coffee to open your eyes, while I'm doing yoga in the morning and watching the sun rise. I'm going to be driving a big mower around the grounds all morning, smelling the sweet Berkshire air. And in the afternoon, I'm going to be cutting carrots in the kitchen. Blissed out."

"Cop-out," said Nina. "Escape."

"Excuse me, but this yoga stuff is a four-thousand-year-old psychology. Do you think there might be just one itsy-bitsy thing we might learn from it?"

Nina rolled her eyes.

"So what about relationship?" Tom asked. "Do you think you'll meet someone there?" They all looked up from their desserts.

"I hate to disappoint you, but the truth is I'm really enjoying this time-out. In fact, at Kripalu they practice yogic celibacy. It's not a moral thing. It's more about working with the sexual energy in different ways. It'll be a relief to have the pressure off for a few months. So forget it, you guys. I'm OK. Really."

Silence.

"All right. Of course it's still about healing from Sean, but it's also more than that. That breakup opened my eyes to something inside me that wants to emerge. It's just not about relationship right now."

"Well, I hope it emerges soon," said Nina. "We want you back in one piece."

"Yeah," said Tom. "Hatch the cosmic egg, already."

"Well, I have another perspective on that," Paula said. She'd been quiet and pensive all evening. "Steve, remember that night at Mark's party last year? Think back over the time since then and all that's happened. You're launching yourself on this personal quest, which I, by the way, think is fabulous. I'm getting ready to start my new company.

"A year ago, our lives were a mess. Falling apart. But look what all of that pain launched us into. It's not about going back to the way things were. That's the whole point. It's about letting life bring you to something new."

"Here's a plan," I said. "Let's agree to meet right here in one year, at the end of my sabbatical, and see where life has taken us. We'll see where Paula's company has come. If I've gone into some deep yoga posture and merged with the One. If Geoff's vow to stay out of big political cases holds. And where another year of psychoanalytic training will have taken you, Nina. If Mark has won a Pulitzer, and if Tom is ready to get out of my chair."

We clinked our coffee cups together in agreement. Tom pointed his finger at me. "But if you come back wearing a towel on your head or any other item of weird non-American clothing, we're building a back door to the office suite."

2

To the Mountaintop

Passage O soul to India!
Passage, immediate passage! the blood burns in my veins!
Away O soul! hoist instantly the anchor!
Cut the hawsers—haul out—shake out every sail!
Have we not stood here like trees in the ground long enough?
Have we not grovel'd here long enough, eating and drinking like mere
    brutes?
Have we not darken'd and dazed ourselves with books long enough?

Sail forth—steer for the deep waters only,
Reckless O soul, exploring, I with thee, and thou with me,
For we are bound where mariner has not yet dared to go,
And we will risk the ship, ourselves and all.

O my brave soul!
O farther farther sail!
O daring joy, but safe! are they not all the seas of God?
O farther, farther, farther sail!

                    —Walt Whitman,
                    "Passage to India"

On my first morning at Kripalu, I stood with my new friend Jeff in the late October sun, surveying the magnificent Berkshire scenery. At our backs was Shadowbrook, the main building at Kripalu, which sits halfway up the side of a small mountain that slopes gently down to a gemlike mountain lake. Layers of gently graded hills and mountains surrounded little Lake Mahkeenac on all sides, creating a circular geological formation, which we later learned was called the Stockbridge

Bowl. On this Indian summer day, the hills blazed with yellow, red, and orange—great waves of color swelling and disappearing into blues and purples at the horizon.

"It's amazing what a calming effect this view has on me," I said. Jeff and I had met the previous afternoon, on our arrival at Kripalu for the four-month Spiritual Lifestyle Training Program. He was a twenty-eight-year-old naturalist who had just finished his Ph.D. at the Yale School of Forestry. We had discovered over dinner that we had both recently ended long relationships and had many other interests in common as well—especially a love for cycling and for the poetry of W. H. Auden.

"You know what anthropologists say," Jeff responded, handing me his binoculars. "The favorite territory of human beings is high ground above water. I guess because those were the topographic conditions that favored our evolution. Gotta be in our cells somewhere."

"Makes sense," I said. Jeff, whom I eventually nicknamed "the professor," went on to tell me his theory that whenever people of wealth acquire land, they unconsciously re-create their primal roots, constructing their châteaus and castles on great high stretches of lawn, looking out on water.

I scanned the hillsides with Jeff's binoculars. With the leaves already thinning, I could see the great mansions of the Berkshires' Gilded Era dotting the shaved hilltops. The Tanglewood estate adjoined Kripalu's property to the east, and I could see the little red house where Nathaniel Hawthorne had written his famous *Tanglewood Tales*. Above it, I saw the mammoth black-green Tappan "cottage" and the summer campus of the Boston Symphony Orchestra.

"It's a power spot," said Jeff, staring intently into the distance. I nodded my assent, as we took another moment to savor the October sun. Finally, I looked at my watch. "Time to go in to the meeting."

We were meeting that morning with the group of thirty-five other spiritual trekkers who would be entering the Spiritual Lifestyle Training Program. For the next several months this "class" would be living together, working, eating, doing yoga, washing dishes, cutting vegetables, plowing driveways, sitting in meditation, talking about our family and friends back home.

The nervous anticipation I felt reminded me a little of my first day at college. I was surprised at the diversity of the group: Addi, a professional soccer player from Iceland; Carla, a young black woman from south central L.A.; a hot-shot thirty-something software designer named Lenny; Carlo, an unemployed actor from New York; Rita, a grandmother from Kansas; a physicist from Stanford named Hampton; and Giles, a member of the Royal Canadian Mounted Police, who had been commissioned by his government to learn yoga so that he could teach it to the Mounties.

Rani (her English name was Catherine, but in those days, most long-term residents used Sanskrit names) introduced herself as the facilitator of the group. She was about thirty-five, with jet black hair, dark eyes, and a beautiful smile. As she took charge of our session, I relaxed. Rani explained that she had been with the community since its earliest days in rural Pennsylvania. She told us, with some degree of enthusiasm, that we would have a special guest at the end of the morning session. Amrit Desai himself (or Gurudev, "dear teacher," as he was known to his students), the founder and spiritual director of Kripalu, would meet with us, apparently a very unusual occurrence in those days. By the late 1980s, Desai spent much of his time traveling, giving talks and yoga demonstrations around the world. There was a stir of excitement in the group.

As a preparation for Desai's appearance, we would be hearing from several senior members of the community, each charged with telling a different aspect of the story of the past twenty-five years. Ramkumar, who looked as though he might have been a successful young investment banker, told us the story of the early days of the community in Philadelphia and rural Pennsylvania. Saradananda, whose bright face I knew from his many yoga videotapes, told us about the daily schedule: up at five AM for an hour or two of yoga; *seva,* or "selfless service," for the morning hours; a two-hour lunch break, which included an optional hour of yoga; seva again in the afternoon; dinner, and then the evening devotional gathering called *satsang;* lights out at 9:30.

Next, a slender, sweet-looking young man named Yoganand got up to tell us the tale of Kripalu's yogic lineage. He had pale white skin, a shaved head, and a calm, focused demeanor, and he was dressed from head to toe in orange, indicating his membership in the renunciate order at Kripalu. I had already heard that Yoganand was one of the most serious yogis in the community. He radiated a kind of equanimity, moving gracefully and sitting in a full-lotus position as he spoke. I watched him carefully. Are these the results of sustained yoga practice, I wondered?

The story Yoganand told was riveting, and, at different points, I thought, altogether too good to be true. I carried on a running dialogue with myself as he spoke. Is this real, or is this a myth? Are these people deluded? Am I deluded for being here? And yet I wanted to be open. I wanted to suspend disbelief, at least for today. As I listened to Yoganand, I found myself on an internal roller-coaster ride, from doubt to credulity, from disbelief to awe.

THE YOGI'S TALE

"At the heart of Kripalu's lineage," began Yoganand, "lies an astonishing tale of transformation—the story of the life of Swami Shri Kripalvanandji, or Bapuji, 'beloved father,' as he was affectionately known to his tens of thousands of devotees in India." Bapuji (1913–1981) had been a lively yet sensitive boy, born into a Brahman family. From an early age, he longed to be an actor and musician. He could pour his heart out in a dramatic reading, or in a *bhajan* (song). In adolescence, after months of searching for work in Bombay, Bapuji discovered that he would most likely be unable to have a life in the theater. He sank into a deep state of hopelessness and depression. In the midst of this crisis, Yoganand told us, Bapuji had become suicidal.

"Now this sounds real," I thought, identifying with Bapuji's ambition, failure, and broken heart. It reminded me of Paula's nephew Matt—also an aspiring actor—and his suicide attempt.

In the grip of this despair, Bapuji made two attempts on his life. He was praying in the Laksmi temple in Bombay, preparing for a third, when he was approached by a holy man who mysteriously knew of his plans and thoughts. The wandering sadhu enfolded Bapuji in his arms, and eventually Bapuji left the temple in the protection of this mysterious saint. He remained with him for fifteen months, learning spiritual practices that included meditation, prayer, fasting, mantra, and the rudiments of yoga postures and pranayama. Shortly after giving Bapuji his first yogic initiation the holy man, who came to be known as Dadaji, or "beloved grandfather," disappeared. As Bapuji later told it, Dadaji was actually one of the great immortal saints of India in disguise. He had entered into the body of a deceased farmer expressly in order to initiate Bapuji into the secret teachings of kundalini yoga—which were believed to lead to transformation of the body and to the development of supernormal powers.

For ten years after his encounter with his teacher, Bapuji led the life of a pilgrim and teacher, wandering through the villages of India teaching the scriptures—the *Upanishads*, the *Bhagavad Gita*, the *Yogasutras*. During this period, he showed astonishing talent as a writer, a poet, a dramatist, and a composer. Finally, in 1942, as Dadaji had foretold, Bapuji took the *sannyasa* vow, donning the saffron robes of the renunciate.

Yoganand's voice was soothing and calm. He spoke in a methodical, precise fashion, almost as though he was quoting from scripture. The group was transfixed. After twenty minutes, I felt as though I'd been meditating.

Eight years after Bapuji took the renunciate vows, Dadaji appeared to him again, this time in the form of his true and immortal divine body, remaining just long enough to transmit to Bapuji the most advanced, hidden teachings of yoga.

Five years later, while visiting the little town of Kayavarohan in Gujarat province, Bapuji was shown a massive *jyotirlinga*, a cylindrical stone column made of black meteoric rock and carved with the visage of a beautiful boy saint. He recognized the saint as none other than Dadaji, and realized in that moment who his mysterious guru really was: Lord Lakulish, the twenty-eighth incarnation of Lord Shiva (one of the holy trinity of Hindu deities, and the "father" of yoga).

The nattering had begun again in my head. Is this story supposed to be taken literally? But in spite of my internal skeptic, I felt some deep attraction to the mystery, the alchemy, the absolute otherness of this tale. Who's to say?, the other side of my mind argued.

Bapuji went on to become one of the greatest kundalini masters of modern India as well as a prodigious scholar and composer. Later in his life, he became convinced that there was a genuine calling for the teachings of yoga in the West, and he gave his blessing to one of his senior students, the handsome young Amrit Desai, to teach in America. Bapuji actually spent the last four years of his life living with the community Desai had founded in Pennsylvania, where he taught and wrote books for his English-speaking students. Yoganand spoke at some length about the community's direct interactions with this amazing adept—and particularly about Bapuji's generosity, sweet temper, and playful, unassuming manner.

When he was finished, Yoganand sat for a moment in lotus, letting his story reverberate and settle. Behind him, above the altar, was a big picture of a smiling Bapuji dressed in saffron robes. And beneath that, a small black statue of the jyotirlinga with the likeness of Lord Lakulish—a replica of the massive ancient original, which now sat at the center of the newly rebuilt temple of Kayavarohan in Gujarat. The room was full of Bapuji in that moment, and I could feel the devotion of these senior students to this astonishing Indian saint.

I thought how strange and remarkable it was to have this little mountain in western Massachusetts marked with the stamp of one of the most ancient and powerful of the Hindu religious sects devoted to the practice of yoga. I would learn later that Lakulish was indeed a historical figure who had lived in the first half of the second century CE. The sect he founded, the Pashupats, was probably one of the earliest groups to refine the physical practices of yoga. But only later would I learn the true mystery and antiquity of this lineage.

Finally, Yoganand got up and moved lithely to the back of the room. Jeff and I looked at each other. I took a deep breath, and he lifted his eyebrows into question marks.

THE QUEST FOR JIVAN MUKTI

Now Sarita moved to the front of the room. She was a slight, thirty-something woman, with a mass of disorderly curls and a fragile-looking face. "Do you guys automatically buy all this stuff?" she asked. Thank God somebody has raised that question, I thought. Even before Sarita shared her story, her wry sense of humor and the deep lines carving the planes of her face suggested a life of suffering.

Sarita had met Amrit at one of his lectures in New York just ten years previously. She had been twenty-eight and had been strung out on heroin for ten years. Largely through his inspiration, and with the support of the community, she'd cleaned up her act. Sarita had set up a slide show to go with her talk. She picked up the tale where Yoganand had left off.

"One of Bapuji's favorite students was the young Amrit Desai," said

Sarita. Desai, she went on, was the son of a poor merchant-caste family in the little village of Halol, in Gujarat province, not too far from the temple of Kayavarohan. Sarita flashed some pictures of the young, handsome Amrit Desai—in one slide, he is dashing in his Indian air force uniform; in another, he looks like Tony from *West Side Story*, leaning against his late-model convertible, black hair cut fashionably and slicked back on the sides. "Gurudev, like Bapuji, was ambitious," said Sarita. (As a young man, she told me later, he adopted not only the *Bhagavad Gita*, but Dale Carnegie's *How to Win Friends and Influence People* as his guiding scripture.) In 1960, Amrit came to America, much as Bapuji had gone to Bombay: to make his fortune.

In America, Desai found his way first as an artist, winning awards for his paintings and textile designs. But he soon found that he had most success as a yoga teacher. It was the late 1960s, after all. Desai was young, lithe, charismatic, and an authentic Indian. It wasn't long before a group of devoted young American seekers gathered around him.

In 1972, Desai founded Kripalu Center, an intentional yoga community, or *ashram,* named for Bapuji and housed, initially, in a rural property in Sumneytown, Pennsylvania. Under his guidance, and over the seventeen years since, Kripalu Center had grown from the small group of young devotees who had known Bapuji directly, to the largest residential yoga community in the United States. In 1981, after some interim moves, the Kripalu community bought the relentlessly plain-but-practical Shadowbrook building from the Jesuits.

Sarita flashed another slide onto the screen. It was the massive new Shadowbrook building just after its completion in 1957. A monument to 1950s Roman Catholic triumphalism, I thought to myself. At the time of the purchase, Shadowbrook, a long, four-story orange-brick structure built as a Jesuit novitiate, had become one of the most infamous white elephants on the Massachusetts real estate market. Designed to comfortably house several hundred budding Jesuits, and envisioned by its architect as "a small self-contained city," it found itself almost empty in the countercultural years of the sixties, as Catholic vocations waned. Finally, to the undoubted chagrin of the local Yankees, the building was purchased by Kripalu.

By 1989, success was written all over the experiment. Kripalu was riding the crest of America's fascination with holistic health, spiritual growth, and wellness. There were movie stars, Harvard professors, international business consultants, prominent athletes, and plenty of dread-locked twenty-somethings. There were yogis from all over the world. It was a big, international community.

There was good reason for Kripalu's success, explained Sarita. Desai and his senior students had worked to create an adaptation of classical, or *raja,* yoga, which they hoped would be uniquely suited to the needs of the Western "householder." Desai was particularly interested in the psychology of yoga, and the application of the ancient psycho-spiritual techniques to the needs of the West. He called Kripalu yoga the "yoga of self-discovery."

Sarita made a helpful digression here. "Even though Bapuji was unquestionably one of the greatest kundalini yogis of the age," she said, "he believed strongly that kundalini was not a practice for most of his Western students." In accordance with Bapuji's wishes, Desai developed a form of practice that, while it incorporated some of the elements of spontaneous energy flows taken from kundalini yoga, was based mostly on what Bapuji called "eternal religion"—the ethical and lifestyle practices laid out in the classical scriptures of yoga.

In the classical traditions of yoga, I discovered that morning, the practice of yoga postures never stands alone, but is meant to be done in a context of ethical practices, lifestyle practices, dietary practices, meditation and breathing practices, chanting, and the repetition of mantra. Together, these practices literally transmute every aspect of daily life into a transformational activity. And it was around these practices that the daily schedule Saradananda had described had been carefully created. It was only that morning that I realized that my practice at Kripalu wasn't going to be about perfecting my yoga postures. Apparently, I had stepped into something much more complicated.

"Most of all," Sarita went on, "Gurudev is interested in creating an intense transformational environment for those Western students who want to go beyond two- or three-week yoga programs, for those who want to live, for some length of months or years, an authentic and slightly more monastic yogic lifestyle.

"In yoga," said Sarita, "the fully alive human being is created on a daily basis by what we eat, how we breathe, how we sleep, how we move, and what we say and don't say. As Gurudev says, 'This is a hothouse environment of spiritual growth, not right for everyone.'"

Desai, it seemed, promised accelerated transformation, growth, and purification to those who stuck with the forms and structures of practice. But what exactly, I kept wondering, did these folks mean by "transformation"? What was going to be transformed into what?

As I was to discover, Desai was obsessed with the notion of transformation and appeared willing to go to any lengths to get it for himself, to provide it for others, and to talk with others who were interested in it. He had a voracious appetite for relationship with the burgeoning world of psychological and spiritual exploration in the 1980s and 1990s. He put Kripalu on the pilgrimage route not just for students, but for teachers as well.

Almost without exception, I would soon learn, Desai was generous in sharing the limelight with others, showing an unfailing spirit of ecumenism: Buddhists, Christians, Sufis, Hindus, Ayurvedic physicians, scientists, and philosophers all held court. There was a steady stream of swamis, yogis, Indian princes, and politicos, and American psychological and spiritual teachers of every description—from the eminent to the not-infrequent New Age snake-oil salesman. At one point during my stay, the whole community did the controversial "est" training (later the Forum) together. At another, the community spent weeks being trained by the Hindu nondualist Rishi Prabhakar in his *siddha samadhi* yoga. Author Lino Stankich taught conscious eating. Bikram Choudry (Beverly Hills' yogi to the stars) spent a couple of remarkable weeks with the community, teaching his particular method of hatha yoga, and Desai built a special heated studio so that we could continue to keep this technique in the Kripalu culture.

A PRINCELY YOGI

As Sarita finished her talk, there was a commotion outside. Everything stopped for a moment. The door opened and in walked Amrit Desai, surrounded by a small phalanx of senior students and attendants, all dressed impeccably in white. Within seconds Amrit's big chair had been placed at the front of the room, a little table next to it with a single rose, reading glasses, and a glass of water.

My first impression was of his sweetness. He was smaller than I had imagined, and he seemed more to float than to walk. This impression was perhaps enhanced by the simple brown velour robe, a personal signature, which hung elegantly from his slender shoulders and flowed with his stride. His face, framed with a well-groomed mane of dark hair, was soft, and was further softened by a huge smile. His demeanor could only be described as princely—unassuming and extremely well mannered, but infused with the carriage of royalty. The guy knew how to enter a room, I thought. At his feet knelt a large Western woman, whom I would later come to know as his "right hand"—Krishnapriya. She wore a white silk sari, a white silk flower in her hair, and a commanding stare.

The energy in the room shifted noticeably. There was a sense of quiet, of reverence, of attentiveness to Amrit's every word and to his occasional needs—a microphone, a magic marker, a tissue, all appeared with lightning speed with a simple glance from Krishnapriya. After a short period of quiet meditation, he launched into a brief but exceedingly inspiring talk, much of which I jotted down in the leather-bound journal Mark had given me at my departure dinner.

Desai talked that morning about the preciousness of a human life. "In the world of yoga," he said, "you must remember there are hell realms and heavenly realms and animal realms and other realms where souls abide." But the human realms, he said, are most precious. Here in the human realms we suffer, but we also have the tools to wake up. And unlike the heavenly realms of the *devas* and *brahmas,* celestial beings, we have the desire to wake up. The human realms have just the right mixture of pleasure and pain to prod us toward taking the path of liberation.

"You have come to live in the guru's house, now," he said, smiling. "This is a very auspicious time, you know. Maybe thousands of lifetimes you wait for this. You must be very careful not to waste it." Amrit talked about the preciousness of taking a period of time to live quietly, deliberately, away from the restlessness of our culture. "There must be movement back and forth, from the mountaintop to the marketplace," he said. "But just now is a moment for the mountaintop. How will you use it, I wonder?" He talked about how yogis discovered the amazing potentials present in the "seed of the self" and challenged us to be yogic scientists, to experiment while we were at Kripalu with those ways of living that helped us to be fully alive. He urged us to tune in carefully to our energy, to listen to it, not to abuse it. "A conscious use of energy is the hallmark of a yogic lifestyle," he proclaimed.

At the close of his talk he spoke personally, and quite movingly, of the transformations he'd seen through the years—the many students who'd learned to open their hearts, their eyes, their minds, who'd learned to live well, creating happiness for themselves and for others. He talked of the friends and students back in India who had been transformed by the practice of yoga. And, finally, he challenged us to be clear about our intention for our stay. "What are you looking for? What do you need—because you need something, or otherwise why would you be here? We will help you create the conditions through which you can wake up from your particular brand of suffering. But get clear. If you don't the time will be gone. You will have missed a precious moment."

And with that he was gone. Just as quickly and dramatically as he'd arrived. Jeff and I sat and looked at each other, digesting what we'd seen. I felt like I'd just heard an excellent baccalaureate address, or a sermon from my Presbyterian boyhood—"There is much to be done! Let's be about God's work while we have time." For all his apparent equanimity, there was a sense of a quietly supercharged energy around Desai. I had heard about his amazing feats as a yogi, and the remarkable spontaneous flow of yoga postures with which he sometimes mesmerized huge crowds.

But some things gave me the willies. I was troubled by the language: guru, disciple, Gurudev. I was troubled by the devotion. Krishnapriya's attentive presence raised all sorts of red flags. What's with the sari? The posturing? The glare? And what does all of this bowing mean? Was I on the edge of getting involved in some kind of cult?

THE SEARCH FOR TRANSFORMATIONAL SPACE

After lunch I found a big elm tree on the sloping west lawn and settled back against its gnarly gray bark, watching the clouds drift slowly across the sky over Lake Mahkeenac. Amrit's question hung in my mind like one of the gathering clouds. I had clearly found a magical space. But what precisely was I looking for from it?

In the months leading up to my departure from Boston I had thought a lot about this. Under the elm that day, I began to pull together some of the ideas that had been cooking in my mind for the previous year.

When any of us gets ready to "hatch out" into the next developmental expression of self, we begin looking for the cocoons that will hold us through the rebirth process. I like to call these cocoons transformational spaces—environments made up of webs of special kinds of relationships, safety, freedom, and challenge. We intuitively search for these spaces at those times in life when we're attempting to align with an internal developmental thrust. At these times of growth we seek out "training environments"—schools, college, the army, a mentor, a psychotherapist, or a spiritual community. The transformational spaces we choose have certain qualities that are essential to the work of development. Without them we truly cannot find ourselves.

Effective transformational spaces create the conditions for our growth and make growth all but inevitable. Once we find them and commit to them, transformation is pretty much a "done deal." But here's the rub. Many environments proclaim themselves to be transformational spaces. But many of these fail to provide the real conditions needed for maturation.

Authentic transformational spaces can only be known from the inside out. No one can tell us precisely which transformational environment would be just right for our needs. But when we find a fit, we know it. Some exceptionally effective transformational spaces—like relationships—may seem unlikely to the outside observer. Surely, my trip to Kripalu had seemed extremely weird to many of my friends and colleagues.

Effective transformational spaces do not have to be explicitly spiritual or explicitly psychological. Authenticity may require that we discover a completely nonspiritual, nonpsychological language to facilitate our "hatching out." But whether spiritual, psychological, or otherwise, really effective transformational spaces have certain qualities in common.

1. They create a quality of refuge. These environments are temporary safe havens from the ordinary demand that we must know what we're doing, or who we are. We are allowed and even encouraged to have "don't know mind." As Socrates taught, "The beginning of wisdom is the acknowledgment of our own ignorance." We are encouraged to empty ourselves of our posturing, of being the "one who knows," so that we can fill up with a new kind of knowing. Only an environment that encourages this "don't know mind" in both the teachers and the students is truly transformational space. Those all-too-ubiquitous training grounds that encourage "don't know mind" only to impose a whole new system of beliefs do not qualify. They only compli-cate the process—or worse.

There is a deep kind of safety in knowing that we are going to be accepted as we are. But as we let go of the pretense of knowing, our vulnerabilities are exposed. For this reason, our entry into this kind of transformational space is often protected by rituals that create a special zone of safety, carefully set apart from other aspects of our lives. We have all experienced initiations, inductions, and graduations that ac-knowledge that a process of rebirth is happening and is in need of protection.

2. They create safety through constancy in relationship. In these environments, a special relationship is created between a mentor or teacher and a student, in which the mentor is constant, reliable, non-abandoning, and nonreactive to the student. In this safe and nonreac-tive relationship, the student, or patient, or trainee is allowed to reveal and experience not only the parts of herself that are already owned and acknowledged, but also the parts that are currently hidden and dis-owned. In this safe zone of relationship, the student can experience her magnificence as well as her limitations. The mentor provides a reliable and constant emotional home base for the student, and as new aspects of the true self emerge in the safety of this relationship, it is the pro-found intimacy in the sharing of these discoveries that promotes matu-ration.

In some cases, this deep emotional safety can be created even in the midst of great external dangers. Soldiers, for example, under the most difficult and traumatic of battle conditions, might experience trans-formational space if the web of relationships in their unit, and with their commanding officers, offers this kind of reliability. When soldiers are held in the constancy of much loved, admired, and trusted friends and commanders, they may find themselves experiencing profound new awarenesses of interiority and selflessness. In these highly charged situations, the whole group relies on the creativity and full capacity of each of its members. Individual capacities may grow by quantum leaps as a result.

3. They encourage creativity and experimentation. These environ-ments promote "out of the box" thinking. Trying on new ways of being, recombining and reorganizing parts of the self, and experiencing intense feelings and sensations previously denied to the self are encouraged. The daily activities of life are seen as a stage on which to act out the drama of human development and maturation. Attachment to the outcome of these activities is less important than the process. In spite of this, the products of these training environments are often well produced as well as remarkably innovative.

4. They are organized around "transitional objects" that are constant and reliable. During the process of transformation, certain people, places, or things become highly charged with meaning, and for a time become symbols of transformation itself. These "transitional objects" are present in different forms at every critical stage of human maturation, from the humblest comforts of childhood to the most sublime consolations of old age.[1]

The classic transitional object of childhood is the favorite blanket or special stuffed animal. When I was four years old I had a soft, blue-and-white checkered blanket with which I slept and cuddled. I desperately needed to cling to this tattered flannel friend—to hold it and suck it at difficult moments when I needed to feel soothed. The blanket was helping me bear the age-appropriate but terrifying discovery that I was a separate human being, and that others in my environment were not just emotional extensions of me, but were separate too. Up until that time, everyone and everything else in the world had still been, emotionally speaking, "me." The blanket partook of this magical world of emotional fusion, because it was also, at times, just an extension of me.

The blanket became, for me, a transitional object *par excellence* because sometimes it could be "not me." At times, I could experiment with letting it be just a blanket, utterly separate. It therefore occupied the intermediate realm between emotional fusion and emotional separateness. It was both "me" and "not me." That little blanket to which I clung—and from which I eventually parted—was an integral part of my process of growing up.

As adults, we have different developmental challenges altogether, but we still need transitional objects in order to negotiate them. Our new "blankies" are usually less concrete and more condensed with meaning. For example, the Buddha often used the image of a boat to describe the role of meditation. Meditation practice is the boat that helps us cross the river of delusion, the river of suffering. When it brings us to the other side, we can discard it. The Buddha was clear about this: "The boat is not the opposite shore—it is just the vehicle we use to get there." When we're in midstream, we must cling to it as if our lives depended upon it. When we get to the other shore, however, it can be completely relinquished.

Marti, a friend in my seminary days, clung to her copy of *The Cloud of Unknowing* for an entire year, reading and rereading it, and practicing the techniques described in it. This extraordinary fourteenth-century mystical text was a constant, reliable mirror for Marti, in which she could see aspects of herself that had previously been invisible. So subtle and tenuous were these newly emerging qualities, however, that she had to go back to the book, and the practices, again and again. Eventually she began to relax her grip a bit. The teachings were inside her. The little frayed paperback, like a bridge, had taken her where she needed to go. It still comes with her in her moves around the country. But it is more inside now than outside.

5. They do not deify these transitional objects, or themselves. The best transformational spaces recognize that the practices and symbols of transformation only serve to set into motion and support the normal development of the human being. The glory, as it were, is given to human nature, or to God, or to the soul, and not to the transformational environment itself (or to its idiosyncratic transitional objects). There is a heightened awareness that it is our inherent potential humanness that is made sacred—not the vehicles that bring these potentials into realization.

It is of utmost importance that teachers not be deified. Nothing undermines the potential of an environment to be truly transformational more than a teacher who is seen to be perfect, all-knowing, or "the ultimate authority." In the best transformational spaces, even brilliant, charismatic, or truly enlightened teachers are understood to be exemplars and guides, not gods. They are simply representatives of our own highest nature, that serve to evoke our own essential humanness. They may for a time become highly charged presences, surrounded with love and respect. This is quite normal. But even these powerful guides are understood to be transitional. They must, finally, set us free to be ourselves.

6. They provide us with a way of finding out who we are. The best transformational environments avoid telling us who we are. Rather, they support us in finding out who we are for ourselves. They do this by providing techniques and practices that give us full, direct, and immediate experiences of ourselves—experiences not necessarily mediated by any preconceived belief or faith. These transformational spaces are concerned with truth and clear seeing, and promulgate not doctrines or beliefs, but ways of exploring reality directly.

7. *They do not have to be perfect.* As the great English psychoanalyst D. W. Winnicott taught, "A good-enough mother will do." So, too, a good-enough therapist, a good-enough mentor, a good-enough spiritual practice, a good-enough school will do. The most effective transformational environments make explicit the view that they are only supporting and facilitating an internal developmental thrust that is completely natural, that is our birthright, and that only needs to be encouraged in order to manifest.

Indeed, when a group, a path, a teacher, a practice, or a community begin to see themselves as having "the perfect way," it is a sure sign that reality testing has been impaired. Though the language of these groups can be infused with a kind of intoxicating idealism, they actually promote delusion and a kind of grandiosity that is counterproductive to the maturing personality. They do not make room for limitations, vulnerabilities, or the dark side of us all.

Ironically, it seems that those moments in life when we're most open to change, to development, to maturation, are precisely the moments we're most vulnerable to giving ourselves away. Unfortunately, more than a handful of snake-oil salesmen have created pseudotransformational spaces that promise perfection, enlightenment, absolute safety, and the corrective emotional experience of the happy family we never had. What could be more compelling? When we're overwhelmed with our suffering, we're sure to find these appeals particularly attractive.

8. *They are open to, and support, other paths to development.* A friend of mine, whom I knew initially as a devout Anglican churchman, and who is also a professor of art and architecture, was telling me one night about his love for the Boston Athenaeum, the elegant old library and cultural center on Beacon Hill. Through a haze of cigar smoke and excellent after-dinner port, he rhapsodized about how the Athenaeum was "the church where he worshiped." I challenged him. "Gee," I said, "I thought All Saints was the church where you worship. Do you have

two Gods?" "Oh, for heaven's sake, Cope," he said, "every mature human being must have more than one church."

I've since discovered how right my friend was. Therapists and spiritual teachers alike often demand that we limit ourselves to one practice. But the best transformational environments support any other learning or self-expressive processes in which we're already engaged, helping musicians make better music, enhancing psychotherapy patients' skills for connecting with self and other, deepening one's faith in one's own religion. We should be wary of any transformational space that claims exclusive rights to our time, energy, or money.

COMMON SENSE, SKEPTICISM, AND OPENNESS

I took a break in my journaling and sat up. The clouds had gathered into a dark knot over Lake Mahkeenac, completely obscuring the sun, and a chill wind had begun to gust. I pulled my parka closely around my neck. For the first time, in that moment, I felt like a pilgrim. I'd left home and family and career behind. I was among strangers. I felt a little bit lonely. Frightened. Excited. Courageous. Proud of myself.

I picked up my journal again and wrote, "The territory of a pilgrimage is not on any external maps. 'We are bound where mariner has not yet dared to go,' says Whitman. What am I on the edge of here? I can't help but remember Jung's admonition that Westerners cannot dive into authentic Eastern spirituality without risking a possibly disastrous disorganization of the personality."

I remembered, too, Jacob Needleman's helpful observation that in order to be successful, the spiritual pilgrim needs three distinct qualities in approximately equal measure: common sense, skepticism, and openness.[2] And these all at the same time. If we're only skeptical, then what's the point? If we truly live "separated by only the flimsiest veil" from vast and unimaginable inner realms of consciousness, as William James declared, our inquiry must require the occasional "willing suspension of disbelief." Surely today's story of Bapuji, Dadaji, and Gurudev had required this quality of openness. But be careful, advises Needleman. It's no good to be only open, either. "Remember," says Jung, "to search also for the dark side of the truth." A good number of paths like the one I was just now exploring had already been exposed as harboring as much greed, avarice, and delusion as any skyscraper in Manhattan. Best not to lose the skeptical view, I coached myself.

Many who knew about these things (Needleman included) advised that the best kinds of transformational spaces to choose were those that were anchored in a long line of teachers and teachings. "Choose classical traditions that have been tested and refined," suggested Needleman. This seemed to make sense.

As I ended my journaling, I realized that I had chosen, in yoga and in Kripalu, a tradition that had in abundance many of the qualities of mature transformational space: powerful teachers and mentors, the constancy of thousands of years of teachings, simple but effective practices and techniques, inspirational scriptures and commentaries, the comfort and companionship of many other fellow pilgrims and practitioners. On that October afternoon in 1989, I knew that I needed the support of transformational space as much as I needed oxygen and food. And, like Whitman, I felt willing to risk nearly everything to find it.

ON SACRED GROUND

"You know what you said this morning about this being a power spot?" I asked Jeff. We had hiked up the ridge behind Shadowbrook and were sitting on a shale wall surrounding an overlook that gave us a panoramic view of the Stockbridge Bowl. "Well, I was thinking about what Margaret Mead used to say, 'There are certain places on the face of the earth where, for no apparent reason, very special things happen, over and over again.' "

Jeff and I had just spent twenty minutes looking at a bulletin board full of old photographs and newspaper clippings that detailed the history of Shadowbrook and the surrounding countryside. We'd both been amazed by the layered spiritual history of the place. Ever since there had been human beings in this neck of the woods, it seemed, this piece of ground had been held as sacred. The Native Americans believed that the unusual circular formation of mountains, with the lake at the center, was auspicious, and it became a center for great councils of local tribes, who perhaps used the high ground of what is now Shadowbrook for sacred ceremonies.

We sat in silence and devoured the view from the ridge.

"You know, Shiva likes to live on mountaintops," Jeff said, showing his teeth in a slightly malevolent smile. "He lives on Mount Kailasa in the Himalayas. Another mountain—Mount Arunchula—is said to be his lingam. Pilgrims make a practice out of circumambulating Arunchula. Dangerous guy, Lord Shiva. His body smeared with ashes. Hair piled up in matted locks. A cobra around his neck. Amazing, isn't it, that he decided to plant his trident on this little mountain in western Massachusetts? A little scary."

3

$\mathcal{B}$RAHMAN: ECSTATIC

UNION WITH THE ONE

Exultation is the going
Of an inland soul to sea,
Past the houses—past the headlands—
Into deep Eternity—

Bred as we, among the mountains,
Can the sailor understand,
The divine intoxication
Of the first league out from land?

—Emily Dickinson

It was the end of my first month at Shadowbrook. I was tucked into my bunk bed, listening to the quiet breathing of the five other "brothers" with whom I shared this cozy (or claustrophobic, depending on my mood) dorm room. It was ten o'clock, and most of the lights around the building were already out. I lay for a while thinking about the day: yoga at sunrise, cutting vegetables with my friends, a hike to the ridge with Jeff, an hour and a half of meditation before dinner, during which I had entered a deep and blissful state of concentration. I was too excited to sleep.

That evening I had had a long talk on the phone with Nina. "I can't believe this," I had said. "I'm just happy all the time." I went on to explain to her how I had found myself thriving in this place. I felt safe. I felt soothed and energized by the yoga and the diet and the friends.

For the first month of my stay, I had been working in the kitchen. Hours of patient slicing. The rich smell of damp vegetables, carrots, broccoli, celery, rutabagas, squash. The silent camaraderie with my fellow slicers. Simple physical work allowed my mind to slow down. I began to feel things more acutely again, to smell and taste. I noticed what a carrot was really like. The sunrise and sunset had again become parts of my day.

"Don't you miss your analyst?" asked Nina, referring to the several years of classical psychoanalysis I had completed just before leaving for Kripalu.

"Oh, my God," I said, "that is the one thing I definitely do not miss." I was relieved to let go of my habitual focus on intrapsychic conflict—my own and others'. I was tired of the too often self-absorbed world of psychotherapy. "No, it's a total relief, Nina. There *is* life after treatment!

"There's something about how these yogic practices work directly with energy. It's like they bypass the mind, or something. At least the intellect. My mind feels so calm. So focused. More and more, I have the experience of complete well-being."

"I don't know, Steve. When we were out there last week I felt . . . it was . . . well, it felt a little bit too much like the *Magic Mountain*. You know, cut off, isolated, unreal. Like Thomas Mann's sanitorium."

"Well, it is a sanitorium, I guess. I finally had to resort to inpatient treatment, Nina. Haven't you always thought I should spend some time in 'the bin'?" We both laughed. But I knew that some of my friends back home were worried about me. Worried that I was running away from my conflicts. That I was running from intimacy, from commitment, from career.

"Nina, now I understand why I felt the need to get deeply quiet. Living like this out here, with so few distractions, I find myself going into amazing states of meditation. My mind goes into these deep stages of concentration that I'd only read about before. It is utterly blissful. And it's as if moving in and out of these bliss states is transforming me in all kinds of ways."

"No, no, no, no, no. Steve, can't you see? You're just going into la-la land. It's artificial. It's just what Freud said about nirvana. It's a regressive attempt to return to the oceanic feelings of infancy, a kind of infantile symbiosis. It's *unreal*. For God's sake, come back."

I felt a kernel of truth in what Nina was saying.

"You're going to end up like Ed Brown's wife, Steve. Remember, she left him after she'd gone away on some retreat and 'fallen in love with the world.' Don't forget what he said. 'The problem was, she didn't love anybody in particular.' People, Steve. Remember us?"

"OK, OK, Nina. Ease up." There was no question that I was avoiding the problem of intimate relationship for now. And yet, at the same time, I felt pulled in by the compelling mystery of these deep meditative states I was finally being given a chance to explore.

A week earlier, while raking leaves in the orchard on a beautiful November afternoon, I'd spontaneously dropped into a deeply concentrated state. Blissful. Transcendent. The effects had lingered for a day or so. As I lay in my bunk, I thought over that experience. I hadn't told Nina about it, of course. But I wondered if she was right. Was it regressive? Or was it just a normal human experience that everyone has? As I thought back, I could remember several similar experiences, one in particular that had happened long before I became enamored of spiritual practice of any kind.

The summer after my junior year in college, I had stayed on at school after most of the other students left, to paint my skiing coach's sprawling white clapboard house and barn. It was a huge job for a lone painter. "Coach" had one of those classic New England frame houses that had sprouted a new wing about every fifty years over the last two centuries. It was a mess: big yellowing blisters of paint on every surface. Everything had to be meticulously scraped, primed, and repainted gleaming white, with shutters of New England green. But it wasn't a problem. I was in no particular hurry. Nor was Coach. I was a perfectionist in my painting, and he liked that. I settled into the rhythm of painting: long, languorous days in the sunlight, with my wiry and ruddy middle-aged mentor or his cheerful wife working on the flower beds around me, or off in the apple orchard trimming and sprucing.

One beautiful June afternoon, as I stood on my ladder, I was overcome with a feeling of what I can only describe as profound and utter well-being. For no apparent reason, I dropped through some unexpected crack in my ordinary mode of consciousness into a state of "time out of time." The most mundane moments were infused with the deepest sense of satisfaction. The enchanting perfume of the iris at my feet; the steady hum of farm machinery in the distant field; the cat curled up in the sun, watching; even the rich oil smell of the paint. It all seemed so completely right. I was utterly OK. More than OK. My senses were alive, and every sight, smell, touch, reverberated with the sublime. I melted into what was. My painting seemed effortless. There was no bottom to my feeling of well-being. No hard edges anywhere. At one point, out of the blue, I sobbed as if with a lifetime of accumulated burdens. And throughout it all I just painted.

I spent the entire afternoon in this altered state, and it waxed and waned over the next several days. What was happening to me? This was a quiet time in which nothing particularly dramatic was going on in my life. I was not in love, I was not taking drugs. I was not trying in any way to have a spiritual experience. I had not yet discovered the Eastern contemplative traditions, meditation, or even "consciousness." I was just painting a house.

In the weeks following this episode, I remembered other versions of this kind of experience: once on an early morning swim in Lake Ontario when I was sixteen; once in a shabby hotel on the Amazon with a group of friends; once lying on the bed in my grandmother's big front bedroom during a snowstorm. These moments were rare, and yet the territory seemed so familiar. Each time it happened, I felt as though I had just fallen out of the sky onto the solid ground of my real home. There was also a sense that "I" had in some way disappeared as I melted into experience. That afternoon on the ladder, there was no more "me"—only painting, breathing, smelling, seeing. Paradoxically, without "me," I felt more real, more present, more alive than ever.

At the time of the ladder experience, I didn't have the opportunity to tell anyone about it, or even the words to describe it as I'm doing now. But in the years since I've moved to Kripalu, I've discovered that almost everyone has had at least one experience like this, and many people have them off and on throughout life. They are ordinary moments of mystic union, which seem to happen when, for whatever reason, we're neither grasping at experience nor resisting it; when for some reason we surrender to the way things are. They are ordinary, because they are simply manifestations of our basic nature—luminous, clear, awake, whole, and living beyond time and effort. They manifest naturally when we are not trying to get anywhere or achieve anything.

These transcendent moments are entirely unpredictable. We can't make them happen. And, surprisingly, perhaps, they happen in the midst of painful as well as pleasurable circumstances. One of my friends remembers having such an experience in the jungles of Vietnam during the war; another friend after a painful childbirth; my twin sister had a life-transforming experience on a particularly terrifying night while she was on a pilgrimage from Paris to Santiago de Compostela in Spain. Another friend remembers such a moment while she was swimming in a local pond: she recounted it to me with relish, saying that she felt "completely one with the pond," and could remember communicating with the fish and the seaweed; she said she "knew directly in her soul" the whole teeming, microscopic life of the pond, and "it knew" her.

A number of years ago, a survey was done that showed that over 40 percent of Americans had had some such transcendental experience at least once in their life; 20 percent said it had happened several times; and 5 percent said it happened often.[1] And yet, because we have no frame of reference within which to hold these experiences of "time out of time," we tend to deny them, ignore them, or minimize them. Respondents to this survey, almost to a person, told pollsters that they had never discussed these experiences with anyone—not even a minister, priest, or rabbi. What was the reason? "They would think I was crazy." Like Scrooge, who discounted the appearance of Marley's ghost as the result of some "undigested bit of gruel," we will rationalize and look away as hard as we can.

And yet, all of us who have had these experiences know, in spite of our denials, that we are changed by them. When we land again in our ordinary state of consciousness, we're not quite the same, not quite so identified with our minute daily concerns. We're vaguely aware that, at least in some parallel universe, we are unutterably fine just the way we are, and that everything is completely OK. "It is," as the poet David Whyte says, "in the self-forgetfulness of meeting some sacred otherness in the world that we both lose ourself and find ourself."

YOGA AND THE "BREAKING-THROUGH" OF OUR TRUE NATURE

The yogic traditions have developed a sophisticated understanding of these enlightenment experiences. Yogis use the general word *samadhi* to describe the entire spectrum of "awake" mind-states,[2] and, as we'll see as we get deeper into this inquiry, yogic sages have gone to great lengths to describe them precisely. Patanjali, one of the greatest of these sages, dedicates the entire first book of his masterpiece, the

Yogasutras, written around 200 CE, to this task. He gives a description of one of the less esoteric forms of samadhi in the third book of the *Yogasutras:* "When nothing but the object is shining forth in that meditative absorption, and when the mind is as it were void of its own-form, this is known as ecstasy *(samadhi)*."[3]

Here Patanjali captures the essence of my own experience on the ladder. "I" had disappeared ("the mind void of its own-form," as Patanjali said) and had become "the seeing without a Seer." I actually had the experience of the solid anatomy of my body dissolving; instead of a frozen form, I experienced myself as a river of energy and intelligence. The essence of the experience was a state of "flow": I was pulsing with the river of life. Life, not "I," was, as Patanjali states, "shining forth." "I" and the "object" (whatever I focused upon—iris, apple tree, paint smell, sun on skin) had become one, and nothing but pure seeing, smelling, sensation, remained.

In the state of samadhi, the mind enters that "divine intoxication" of which Emily Dickinson speaks, the "exultation" of complete freedom. As Ramakrishna, the great "god-intoxicated" nineteenth-century Bengali saint, describes it: "When entering samadhi, or absorption in God-consciousness, one feels like a fish released from a small jar into the vast, powerful current of Mother Ganga. One swims everywhere with perfect freedom and spontaneity. There are no partitions, no boundaries."[4]

This is the quintessential liberation experience of mystics in all ages and of all faiths—Christians, Jews, Muslims, Buddhists, Sufis, Taoists, Hindus. The thirteenth-century Christian mystic Meister Eckhart, for example, wrote about what he described as "the breaking-through of (his) true nature" into his daily life: "In this breaking-through, I receive that God and I are one. Then I am what I was, and then I neither diminish nor increase, for I am then an immovable cause that moves all things."[5]

The eighth-century Hindu mystic Shankara expressed his understanding of awakening like this: "I am reality without beginning, without equal. I have no part in the illusion of 'I' and 'you,' 'this' and 'that.' I am *brahman,* one without a second, bliss without end, the eternal, unchanging truth. I dwell within all beings as the soul, the pure consciousness, the ground of all phenomena, internal and external. I am both the enjoyer and that which is enjoyed. In the days of my ignorance, I used to think of these as being separate from myself. Now I know that I am All."[6]

The literature of mysticism is replete with stories about this particular mind-state, but it's important to lay hold of the fact that not only acknowledged mystics have these experiences. Most of us ordinary folk have tasted these moments of "union"—on the ladder, in the pond, in the jungle, on the hospital bed. In the yogic view, it is in these moments that we know who we really are. We rest in our true nature and know beyond a doubt that everything is OK, and not just OK, but unutterably well. We know that there is nothing to accept and nothing to reject. Life just is as it is. It is in these moments that we awaken from the dream of separateness in which we usually live.

The whole path of yoga begins with these little daily experiences of waking up. Awakening comes, in yoga, not at the end of the path; rather, it is present from the very beginning. Ramakrishna, perhaps the greatest Indian mystic of the last two centuries, was fond of saying, "Only the divine can worship the divine." In the experience of samadhi, in other words, it is our awake nature that recognizes itself in the mirror of consciousness. In these moments, we are dissolved back into the One that is our source.

BORN DIVINE

Yoga puts our experiences of enlightenment at the exact center of our being. Amrit Desai had a concise summation of this view: As he so often said, "We are all born divine." This is the classic statement of the perennial philosophy of yoga: Each human being is at core a soul (*atman*) that dwells eternally in the changeless, infinite, all-pervading transcendent reality of brahman—the supreme essence from which all creation derives.

In this view, all beings are members of a single holy family, proceeding from the one and only divine substance. The belief that "the whole world is one family" was central to Bapuji's practice and work in the world. Though we may appear separate from one another, we are no more separate than the wave is separate from the sea, or than the air in a glass jar is separate from the surrounding air. We are pervaded by and animated by the same spirit, the same nature, and that nature is constant through the manifold changes of birth, growth, and dissolution; it cannot be wounded, or separated from itself.

"Born divine" is a notion that fairly saturates Indian philosophy and spiritual practice. It was first systematically articulated in the tradition known as Vedanta, which arose on the Indian subcontinent as early as 600 BCE, and has been a powerful force in Indian spiritual history even to the present day. Most of the branches of Vedanta hold one fundamental view in common: all individual souls are one with the ground of being, the Absolute. Because all beings are one with the great river of life, we are all, in effect, just a single soul. We are, in the classical dictum, "One without a second."

The metaphysics of Vedanta were laid out in the Indian gnostic scriptures called the *Upanishads*—perhaps the Indian literature most familiar to Westerners. There are over two hundred *Upanishads,* composed in both poetry and prose, some of them written as early as the middle of the second millenium BCE, and others as recently as our own century. This body of mystical writings includes some of the most inspired and sophisticated scripture in human history, including the scripture perhaps most widely known to Westerners, the *Bhagavad Gita* (The Song of God). Most American yoga students are at least vaguely familiar with the three great maxims of the Upanishadic sages: "Thou art That" *(tat tvam asi);* "I am the Absolute" *(aham brahma asmi);* and "All this is the Absolute" *(sarvam brahma asti).*

In other words, what we are seeking is already at the core of our nature. "We are that" which we seek. We are already inherently perfect; we have already arrived; and we have the potential in each moment to wake up to our true nature. In the words of one extraordinary teacher whom we'll meet later on in the book, "Everything is already OK."

The notion strikes us as radical, and it surely is. What it means is that in our essential nature we are already fully awake and enlightened; it means that God is available to us fully in each moment, simply because God is our true nature. We simply have to stop resisting. There is no distance to travel, nothing special that we have to do to earn God. It's a "done deal."

In order to get inside the yogic view, it's important to understand that the "divine" being referred to is not the creator God of deistic religions like Christianity, Judaism, or Islam. Rather, God is the transcendental ground of being itself, the essential nature of all life, pure consciousness. The divine nature is often referred to as manifesting three indivisible aspects: *sat-chit-ananda*—or being, consciousness, and bliss.

When we begin to see clearly who we really are, according to this view, we feel a natural friendliness toward all beings. Beneath the surface of our separation, we feel the hidden, unseen threads that link us. We know that we're exactly alike inside. We're the same being. As author John Welch says, "We are each like a well that has its source in a common underground stream which supplies all. The deeper down I go, the closer I come to the source which puts me in contact with all other life."[7]

Our everyday ladder experiences, then, are perfectly predictable. If awakeness is our true nature, why is it surprising that we should have powerful moments of direct realization of awake mind? Why shouldn't enlightened mind break through in the oddest moments, precisely when we're not looking for it? And why is it surprising that we should experience in these particular moments a deep sense of coming home?

THE BIRTH OF THE DIVINE CHILD

Inevitably, after we have these moments of recognizing who we really are, we fall asleep again. But some of us are never the same. We're haunted by what we've experienced. It echoes in everything we do. Having experienced it once, we quicken to our truest nature when it is revealed to us again—as it inevitably will be. We feel the alienation from this way of being when we're not living from it. We feel homesick for our true nature. We begin to long for it.

All mystical paths have taught that the union with God, or with the Absolute, subtly transforms the self. Each time we penetrate into samadhi, we have a small death-rebirth experience. Samadhi destroys the world as we know it—its boundaries and categories. The deeper into union I penetrate, the less I am "I," and the more I am "we." For this reason, the merger with the One is known to create psychological upheaval and world-shattering shifts in perception. "No one should speak glibly about attaining ecstatic union," says one yogi, quoted by author Lex Hixon.

This love is so overwhelming that you will lose consciousness of the conventional world. You will not be able to entertain the slightest feeling of personal ownership, not even toward the body, which is the most precious and jealously guarded possession of most persons. There will no longer be any instinctive notion that the body or the mind constitutes your being.[8]

These are the deaths that are necessary for the birth of what Carl Jung called "the divine child"—the deeper layers of the spiritual self. Each time the self enters the cocoon of samadhi, the inner "divine child" is awakened a little more, and the self emerges as a butterfly from the cocoon. The sixteenth-century Spanish mystic Teresa of Avila used this image to describe the birth of the new self:

When the soul is, in this prayer, truly dead to the world, a little white butterfly comes forth. O greatness of God! How transformed the soul is when it comes out of this prayer after having been placed within the greatness of God and so closely joined with Him for a little while—in my opinion the union never lasts for as much as a half an hour. Truly, I tell you that the soul doesn't recognize itself.[9]

In yoga, it is believed that once the soul has been awakened to the presence of its source, consciousness of source can be cultivated through a cornucopia of practices—ethical and lifestyle practices, meditation and postures, mantras and breathing, purification and diet. The classic guide to yoga practice—the eight-limbed path, or *ashtanga* yoga—is entirely organized around the systematic penetration into deeper and deeper states of samadhi. The word *yoga* itself means, literally, to be "yoked"—or to be in union. Eventually, repeated penetrations into mystic union transform the physical structure of the body, the personality, and the mind. At the highest stages of practice, *nirbija* samadhi (or samadhi "without seed"), the soul is constantly in union with source—at one with the Absolute, with brahman, God, the transcendent ground of being. The classical practices of yoga are believed to methodically create a state of permanent union with the One.

THE UNKNOWN

From my perch on an upper bunk I could see Lake Mahkeenac, and the mountains in the distance, illuminated by the moon. The dark waters of the lake shimmered with light. The sweet smell of mountain air flooded the room from the two open windows at the foot of my bunk. For now, at least, my complicated life in the city seemed far away, and I was content to leave it there. I could sense the spirits of the Mahican ancestors moving silently across the lake, along the ridge in the distance, and in some ceremonial act at the center of the high ground of the mansion lawn. I could imagine, too, the spirits of the Jesuits at prayer, moving in monks' cloaks down the marble stairs at the base of the old mansion. I lay on my bunk, remembering the Sanskrit chants and the wailing of drums from the main chapel, mixed with the sweet, cloying smell of incense and the ever-present spirit of Bapuji.

In my mind's eye, I had an image of brahman as the oceans of the world, and I imagined myself as the tiniest wave on that ocean, a brief flash in the unending rising and falling away of ephemeral forms. "I am nothing, and I am everything," I thought. Just part of the divine play of God. Majestic with all the majesty of nature, and with all the attributes of the divine. And yet hidden in the vastness of it all, a spark, a mere nothing, mystically one with the maelstrom of the world.

As I drifted off to sleep, I thought again of a poem by Emily Dickinson, a poem that had been written in Amherst, only blocks from Coach's house. "Can the sailor understand, / The divine intoxication / Of the first league out from land?" In another place, Emily had written, "The deepest need of man, is for the unknown—for which we never think to thank God." Penetrating this unknown seemed to me like the most important thing in the world. Why should we not live in this mystery all the time? I fell into sleep with thoughts of gratitude.

4

SHAKTI: THE PLAY OF
THE DIVINE MOTHER

Who in this world
can understand what
Mother Kali really is?
The six systems of philosophy
remain powerless to describe Her.
She is the inmost awareness
of the sage who realizes
that Consciousness alone exists.
She is the life blossoming within
the creatures of the universe.
Both macrocosm and microcosm
are lost within the Mother's Womb.
Now can you sense how indescribable She is?

The yogi meditates upon Her
in the six subtle nerve centers
as She sports with delight
through the lotus wilderness
of the pristine human body,
playing with Her Consort,
Shiva, the Great Swan.

When anyone attempts to know Her,
the singer of this song laughs.
Can you swim across
a shoreless ocean?
Yet the child in me still
reaches out to touch the moon.

—Ramprasad,
Translated by Lex Hixon

The first time I heard Amrit Desai give a talk about the "born divine" scenario, I felt a silent screech of fingers on the blackboard of my Protestant psyche. It was a compelling notion, yes. But I was skeptical. As a good Episcopalian (having converted from my boyhood Presbyterianism in college), I had been taught that I'm "born in the image and likeness of God." But what about the part where I'm a "miserable sinner," essentially separate from God because of my fallen nature? What about that line I repeated every Sunday morning in church for quite a few years of my life: "We are not worthy to gather up the crumbs under Thy table"?

During the first couple of months at Kripalu, I was nervous about confronting Amrit with my questions about the yogic belief that we're all "born divine." I was an eager learner. I wanted to understand what I was getting into. So, often during his evening talks I would sit right up front, listening intently. It took Desai many months to learn my name, but from early on he noticed my interest, and, never quite able to summon up my name, he came to refer to me as "the brother with the glasses." (In an adaptation of an Indian monastic tradition, men at Kripalu were called "brothers" and women, "sisters.") Not that there weren't dozens of other "brothers" with glasses. One evening I took a deep breath and raised my hand. Desai smiled in recognition and said, "Yes, the brother with the glasses."

I walked up the steps to the top of the raised altar in the main chapel, where he was so regally seated. Protocol was incontrovertible in these moments: one bowed and knelt on a cushion next to his big thronelike chair. This was truly uncomfortable for me, but I understood that this gesture of surrender, called *pranam*, which placed the head beneath the heart, was meant to symbolize devotion not to this man, but to the "inner guru." I forged ahead. "I have a problem with this notion of 'born divine,'" I said. "I mean, I *like* being a human being. I don't want to be God. I don't want to live in some transcendent realm with the angels. I want to live here. On Earth. In my body. I thought that was what yoga was all about."

"You see," he said, chuckling as he often did, and addressing the whole group, "this is such a good question. Because there's really no problem here. We can be absolutely human and divine at the same time. Is God only in some aspects of life, and not in others? No. You can't split God. Can you split God? If God is anywhere He is everywhere. Not just in the transcendent realms. But in your body. In human foibles. In the dung heap as well as the great banquet hall. This is the teaching of the greatest yogis."

He paused for a moment, leaned toward me, and put his hand on my shoulder. In that moment I was quite won over by his warmth. In fact, the energy of his physical presence was almost overwhelming. His smile was beatific and mischievous all at once. "In Christianity, don't you have this understanding: God is both—what do you say—immanent and transcendent? God is both here, within, right now, and is also everywhere? At the same time? It is the same God, the same Reality. Just our language has trouble capturing it. This is the wonderful thing about yoga. You find God right here, right now. In the body. You become a fully alive human being. You become jivan mukta—awake in this lifetime. As a human being. Not in, what did you say? Transcendent realm with the angels. No. Not at all. You see, you *are* an angel."

His beautiful words brought a surprising pulse of energy into my heart, and for a moment I felt as though my sternum was going to crack open. My rational mind seemed momentarily incinerated. I had to catch my breath. And I sat quietly for a moment, just looking at a smiling Amrit.

"Well," I said. "When you put it like that, I guess there isn't a problem. But isn't it really more like 'born human and born divine,' then?" "Yes," he said, displaying his famous broad, gap-toothed smile, "that is a good corrective. I like it."

I walked back to my seat with my heart pounding. I had made a very warm connection with the great yogi. He'd touched me! For the next fifteen or twenty minutes, I felt a profound tingling in my spine. Was I just imagining this? A sense of well-being flooded my body, a deep sense that all was well, that I was utterly OK. This lasted for an entire day. Was this some special power of his? Was he transmitting an energy that actually made me feel "born divine"? Had he just given me a secret transmission? Or was it my own self-esteem burgeoning in response to finally having a public dialogue with him? I remembered my intention to be both open and skeptical. But I could feel how much I really wanted him to be a magician.

THE DRAMA OF THE DIVINE DESCENT

As I learned more about yoga philosophy and psychology, I discovered that for millennia, yogis have been preoccupied with questions about the relationship between the human and the divine, matter and spirit, the immanent and the transcendent, the phenomenal world and the unmanifest realms, the One and the many. Indeed, most archetypal yoga stories emerge somehow out of the tension between these two polarities. One of the classics of this genre is the story of the divine descent, told in the ancient scripture the *Puranas*.[1]

Lord Vishnu, Sustainer of the Universe (and one aspect of the Hindu trinity, Brahma, Vishnu, and Shiva), decides to leave his heavenly abode and incarnate in the phenomenal world as a ferocious sow, a powerful embodiment of "mother-protectress," in order to defeat a particularly virulent strain of demonic energy. Having triumphed over this demon, Vishnu discovers that he doesn't want to return to his transcendental existence in the unmanifest realms. He is delighted to be incarnate in the play of space and time. Even though it's a more unrefined, gross existence than he's used to, it has its rewards. As the sow, Vishnu finds delight in suckling his little piglets, in caring for and protecting his young.

Now it happens that the other divine beings, stuck in the heavenly realms and bound by their heavenly conventions, become greatly disturbed by Vishnu's play in the earthly realm. Finally, peeved, they request the assistance of Lord Shiva, the destroyer, and the quintessential expression of divine transcendence. Shiva appears to the incarnated Vishnu in all the majesty of his divine body and implores him to return to the transcendent realms. But the sow calmly continues to suckle her young. Shiva, angered, strikes the sow with a thunderbolt, and swiftly and painlessly kills her. Vishnu springs forth, "like a bright sword from its dark sheath," laughing in ecstasy at his divine play, and immediately manifests himself again in the abode of pure consciousness.

Vishnu, still laughing, makes it clear to the other transcendent beings that he never really abandoned the state of pure being. His experience in the phenomenal world was simply the play of energy and consciousness, of matter and spirit, in which he took momentary delight.

What is revealed in the drama of the divine descent is the creative tension arc between the human and the divine that saturates much of Hindu cosmology. The divine longs to express itself in the power and energy of the phenomenal world. The human longs for the pure being and consciousness of the divine. The two polarities strain and arc toward each other: God at play in human form, human form straining toward God.

THERE IS ONLY THE DANCE

It was a wintery morning in early December. The main chapel was utterly still. Four or five hundred yogis sat quietly around the perimeter of a large, empty circle of carpet. In the center of the circle sat Amrit Desai—meditating, absorbed. Almost everyone's eyes were closed, and there was a sense that we were all breathing together, joined in a deep silence, all dropping quietly as one body into the still point of consciousness. Big sections of the carpet were washed in yellow sunlight. Outside, the wind howled and blew the snow in drifts against the side of the building.

Amrit began to move. Subtly at first. Just a finger tracing a slow path along the carpet, then an arm, rising effortlessly overhead. All eyes—open now—concentrated on his moving form. For the next twenty minutes, an ecstatic dance seemed to take over his body, drawing him down slowly, pulling him up gracefully, flinging him across the room violently. He shook, he reached, he strained as if to touch some unseen partner in the dance. His body entered spontaneously into postures I had never before seen. He was powerful, graceful, and uncannily lithe for a sixty-year-old man.

As Amrit entered deeper into the dance, the entire room seemed to be pulled down by a deep undertow of absorption. We were lost with him in the dance of energy. At the center of this dance was a profound state of stillness, of quiet, that seemed to deepen with each passing minute. The room was both electric with energy and completely still at the same time.

Ten minutes or so into the experience, I noticed a change in my perception. Colors had become brighter, bolder. The blue and gold tiles behind the altar were fairly pulsing with flashing hues. Light itself had become a palpable golden presence. At moments the whole room dissolved into waves of light, particles of energy. And all the while, I felt the whole room breathing together and somehow moving together, pulsing and expanding and contracting. At one point, I had an experience of energy rushing up and down my spine, as I'd had when he'd touched me, a tingling at the crown of my head, my whole body suffused with an intense heat.

Amrit's movements reached a peak in a moment of quiet frenzy that seemed remarkably like an orgasm and then slowly dissolved. His body entered a deep quiet as he came back into lotus pose for meditation. The room was drawn deeply into a state of absorption by some subtle ineffable pull. Down, and down.

When at last Amrit opened his eyes and looked up, the room was still. Several people sobbed quietly. Others had discovered their own bodies entering into spontaneous postures. I found that I had spontaneously entered the child pose, my forehead on the floor, arms at my side holding myself. My belly pulsed with energy.

Finally Amrit stood, walked to his chair at the front of the room, and beckoned for his harmonium. The instrument was set in front of him, and he began to play a low drone. Over the drone, and almost as a continuation of his dance, emerged a hauntingly beautiful chant to the divine Mother.

LILA: THE PLAY OF ENERGY AND CONSCIOUSNESS

After the posture-flow demonstration and the chanting were over, I grabbed my friend Bruce, a longtime resident at Kripalu. "Let's go for a walk."

We bundled up in our parkas and boots and walked up the long east drive in the bitterly cold, clear morning. Before coming to Kripalu six years earlier, Bruce had had a successful career as an actor, producer, and director, and he had founded a large regional repertory company. As much as anyone I knew in the community, he had his feet on the ground. When I bumped up against something complicated or esoteric, I often relied on his evenhanded view.

"What just happened in there?"

"That was *shakti*," laughed Bruce. "And you've just seen a classic Amrit Desai demonstration of the essence of hatha yoga."

We walked briskly up the drive and, finally, the entire four miles into the little town of Lenox. Over the next two hours, Bruce explained the meaning of the events of the morning.

In the yogic view, he said, shakti is the energy essence of the phenomenal world, the purely active force in the manifestation of the universe. Shakti is seen as the divine Mother, the essence of the feminine principle, because she brings the world into being. She is matter, or *mater*. She is also energy, the primordial power that is always at play, creating, preserving, destroying the world of form. There is no object or event that does not disclose the presence of her power. But the body of a yoga adept is a particularly open channel for the play of pure energy. It was shakti that was moving Amrit's body in the posture flow. (Shakti, when capitalized, refers to the goddess—Shiva's consort—who is the embodiment of the feminine principle; in lowercase, shakti refers to the nonpersonalized principle of pure energy itself.)

"Shakti," said Bruce, "is the archetypal feminine. That's why Gurudev chanted that hymn to the goddess Kali, a particular form of the divine Mother, afterward.[2] His experience of the pure energy of shakti in his body during that posture flow aroused his devotion to the Mother. But the thing is, you can't really understand the action of Shakti in the world without understanding Shiva, Shakti's consort."

"OK," I said. "Lay it on me."

"Shiva is the masculine principle in creation," Bruce said. "He is pure witness consciousness, the archetypal seer. He is the formless brahman, pure spirit, transcendent, and without any attributes."

"Now I'm confused. Shiva and brahman are the same?"

"Well, yes. In this path Shiva represents brahman.[3] You might think of Shiva as the still point, the absolute subject, the One," said Bruce. "And shakti as the dance. It's like T. S. Eliot said—'Without the still point, there would be no dance.' In the yogic view, the entire universe moves between these two poles—*shiva* and shakti. Pure consciousness and pure power. Pure being and pure becoming. The still point and the dance. Always arcing toward one another.

"Here's the really cool thing," Bruce continued. "In hatha yoga—the practice of postures and yogic breathing—the whole drama of the universe gets acted out right within this very earthly body. In this drama, all the condensed powers of shakti lie coiled at the base of the spine. This is what we know as kundalini, the essence of divine goddess energy. The kundalini shakti longs to rise up to meet her consort, shiva, pure witness consciousness, who resides in an energy center at the crown of the head, the so-called crown chakra. The union of shiva and shakti, which is the goal of hatha yoga, is accomplished when shakti moves up through the central energy column in the area of the spine—called the *shushumna*—and arrives at the crown. On its trip to meet shiva, this highly condensed energy of kundalini shakti awakens all of the latent energy centers in the body, and as this happens, the body moves spontaneously into hundreds of postures.

"The dance that results is the interplay of energy and consciousness, or what yogis call *lila*—the divine play. The posture flow you saw this morning was just lila. Gurudev knows how to turn his body over to the forces of pure consciousness and pure energy, letting the two dance and play."

We walked in silence for a while, the wind blowing snow in our faces. And I thought to myself. All this time, I'd been doing postures and nobody ever told me what it was really about. But I could feel the rightness of Bruce's explanation. I could feel the interplay of consciousness and energy in the experience of the morning. Gurudev's body reaching toward something ineffable. The whole room entrained in his powerful state of samadhi.

"OK, now I understand, but then if all of that was happening in him, why was my spine tingling?"

"Well, that's easy. The body of a yoga adept, like Gurudev, becomes very refined. He's learned how to tolerate intense amounts of energy—kundalini shakti—moving through his physical form. His body actually vibrates at a higher rate than yours or mine. And so when you touch him, or get near him, you can feel that powerful energy charge. And just in the subtlest way it begins to awaken your own kundalini. That's all. It's very simple. It's not like he's intentionally trying to zap you or anything. He used to do that. And believe me, when he wants to concentrate that energy and send it toward you, it can be intense. Even unbearable. But he doesn't do that anymore. As far as these little charges of energy go, like the ones you got, he can't help it. It's just the nature of the energy."

I gave Bruce my most skeptical look. He just laughed. "Well, you're the one who had the energy experience. What do you think it was?"

When I got home from our walk, I jotted down some notes in my big leather notebook, a simple schematic that to this day helps me to organize my understanding of the two poles of energy and consciousness.

SHIVA	SHAKTI
The archetypal masculine	The archetypal feminine
The Seer	The Mother
Pure witness consciousness	Pure embodiment
Pure being	Pure becoming
The One	The many
Transcendent	Immanent
The still point	The dance
Spirit	Matter
The unmanifest	The phenomenal world
The sun	The moon
Light	Dark
Nirguna brahman	*Saguna brahman*
Unity	Multiplicity
Wave	Particle
Consciousness	Energy

BRAHMAN AND SHAKTI ARE ONE

With this understanding, the parable of Viveka began to come into focus. On his journey home, Viveka would have to encounter both the archetypal masculine and the archetypal feminine. On the mountaintop, he would encounter the ascetic form of Shiva—the seer, pure witness consciousness, akin to the transcendent, formless brahman without attributes (*nirguna brahman*) that is the essence of wisdom. And in the marketplace, he would encounter the Mother (*saguna brahman*—or brahman with form), who is really the mother of the phenomenal world in disguise, pure becoming, pure energy, the embodiment of compassion, the sow suckling her piglets.

In order to come into union with his true self, Viveka would have to come to understand the essential unity of these polarities. He would have to understand the words of Ramakrishna:

Supreme Reality alone exists—as *brahman*, the Pure Consciousness within and beyond all finite forms of consciousness,

and as *shakti,* the primordial, evolutionary Divine Energy. They
are not two. *Brahman* and *shakti* are like the snake and its
smoothly flowing motion, like milk and its whiteness, like water
and its wetness. When considering water, one inevitably thinks
of its wetness. When contemplating the wetness of water, one
inevitably thinks of the water itself. Precisely the same is true of
the Absolute and the relative, which are indifferentiable in essence. The Absolute is inevitably expressed by the relative, and
the relative is inevitably contained by the Absolute. *Shakti* is
the creative Mother-Father-God, the fount of revelation. *Brahman* is the inconceivable, indescribable nature of Reality. . . .
brahman and *shakti* are one.[4]

What this means for us, I understood, is that we don't have to leave
the body to find the One in some transcendent realm. The body is the
field of brahman. The earth is the field of brahman. In the yogic view,
the body is just the outward and visible form of an infinite interior
world of consciousness, intelligence, and compassion. "Deep eternity,"
in Emily Dickinson's phrase, is right here, right now. It is the subtle
interior anatomy of the body—and the subtle interior anatomy of this
entire world of form.

"The goal of human life," says Ramakrishna, "is to meet God face to
face." But the magic is this: if we look deeply into the face of all
created things, we will find God. Therefore, savor the world, the body.
Open it, explore it, look into it. Worship it.

TANTRA

I would later come to understand that Desai's teaching—and the lineage from which he issued, the ancient *Pashupat* tradition—was saturated with a sophisticated version of Indian spirituality known as
Tantra, a metaphysic that espoused a reaffirmation of the world. In the
Tantric formulation, *spirit is co-essential with the phenomenal world.* If
the Absolute is anywhere, it is everywhere—equally present in the
body as in the soul, in sexuality as in celibacy, in the profane world as in
the sacred.

The body, in this view, is *devata*—the visible form of brahman. The
Tantric student, or *sadhaka,* comes to believe that we are one with the

divine here and now, in every act that we do. Liberation, in the Tantric traditions, is gained not through renunciation, but through entering fully into the play (lila) of energy and consciousness. Says Heinrich Zimmer, one of the great scholars of the Tantric traditions:

> The candidate for wisdom does not seek a detour by which to circumvent the sphere of the passions—crushing them within himself and shutting his eyes to their manifestations without, until, made clean as an angel, he may safely open his eyes again to regard the cyclone of *samsara* with the untroubled gaze of a disembodied apparition. Quite the contrary: the Tantric hero *(vira)* goes directly through the sphere of greatest danger.[5]

The Tantric teachings, which arose in medieval India, provided the metaphysical soil for the growth of a remarkable path of experiential knowledge. The supreme reality in this view cannot merely be described or understood. It must be realized. Out of this metaphysic arose a view of life that framed the whole of human existence as a process of identifying with the creative source of the cosmos. The whole of life is a pilgrimage back to the center, where energy and consciousness spontaneously arise together.

THE WHOLE WORLD IS ONE FAMILY

Two days after Bruce gave me his teaching on shiva and shakti, Jeff and I took a mountain-bike ride up the trail behind Shadowbrook. It was a warm day for early December, the sun shining through several drifting islands of fluffy white clouds. The snows of previous days had burned quickly away in the heat of the sun and mild temperatures. We pulled nylon caps over our heads, our bike helmets on top of those, and hopped on, pedaling hard for ten minutes or so, angling up the side of the mountain behind Shadowbrook, through a craggy old apple orchard, and up the road to the crest of the ridge. The trees around the Stockbridge Bowl had long since lost their leaves, and the landscape had begun to adopt its winter hues, moody soft grays and maroons. The air was cold and clean. After we hit smooth sailing on the road, "the professor" began to describe what he'd discovered about the original inhabitants of the land.

The Mahicans and their ancestors had fished the glacial lakes and streams of the Berkshires as far back as twelve thousand years ago. Apparently these tribes of the eastern woodlands had a rich and vital culture. They were expert farmers who cultivated vegetables unknown in Europe. They called their corn, beans, and squash the "three life-giving sisters." To the Mahicans, hunting was both a science and a religion. They felt the animals they hunted to be their relatives and teachers. Moose, deer, fox, and fish were described as "cousins," and given personalities and spirits, all of which were recounted in their songs and dances. It's not unlikely that a site like Shadowbrook was used for their religious theater of praise and thanksgiving, rituals in which they gave thanks to the animals and plants who sustained them.

Jeff and I found an ideal seat on two big slabs of shale at the crest of the ridge. We were in a sea of brown wood ferns and scrub oak. The woods were still damp, and the December air was filled with the smell of rotting maple leaves. Jeff told me how the Mahicans had learned to tap the maple trees for sap in the late winter, and how the early European explorers reported home that they'd found a paradise where the "trees gave honey without the intervention of bees."

This particular tribe, Jeff went on, had a reverence for countless beings in realms other than human. Not only the animals, but trees, rocks, and running rivers all had spiritual natures. There was a sense of the One Spirit infusing all of creation. "I think the Mahicans would be pleased that the land has been reclaimed by another tribe that reveres it," mused Jeff.

We lay on the big slabs of shale, pulling off a layer of fleece to better soak up the uncommonly warm early winter sun. The heat was soporific. We dozed. When I came to, I had the sense that I had just arrived, that all the cells of my body had just landed, together, on this particular rock, in this particular woods. My mind had quieted and stilled deeply. I had a sense of great well-being. I felt completely at home in these woods, I thought. Utter relief.

Buddhists and yogis, I was thinking, are always talking about being "here" and "now." But how often do we really know where "here" is? How can we really be "here" without knowing the spirit of the place? Without knowing its animals and insects and trees and rocks? Without knowing how the shadows fall in autumn, and on a crisp winter's day like this one?

"The whole world is one family," taught Bapuji. We're all so deeply connected. Yogis see the world saturated with the spirit of the divine. In this view, all aspects of the divine manifestation are celebrated. All are listened to. When we pay close attention to the world of the many, we inevitably discover the One.

As I sat musing, I remembered that on the night of his final enlightenment, even the Buddha had to call on the power of the Earth goddess, the divine Shakti, for help in his struggle with the forces of Mara, the dark powers of delusion. He touched the ground where he sat. "This earth," he said, "is my witness." Yogis, and Mahicans, might take that statement even further: this earth is my family member, my sister, my self.

Finally I woke Jeff out of his reverie, pointing to a large red-tailed hawk hanging just above us in the cold blue sky. "The goddess in one of her disguises," I said.

Jeff trained his binoculars on the bird for a moment, then took a deep breath of mountain air. " 'There is a moment in every day that the devil cannot find,' " he sighed, quoting William Blake.

"Seems like I've been having more than my share, then." We laughed and hopped back on our bikes, riding down the mountain at full tilt, Jeff calling to the hawk still circling overhead.

Part Two

THE SELF IN EXILE

5

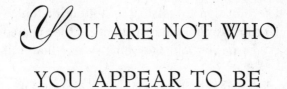OU ARE NOT WHO
YOU APPEAR TO BE

Oh, I could sing such grandeurs and glories about you!
You have not known what you are, you have slumbered upon yourself all
    your life,
Your eyelids have been the same as closed most of the time . . .

Whoever you are! claim your own at any hazard!
These shows of the East and West are tame compared to you,
These immense meadows, the interminable rivers, you are immense and
    interminable as they.

—Walt Whitman,
"To You"

As my four-month stay at Kripalu wound to its close I began to feel
anxious. I had had several months of comparative bliss—hours of yoga
and meditation each day, cutting vegetables with an extraordinary
group of people from all over the world, a renewed relationship with
nature. But something else had happened. Something I didn't yet understand. I felt both compelled and annoyed by the mysteries of Indian
spirituality. Doing postures was almost pure delight. Breathing practices. Diet. Lifestyle. It all worked to calm and soothe, to energize. But
as I tried to look under the surface of the daily practices, I discovered a
maze of incomprehensible metaphysics. Vedanta, Tantra, Samkhya, Advaita Vedanta, Veda. Huh? I tried reading some of the most basic scriptures, but I couldn't understand what any of them really had to do with

my life. My confusion and the anxiety of my impending departure made me feel bold with Amrit. I was like a dog with a bone.

I would raise my hand. He would smile. "Stephen?" Finally, he'd learned my name. Up I would go, to kneel next to him. As I felt my own strong determination to get to the bottom of things, I couldn't help but think of my psychotherapy patients as they neared the end of their therapy, how newly bold they often were, how willing to take risks.

"I don't understand this. If 'everything is already OK,' as you say, and if we're born divine, and if the whole world is God, and the Divine Mother is our energy, then why are we suffering? How is it that we create pain for ourselves and for others? Why don't we live in sat-chit-ananda all of the time? I have to go back and face thirty-five suffering patients a week. Does yoga have anything really important to say about their suffering?"

This time he studied me. Then he broke out laughing. He turned to the gathering. "When the soul wakes up, it's thirsting for knowledge. Like brother Stephen, here.

"You're a *jnana* yogi, you know that?" he said, turning back to me. "A yogi who finds liberation through knowledge. The jnana yogis explore the whole world with discriminating intellect. '*Neti,* neti.' Not this, not that, they say, sifting to find what is God and what is not God. What is truth and what is not truth.

"Did you know, yogis teach that the individual soul, the *jivatma,* wanders for eons through creation. Birth and death. Rebirth. Death again. Over and over again, chained to the great wheel of suffering by the great affliction of desire. And finally, just at the darkest hour before dawn, the soul awakes to an awareness of its own suffering. Just as yours has.

"Have you read, yet, the *Bhagavad Gita*—the story of Arjuna and Krishna? The greatest scripture in all Hinduism?[1] There you will find the answer you seek. And here is the lesson you will learn there: The fundamental experience of human suffering is the experience of alienation from the self, from the source—from God. Unlike your Christian religion, for example, we don't believe the problem is sin, or guilt, or wrongdoing. It's simply misidentification!"

Desai then proceeded to tell the story of the *Bhagavad Gita* to the rapt audience. He set the scene: Arjuna, the warrior, and his charioteer, Krishna, avatar of the Hindu god Vishnu, drive onto the battlefield of Kurukshetra and survey the forces arrayed against them, which include many of Arjuna's family members. Arjuna's first response to the scene is desolation and despair. "I will not fight this battle," he says. He retreats to the floor of the chariot in the face of a seemingly impossible choice between dereliction of his sacred duty (dharma) and the killing of his kinsmen.

Amrit grew more and more animated as he got more deeply into the story. "Krishna," he continued, "pulls Arjuna up from the floor of the chariot and begins his teaching, which proceeds through eighteen sublime chapters. Krishna explains to Arjuna how ensnared he has become—ensnared in the material world, ensnared in ego. And he says to Arjuna, you know the real problem here is that you don't know who you really are.

"Pay attention to this," Amrit said. "You don't know who you are. Who you think you are, you are not."

THE PSYCHOLOGY OF SELF-ESTRANGEMENT

Desai proceeded to give a brilliant description of Arjuna's dilemma—and our own. After eons of wandering through incarnation after incarnation, we've gradually forgotten who we are. We've forgotten that we're simply the fantastic play of consciousness and energy, of shiva and shakti. Like Viveka, and like Arjuna, we've become ensnared in first a subtle, but then an increasingly gross misidentification.

Now we have become exclusively identified with our physical bodies, with our possessions, with our thoughts, with our personalities. We think we're our ideas, our careers, our families, our countries. We live our lives in utter ignorance of the vastness of our real nature, estranged from our true selves. This is the source of our suffering.

In yogic philosophy, the source of this alienation from the true self is not sin or wrongdoing of any kind. It's simply ignorance—*avidya*. As they awaken to themselves, Viveka and Arjuna's fundamental problem is not guilt. It's delusion. The Upanishadic sages described this ignorance as a "veil of illusion" that obscures the truth and confuses the mind so that it cannot discriminate between reality and appearance.[2]

In the yogic view, suffering has its origins in a process called extroversion (*unmesha*). The soul gradually becomes completely identified with the material plane of existence, even though this "gross material plane"—the physical body and the personality—is only the most outward and visible aspect of her true home. This is a disastrous misidentification because, in addition to the body, mind, and personality, yoga teaches that the true home of the soul is also beyond time and space, in the eternal now of consciousness. When we live disconnected from these vast roots of the Self, we suffer.

Self is capitalized here because it refers to the divine, awake, free self. Given the yogic view of our predicament, it's not surprising that we so often feel estranged, that we feel unreal, that we feel disconnected from our center. That is precisely our condition.

Yoga psychology gets very specific about the exact nature of the conditioning that keeps us ensnared in delusion about our true nature. The classical scriptures identify five "afflictions" or *kleshas*—five conditioned beliefs and behaviors that keep us bound to "gross apparent reality." They are:

1. *Avidya:* Ignorance
2. *Asmita:* "I-ness"
3. *Raga:* Attraction
4. *Dvesha:* Aversion
5. *Abhinivesha:* Clinging to life and fear of death

These five afflictions are seen as being in a kind of cause and effect sequence and are listed in the order in which they arise. Ignorance is the ground from which all the other afflictions spring. Out of ignorance arises "I-ness": the belief in and clinging to a separate, solid, "small *s*" self. Out of "I-ness" arise attraction and aversion—our complete identification with our likes and dislikes. And out of this inevitably arises clinging to life and fear of death—a deluded and desperate desire for life to be small, neat, permanent, and solid rather than vast, incomprehensible, impermanent, and discontinuous, as it really is.

In addition to the five afflictions, the scriptures also identify four erroneous beliefs that sustain the delusion of the kleshas. These are:

1. The belief in the permanence of objects
2. The belief in the ultimate reality of the body
3. The belief that our state of suffering is really happiness
4. The belief that our bodies, minds, and feelings are our true Self

When our vision of reality is colored by the five afflictions and four erroneous beliefs, we live in delusion: the atman is no longer able to recognize home as the safe and commodious reality of brahman. "As the waters of a clear spring screened by vegetation cannot be seen," says author and teacher Rajarshi Muni, "so also the human soul concealed within the material bodies cannot shine forth, and its real nature remains beyond comprehension."[3] In the thrall of the afflictions, we see the world totally distorted by what Deepak Chopra calls the myth of materialism, the deluded view that "gross apparent reality" is the whole shooting match.

ONE PROBLEM, ONE SOLUTION

At the end of his long disquisition on Krishna and Arjuna, Amrit gave me a warm, welcoming look, and spontaneously opened his arms. I dove into them and lay across his lap as he gave me a kind of whole body hug. No one was more surprised than I. After a few moments, heart pounding in my chest and slightly dazed, I took my seat again. As I sat down on my cushion at the front of the room, I was overcome with emotion. I felt an upwelling of love. Tears streamed. My body was incredibly hot all over. My belly was on fire. My face felt bright red. And for a moment my whole body felt as though it was melting. I wanted to melt into him. The feeling was sensual, almost sexual, but not quite. I felt in a swoon, or what I imagined a swoon might be. It was like being in love, only it seemed to be happening in some wholly new place inside. I had the sense that some ancient internal barrier had been broken down. Everything was completely OK.

Meanwhile, Amrit talked on for another hour. For me, the whole room was alive with energy. I saw bright lights. My heart pounded. My mind tuned in to the talk and then out again. "In yoga," I heard him say, "there is only one problem and one solution: the problem is that we've forgotten who we are; the solution is to remember who we are, to reidentify with the entire reality of atman.

"We are like people walking around in a room with the lights off." I had heard him use this analogy before. "We are attempting to move around and live in this room without light. So naturally we bump into things, and into each other. We continually hurt ourselves and others. And we feel a sense of dissatisfaction and pain.

"We are deluded because we think that our fundamental dilemma is that there is something wrong with this place that we're in. Even more painfully, we think there is something wrong with ourselves. Actually, there is nothing wrong. If we could simply turn on the lights, we would see reality more clearly. The solution is so simple: illuminate the landscape. With the light of *vidya* (knowledge, or the opposite of *avidya*), we might align our movements and our behavior with the way things really are and we could be quite content and effective in living life with ourselves in this very same reality. Cutting through avidya is simply turning on the lights. One problem, one solution."

Even though I was in a daze, I got the gist of the rest of the lecture. The good news is that this reidentification with the true Self is not so difficult. It is happening all the time. Indeed, everything in life is continually pointing us back toward our true nature. Yogis discovered that when avidya is seen through—when we have a direct experience of the reality of atman, like my experience on the ladder, the entire chain of the kleshas and the erroneous beliefs is cut. We wake up again, in that very moment, to our true nature. In this view, direct knowledge of the reality of atman is all the healing we need. This knowledge, or vidya, in itself immediately cuts through the sting of human suffering.

THE DIVINE EYES

After the talk I found my way back to my bunk, still rather in a daze. My body was abuzz with energy, so I knew there was no immediate chance of falling asleep. I took out my copy of the *Bhagavad Gita*, and opening at random, found myself in chapter 11, "The Vision of the Cosmic Form." In this chapter, Arjuna asks to see Krishna's divine form. Krishna grants his wish, and gives him "divine eyes," so that he can see into the unmanifest realms.

Immediately, the secrets of the transcendental atman flash into view. Arjuna experiences a kind of psychedelic light show, in which all the boundaries of the self are melted down, Arjuna sees the gods, the *maharishis* ("great seers") and the *siddhas* ("perfected ones"), Buddha, Krishna, all the enlightened beings. All forms dissolve, and both life and death vanish into the light of the eternal. He sees the seven great cosmic planes, and he knows that all realms—earth and the heavenly realms and the hell realms below—are all holy and that all beings in both the manifest and the unmanifest worlds shine with the same light of the one transcendent Self.

Finally, Arjuna says "enough." He cannot bear the blaze of light and heat, of consciousness and energy, which threatens to dissolve his human body and mind. He must return at once to the world of space and time, to his accustomed form. Krishna grants his wish: just as quickly as the experience began, it is over. But Arjuna will never be the same. He apologizes to Krishna: "I didn't know who you were," he says. And his soul now reaches out with love toward his divine guide.

I wondered. Was my experience in the main chapel a moment of *atmavidya*—direct knowledge of the soul? Was Desai intentionally revealing these things to me? Was he destined to play the role of Krishna in my life? And would my contact with him give me the divine eyes? Or was I becoming ensnared in a dangerous delusion?

INTROVERSION: FINDING THE WAY HOME

In the weeks that followed this experience, my inquiry heated up. I had only limited contact with Amrit, so I took my questions to Bruce and to Yoganand and to Rani, eventually cobbling together a basic understanding of the yogic pilgrimage back to the center, the path to the true Self.

Through millennia of practice, yogis learned to reverse the process of extroversion. They discovered that they could unwind the painful misidentification, retracing the steps of the human self back through the layers of reality, from the most gross, physical plane with which we now exclusively identify, to the most refined planes of pure consciousness. They mapped this process, and called it, not surprisingly, introversion *(nimesha)*. The process of introversion required the use of practices that worked directly with both consciousness *(chitta)* and energy *(prana)*, and included the development of deep states of concentration (samadhi) as well as the refinement of energy through postures *(asana)* and yogic breathing *(pranayama)*. This path eventually came to be called yoga.

Practitioners of yoga developed a phenomenally detailed description of the layers of reality that must be retraced in order to find "the way home." In the resulting yogic cartography, the energy of each embodied human soul is understood to be organized in increasingly subtle levels of energy organization, or "sheaths"—*koshas* in Sanskrit. The gross physical body that we can see and touch is only the most outward and visible form of a whole layering of energy realities that exist at increasingly refined and less tangible levels. In the yogic mapping there are three "bodies" *(shariras),* and within these three bodies, five "sheaths" (the koshas).

The Three Bodies (shariras)	**The Five Sheaths (koshas)**
sthula (gross body)	*annamayakosha* (sheath of food)
sukshma (subtle body)	*pranamayakosha* (sheath of vital airs) *manomayakosha* (sheath of mind) *vijnanamayakosha* (sheath of causal intellect)
karana (causal body)	*anandamayakosha* (sheath of pure bliss)

The physical, or "gross," body is known as the sthula sharira. It is also the first sheath, the annamayakosha—literally the "sheath of food." Underlying our physical body, yogis identified a subtle body, the sukshma sharira, composed of three overlapping sheaths. The first of these sheaths, and the closest to the physical body, is called the pranamayakosha, or the "sheath of vital airs." This is an energy organization that most of us can connect with quite directly through pranayama—yogic breathing practices. The next and more interior sheath is called the manomayakosha, the "sheath of mind," the subtle organization of thoughts and will. Even more refined is the vijnanamayakosha, the sheath of so-called causal intellect, which is far more subtle than what we think of as intellect. Finally, we come to the third, the causal body or the karana sharira. This is composed of the anandamayakosha, the "sheath of pure bliss," which is closest to atman.

This notion of subtle planes of reality existing beneath the threshold of "gross apparent reality" is not by any means unique to Indian spirituality. Teresa of Avila, for example, in her classic work *The Interior Castle,* described the self as a castle with rooms arranged in seven concentric rings or circles around the center. The pilgrimage to God required the systematic penetration of increasingly subtle, spiritual inner rooms, until the soul reached its source in the seventh room at the center of the castle.

Most of us consider the physical body to be our true body and think of the subtle levels as more or less imaginary. But yogic practice holds that, in fact, these less tangible levels are just as real as the physical body, and, indeed, we cannot connect with our true selves without a full identification with all of the sheaths simultaneously. This is emphatically not to say that the body must be denied. Rather, the gross body must be experienced in its holistic connection with the energy bodies, the mental bodies, and the bliss body.

While the tendency is strong to want to map the sheaths as concentric and nested layers of a spatial structure with a "core" of atman, or God—as Teresa did—this is clearly, from the yogic view, an oversimplification. The sheaths are no more inside one another than the mind is inside the brain. Their nature is closer to that of a hologram, wherein all the aspects of reality exist at the same time and the same place, completely. The sheaths exist as an energetic whole that manifests within space-time, yet they also exist outside the physical space-time continuum.

The world of gross apparent reality is not even remotely what it seems to be. What we think of as our "self," separate from other selves, distinct, continuous, and to some degree under its own power, is not a separate object at all. In our essential nature we are a Self that lives in union with the whole realm of mind and matter.*

THE WHOLE WORLD IN MYSELF

It was eight o'clock on a blustery night in late February. Snow beat against the big windows of the main chapel. I was sitting at the front of a group of a hundred guests and residents, listening to a talk by Gitanand, a warmly engaging man in late middle age, dressed in saffron robes. I didn't know much, yet, about this American yogi, except that in order to pursue his practice, he had left a coveted tenured position as a physics professor at a prestigious university. He had a certain glow about him, as though he were exuding some particularly subtle light. Perhaps his shaved head and exceptionally slender frame added to the quality of lightness. He was a member of the small renunciate order at

---

* Readers wishing a more in-depth examination of yoga metaphysics will want to turn at any point now to the appendix, "Yoga Metaphysics with a Light Touch."

Kripalu who had committed to a particularly rigorous practice, follow-ing classic monastic training precepts of poverty, chastity, and obedi-ence.

At that point, I was still both suspicious of and intrigued by people who took on Sanskrit names. And I wasn't wild about his costume. But I could relate to this man. His talk was reasoned, articulate, and even elegant—befitting any high-octane graduate classroom. I could imagine him wandering around Cambridge with a pocket protector and the focused gaze of someone spinning out complex equations in his head.

Gitanand was telling the story of a dialogue between a Vedic master and a Western student. "The student, confounded by the radically dif-ferent worldview embodied by his teacher, asks, 'Do we live in the same world?' Replies the teacher, 'Yes, we do. It's just that you see yourself in the world, and I see the whole world in myself.' Yogis insist on seeing the world from the inside out."

The yogic worldview is radical, Gitanand went on. We can experi-ence the entire reality of the universe directly through a full explora-tion of the phenomena of our own bodies, feelings, minds. There is nothing that is "out there" that is not also "in here." Any part of the universe (the many—*bahu*) is a holograph, containing the entire uni-verse within it (the One—*eka*). Whatever is found in the human organ-ism (*pindanda*) is also found in the universal organism (*Brahmanda*). Universal laws apply equally at all levels of reality. As above, so below.

Physics is just beginning to provide us with some Western scientific support for this enchanting view, Gitanand told us. Quantum theory makes clear, for example, that our experience of the body as a frozen anatomical structure is a profound misperception. I had recently heard Deepak Chopra in an evening talk at Kripalu make the same point. The well-defined edges to the physical body are artifacts of sensory percep-tion. Our bodies are just part of a cosmic body that is in constant interchange with itself. Chopra had gone on to describe how this inter-change happens even at the most gross plane of the annamayakosha: "Ninety-eight percent of the atoms of this body," he had said, "are exchanged every year for new atoms, atoms that were formerly part of another structure—perhaps the Buddha, or the Christ, or Genghis Khan."

All of this stands our worldview completely on its head. Our civiliza-tion and technologies are still deeply saturated with Newtonian materi-alistic dualism, predicated on the belief that there is an "objective

reality" that we can know through a scientific method based upon observation and inference.

In many ways, I realized that night, the yogic view of reality is similar
to the one that prevailed in the West before the scientific revolution
separated our inner and subjective world from a supposedly external
and objective one. Prior to this fracturing, our experience of life was
seen much more as yogis still see it: "as manifestations of one indivisible reality appearing in its visible and invisible forms. The condition of
the human body was (in the medieval world) considered the visible
appearance of one's mind and spirit, just as mental activity was an
expression of the individual's way of sensing his physical embodiment."[4]

During the question period, I raised my hand. "It would seem that
the leap from the world of postmodern physics, with its curved space-
time continua, antimatter, and hyperdimensionality, to yoga might be
very natural in a way. After all, doesn't physics seem to be edging closer
and closer to rediscovering the yogic worldview?"

"Good question. But the difference is that the yogic traditions teach
that the entire field of mind and matter can be known directly through
the experience of the self—and indeed, that that is the only way they
can be authentically known. Whereas knowledge in our Western traditions is gained through inference, the Eastern contemplative traditions
have developed ways of knowing the world directly through the text-
book of immediate experience."

Yogis' direct experience is that there is an inner dimension to the
universe—what we see as gross material reality has a wonderful but
invisible depth. Their discoveries have pointed the way home—the
process of introversion as a way to reverse the condition of Self-
estrangement. They created a map to the true Self. And the goal of all
yogic knowledge and practice became the reunion with this Self.

So Paula and I were right, I thought! We have been living in exile
from our true home. We have not been living as fully alive human
beings. We have been alienated from our source. Once I understood
the real import of this yogic view, I felt deeply relieved. I had trusted
my hunches, my intuition. Here was a worldview that actually did have
something to say about my psychological reality.

The yogic view in every way confirms the hunches of the human
being in the process of "waking up" to her true nature—the unrelenting call of an interior life, the haunting suspicions of inauthenticity, the

longing to hear the true voice of the Self, the renunciation of extrinsic sources of satisfaction, the call to the kinds of contemplation that allow us to subtly examine our cognitive and perceptual capacities so that we may transcend them.

We were right, too, at least according to this ancient view of things, to trust the relentless, puzzling, beguiling, troubling call of the unknown. It is this call of the unknown, after all, that is announcing the presence of the "seed of the Self" and all of its potential mysteries. And for this haunting call of the Self, as Emily Dickinson said, we must be grateful. Life is always on the verge of waking us up to the huge mysteries at the heart of this world of flux and time.

HOOKED BY THE DIVINE FISHER

In concluding his talk, Gitanand told a little of his personal story. He said that after achieving a certain level of mastery in his scientific pursuits, he had finally decided to dedicate the next portion of his life to practicing yoga. "I decided," he said, "that at the end of my life I would be more satisfied having been the data than having been the scientist who analyzed the data." He described how the pursuit of theoretical knowledge had become empty for him, then told of his growing hunger for an experience of knowing himself—directly, viscerally, immediately.

As I sat listening to the February wind howl through the big pine grove behind the main chapel, I felt the risk in Gitanand's decision. I felt the excitement of it. I felt the largeness of it. In fact, I couldn't deny that in some ways I felt called to it myself. There was something momentous happening to me. I didn't understand it yet. But I knew in that moment that I wasn't going anywhere. Even though I had been preparing to leave, to move on to the next destination of my sabbatical, it was now apparent to me that I had been inwardly preparing to stay. The decision, I realized, had already been made.

The next day I canceled my travel plans. That night I wrote in my journal, "Gitanand was right. Why not throw my lot in here? There's no point in looking for some ideal 'generic brand' of spirituality. If I'm going to explore it, I'm eventually going to have to take on a particular view. This place isn't perfect, but it seems better than most. Why not let myself dive into Kripalu's lineage, its local saints, idiosyncratic tastes, smells, personalities, myths, and genius, and its weaknesses and peculiar blind spots? My only worry is—who will I be, coming out the other side?"

When I told Gitanand, he laughed his big, friendly laugh. "You've been snagged on the line by the divine fisher. You can pull against it. You can resist. But once you've been hooked, your life can only go in one direction. Relax. Enjoy it."

"Oh, yeah? Who's snagged me? What do you mean, 'divine fisher'?"

"You'll find out."

6

A HOUSE ON FIRE:

THE IDENTITY PROJECT

Before I built a wall I'd ask to know
What I was walling in or walling out,
And to whom I was like to give offense.
Something there is that doesn't love a wall,
That wants it down.

—Robert Frost,
"Mending Wall"

After making the decision to stay on at Kripalu, I had settled comfortably into the rhythm of life on campus. My yoga practice deepened in astonishing ways. My friends back home had their reactions, of course. Nina stopped talking to me for a while. And, my own mind, too, gave me considerable flak: Are you crazy? What about your career? Financial security?

Acculturation, however, set in quickly. Before long, I, too, had a Sanskrit name. For me, Desai (or his minions) had chosen "Kaviraj"—meaning "king of the poets." Outwardly, I laughed at the pretense of it all. But secretly, I loved it. With my new name, I felt that I finally belonged. I was liked and respected. I was given responsible jobs to do. I was having fun. I felt great.

The one thing I did miss quite a bit, however, aside from my friends, was my meditation practice. Many yogic lineages (Kripalu's included) do not stress meditation nearly as much as yoga postures. So, at the first opportunity, I had signed up for a meditation retreat to be given at

Kripalu by a distinguished visiting teacher from one of the yogic lineages that specializes in meditation techniques.

Day one of the three-day retreat—on a weekend in late June—
dawned unseasonably hot. As I sat on my meditation cushion, rivulets
of sweat wound their way lazily down my back, collecting at the base of
my spine into what began to feel like Lake Ontario. "Don't get involved
with it," I thought, repeating back to myself the instructions I knew so
well. "Just observe it and come back to the breath." The woman seated
on the big red mat in front of me kept a small hand-towel next to her
and occasionally mopped her brow and neck. Three rows ahead of me I
could see the back of Paula's head. She had come to join me for this
three-day guest retreat, and occasionally I sent a little silent prayer of
good wishes to her. In truth, I wanted to be someplace else. My body
was screaming. I wanted to be up to my neck in cool water. After a
couple of hours of struggling to stay present with the rising and falling
of my breath, my mind gave up, exhausted. "That's it. I'm toast." Then
I watched as my mind devised a grand strategy for entertaining itself.

Several months earlier, my grandfather had died. The week after the
retreat I was to drive to upstate New York to pick up a truckful of
family antiques he had left to me—furniture, paintings, and little treasures of all kinds. These were certainly not things of immense value.
But I'd grown up with them in Gramp's rambling Victorian house, and
they were packed with meaning for me. I was completely obsessed with
redesigning the interior of my house back in Boston in order to integrate all these treasures. After a while, I noticed that I was spending a
healthy chunk of my time on the meditation cushion perfecting my
design for several of the rooms—colors, carpeting, furniture arrange-
ment. In flagrant violation of the rules of the retreat, I was studying a
book of color swatches between sits. My mind was taken over by the
project. But I was not particularly unhappy with this. I was getting a lot
of decorating done there on the meditation cushion.

The second day of the retreat was even hotter than the first. I was
seated in the front row near the meditation teacher, and when I was
not obsessing about my house, I was looking at him. He was a short and
compact Indian man, with a handsome, olive face and curly black hair
that had developed a life of its own in the heat and humidity. He sat
perfectly still, and was astonishingly motionless for hours on end.

When I went in for my interview on the second day of the retreat, I
told him about the obsession I was having. The teacher looked directly

at me and smiled, cool as a cucumber. Without a trace of humor or irony, and in a thick Indian accent, he said to me, "This furniture. This fabric. This is chickenshit."

Of course, I knew he was right. He was attempting to cut through my chickenshit clinging with the sword of discriminating wisdom. I admired him even more for being so clear. But I was soon to discover that the "sword of Manjushri," which he was wielding, was no match for the powerful clinging of my mind to the beauty of my things, my self, my image. The river of obsession continued, unabated, like the mighty Mississippi.

I didn't stop fantasizing. But I did begin to watch this internal drama a bit more closely. And as I tuned in, I began to hear a lot of new voices screaming, just underneath the fantasy. There was a desperate, panicky, craven quality to their chatter, which I had not noticed before. They were saying things like, "My furniture. My house. My image. My treasure. Me." They were obsessed with how this new stuff would make me look, with how it would make me feel—better, more interesting, more whole, more real. It was frightening to see the kind of hold this stuff had on my mind. In some way, as I began to see that day, my stuff *was* me.

ASMITA: CLINGING TO "ME" AND "MINE"

As we saw in the last chapter, yogic philosophy holds a magnificent view of our human nature and potential. Born divine. But if yogis are correct about our true nature, then why don't we experience our awakeness most of the time? What is blocking our capacity to realize all of the subtle bodies and to remain connected with the quantum field of mind and matter? Why was it so hard for me just to sit and be with myself in the heat?

In the yogic view, the answer lies in an understanding of the second affliction, asmita, or "I-ness." We cling desperately to every outward and visible representation of "me" and "mine," building our lives around the most gross apparent realities, which are by their nature the most impermanent aspects of the whole enterprise. "Upon mistaking a tree stump for a thief," says the sage Sureshvara in the *Naishkarmya-Siddhi,* "one becomes frightened and runs away. Similarly, one who is deluded superimposes the Self upon the mind and the other aspects of the human personality, and then acts on the basis of that mistaken view."[1] We construct our lives as solidly as we possibly can around those ideas in our minds of how our lives should be. As we build our lives around these images we inevitably suffer.

As I looked more closely at this process through the rest of the retreat, I could see in fact how my overweening attachment to my stuff was causing me to suffer, right in the moment of the obsession. I began to be able to feel in my body the pain of clinging, of craving, of greed, holding on so tight to this stuff that I didn't yet have. I noticed the intense restlessness in my mind, and the sense of heat and pain that were associated with this obsession. In fact, the heat of the day was nothing compared with the heat of my clinging and craving. I thought my stuff was making me happy. But when I looked deeper, I discovered a much more complicated reality.

After a while, I understood that the attachment to myself and my image and my furniture was actually taking me away from my self, away from this wonderful opportunity to just sit, just breathe, just feel the warm animal of my body, just feel the soft, sultry heat of June. The density of my attachment was making it impossible for me to have a truly satisfying experience of life in my body just as it was in the moment. When under the sway of this obsession, my mind's attention was always in the fantasized future, or the idealized or devalued past—never present to the reality of the moment.

In the process of this retreat I could see how a systematic examination of my immediate experience led inexorably to a realization of the afflictions and the four erroneous beliefs. Not only did I see the machinations of the first and second afflictions, avidya and asmita, at work, but I was stunned to see the truth of the third erroneous belief, "the belief that our state of suffering is really happiness." I had thought that my decorating schemes were making me happy. I saw, however, how much suffering there really was just beneath the surface of this "happiness."

As painful as this particular retreat was for me, it opened my eyes to the extraordinary amount of time my mind spent in monitoring and evaluating my success or failure, and in making reality match my ideal image of myself. With my newfound awareness, I would notice how there seemed to be an endless tape-loop in my mind that evaluated my progress: "OK, now I've accomplished this, and this, and this. Now I have this much money in the bank. Now I've made this progress in my career. I'm doing alright." This compulsive internal dialogue is quite normal in a culture that rewards achievement, wealth, beauty, and success above all things, and especially in a culture that rewards the achievements of the highly individuated, separate "self under its own power." In this milieu, the internal dialogue is actually a form of self-soothing, of reassuring ourselves that we're really OK. When we can stand back from this compulsive internal dialogue just a bit, we can see the intensity of the craving for solidity and security that drives it.

It turns out that when we lift the lid just the tiniest bit on our internal dialogues, we discover that we're constantly trying to shore up our "sense of self," reassuring ourselves that we're actually real, solid, and continuous, reassuring ourselves that indeed there is a me, and that this me that woke up this morning is the same me that woke up last week, or the same me that woke up twenty years ago in a college dorm. All of these objects that are "mine" say there is a me, don't they? Not only do they say there is a "me," but they say who the "me" is. As I see my wonderful new antiques in my house, they tell me who I am every day. They tell others who I am. I feel reassured by this. I feel safely held and soothed by this. Isn't this OK? Isn't this just how it is being a human being?

MANSIONS OF THE SELF

At lunch break on the third day, Paula and I sauntered mindfully up the winding east drive toward the site where the original Shadowbrook mansion had stood—an enormous expanse of terraced lawn, edged by rough-hewn granite walls and decaying marble stairs that appeared like ruins from a long-lost civilization. We walked out onto the huge stretch of manicured green.

"Makes me want to do a scene from *The Sound of Music*," said Paula, making a dramatic twirl. "The hills are alive!"

"Hard to believe that a single house filled this entire expanse, isn't it?" I went on to describe in some detail what I'd discovered about the house. The Shadowbrook mansion had been built by Anson Phelps Stokes, an American inventor, merchant, and real estate investor. At the time the rambling Tudor "cottage" was completed, in 1893, it was the largest home in America, boasting over a hundred opulently furnished rooms. It took over two years, five hundred workers, and close to one million dollars to build and furnish.

"Talk about me and mine!" Paula responded. "If you're crazed about your truckful of antiques, imagine the suffering that was going on in *this* family's mind."

According to a newspaper article of the time, which Jeff and I had read on our second day at Kripalu, Shadowbrook "represented the very pinnacle of luxurious living." The ballroom, for example, was said to have been so large that a driver could "turn a coach and four horses clean around in her." The lawns and gardens were laid out by Frederick Law Olmsted, designer of New York's Central Park and Boston's famous Emerald Necklace park system. The 738-acre estate had also included a working farm, gardens, stables, and riding trails.

We walked down one of the great marble staircases of the old mansion, through a little woods, and out along a long row of stones whose purpose could no longer be discerned. Was it a wall? A stairway? "'Something there is that doesn't love a wall,'" I murmured. "We build these great mansions, these big self-images, trying so hard to create solidity, continuity, even immortality. But every single force of nature conspires to tear them down."

I remembered something that Bapuji had once said. "Oh, my dear students," he commented. "You build such big mansions of the self. But it's fine, really. Because when you clean them out of all your many belongings, you're going to find that they're just great big spaces in which God can live."

As time approached for the afternoon sit, Paula and I headed back toward the building. "You know, there's one thing I don't get," I said. "The teacher said that I should 'just drop it.' Just drop it? Like, 'Just say no to drugs'? It can't be that simple."

SOMEBODY OR NOBODY?

Actually, the meditation teacher had instructed me to drop the obsession with "me" and "mine" every time it came up and to come back to the breath. I understood that there was nothing wrong with the antiques. It was my immoderate attachment to them that was the source of suffering for me. But the "it" that he was asking me to drop seemed too central to the whole project of my life—to the entire project of creating an identity for myself. And all of my psychological training had taught me that we need our identities as much as we need oxygen.

In the Eastern contemplative traditions, there is a lot of talk about becoming nobody—*anatta* (or "no-self"). And even though it is axiomatic now that "you have to become somebody before you can become nobody," still one always gets the sense that "nobody" is really the preferable state. Well, even after many years in the spiritual practice scene, I don't know anybody who's become nobody.

There is a paradox here. We all do need to develop a sense of a self that is continuous, cohesive, and integrated. Indeed, the achievement of this very sense of self is, according to Western psychology, the major parameter of maturity and mental health. Becoming emotionally separate beings, knowing the difference between self and other, inside and outside, subject and object, is central to our capacity for healthy relatedness to others. Indeed, one of the primary sources of suffering in our modern life is the shakiness and fragmentation of the foundations of our sense of self. This lack of a core sense of self can be the result of trauma, inadequate parenting, or an environment empty of love objects. The goal of treatment in so many of our contemporary psychospiritual techniques is precisely the solidification of this sense of self, and of self-esteem, self-love, and self-concept.

And now I'm supposed to deconstruct this hard-won identity? Now that I've built my personal Shadowbrook mansion, I'm supposed to take it apart? How will that help? Can we find a perspective on anatta that really makes any sense for us, that's not just spiritual idealism?

THE TERROR OF "NO-SELF"

When we were in high school my twin sister, Sandy, took me aside one afternoon to a quiet corner of the library. "Steve, how do people know for sure what to believe in?" she asked in the conspiratorial tone we reserved for our most important talks. "How do other people know who they are? Everyone else seems to know their own mind. But I don't." Sandy risked telling me that her seemingly well considered and articulately expressed opinions were a sham. She was simply saying to others what she thought she should. She was worried that there was some deep inadequacy in her. "Do you ever wonder about this?" she asked. "How do you know who you are?"

At first I pretended I didn't share her experience, savoring a moment of superiority with my twin, whom I always thought smarter and better than me. The longing for the relief of self-revelation finally won out, however. I told her I shared the same fear and confusion. And yes, I, too, thought I was the only one who had these feelings. For some reason, we had both assumed most everyone else experienced an inner authenticity about which we could only dream.

Much later, I discovered to my profound relief that this was not so. And today, after decades of both psychological and spiritual practice and training, I know that the questions "How do I know my real self?" and "Am I aligned with my truest self right now?" will haunt my life, all of our lives, on many different levels across the whole trajectory of our years.

Many of us remember the experience of emerging interiority in adolescence—the birth of the introspective self with which Sandy and I were wrestling that afternoon in the library. Suddenly, in our teens, we're drawn into a completely unexplored inner world. We begin to struggle with the truth of our reality at a more internal level than ever before. Who am I, really? Who is this inner "me" that I'm discovering? How do these thoughts, fantasies, wishes, memories, all fit together to make a congruent sense of a whole person? There is for the first time a distinct apprehension of a self—a self as an active agent in the world. We make discoveries of immense importance about who we are, and we may become, for a while, exhilarated with a new sense of meaning and purpose in our lives.

But there is also a shadow side to this wonderful new capacity for introspection. For from the very first awakening of this introspective self, there arises a sense of anxiety and distress, and a deep concern about authenticity. Who am I *really*? How do I know for sure?

The unsettling truth is that the self as object cannot be found anywhere.[2] It cannot be seen. It cannot be directly experienced. It cannot be located in any concrete sense. And this is deeply disconcerting. "Introspection," psychologist Michael Washburn says, "reveals only thoughts, feelings, images and not the *subject* that is assumed to experience these contents. The . . . subject is, then, inaccessible to introspection, and this inaccessibility—this absence—is as disturbing to the adolescent as the self-certainty of introspection is reassuring."[3] The underbelly of this new sense of self, then, is the fact of no-self and its harbinger, the anxiety of nothingness.

When my sister came to speak with me that day in high school she actually had her fingers under the edges of a profound existential truth: the self cannot be known directly. It can only be known obliquely, reflected in the mirror of our relationships with our external world and the relationship we carry on with it in our own internal dialogues. This is the terror into which we emerge in adolescence. This is why we so often feel insecure, anxious, doubtful, and fragmented.

In adolescence and early adulthood, we set out to master these feelings. We enter into what Washburn calls the "identity project"[4]—the project of constructing a continuous sense of ourselves that feels abiding and reliable. This identity is the platform upon which we stand in negotiating the storminess of both the external and internal world. In an attempt to develop a sense of self that gives us secure, consistent, and recognizable feelings of internal wholeness, we'll use whatever raw materials we have at hand: college degrees, monogrammed towels in the bathroom, our own pew in the synagogue, financial status, sexual attractiveness—or an enormous Tudor mansion.

THE IDENTITY PROJECT

One of the strategies we use to hold our sense of self together was dramatically revealed to me that steamy June day on the meditation retreat. Just under the surface of awareness, I discovered a compulsive internal dialogue about the state of my self. "How'm I doing? Well, OK. I did pretty well with these instructions. I seem to be just about as quiet and attentive as everybody else. I think the teacher smiled at me—does that mean he likes me? How do I look today? I wonder if my hair looks like hell. Better go check in the mirror." As I watched, I saw how tenaciously I clung to this dialogue, and how essential it seemed to be in my strategies for feeling good about myself. In order to assuage the anxiety of nothingness, we look everywhere for mirrors to confirm our existence. And if we cannot see this "self," well, perhaps we can at least hear it.[5] Along the way, this ongoing dialogue actually helps us construct an identity for ourselves, serving as a kind of glue for the self.

The identity project has other effective means, as well. We seek the reflection of ourselves not only in the mirror of our soothing self-talk, but in the eyes of others. As adolescents, we become acutely aware of how we are seen. As Jean-Paul Sartre has it, "I am seen: therefore I am." We are impelled to search for a sense of being from without, seeing ourselves mirrored back in the reflection of our "doing" in the world.

A client of mine named Bill came back from a trip to Mexico in a severe depression. He and his lover, Maureen, had spent six months in Oaxaca working on their various writing projects. Maureen spoke fluent Spanish, but Bill didn't speak a word of the language. After a month or two, Bill began to experience a profound sense of isolation. The sudden loss of all the "mirrors" in his life showed him just how much he relied upon external reflections to maintain his sense of self, despite decades of living and traveling alone, and many years of spiritual practice.

As Freud pointed out, we mostly look for ourselves in two places: work and love. In early adulthood we experiment with relationships and commitments. We may try on a number of different roles and functions, a number of different relationships, to see both how we do, and whether they enhance our sense of being who we think we are. In these years, being recognized as a "this" or a "that" is critical to confirming our own sense not only of being but of value.

My friend Amy's adolescent daughter, for example, latched on to Orthodox Judaism in order to define herself in her world; while her mother saw this as a narrowing down of her daughter's options, she also understood that it helped to soothe her internal uncertainties about who she was. A former client's adolescent son, Brian, made an outright commitment for several years to a gang of his peers, the so-called Bad Boys, who had decided upon rebellion and challenging parental expectations. Brian's father was horrified, but Brian managed to use participation in the club in an effective self-building fashion, developing autonomy from an intrusive and enmeshed family. Whether it is a "positive" or a "negative" commitment may not be as important as the fact that it lands us somewhere that feels solid, predictable, continuous, and stable.

As Jung noted, all of the early milestones in creating a personal identity are celebrated and acknowledged in our culture—departing home for college, marriage, or commitment in partnership, the first child, the first house. They are appropriately seen as "initiations" into deeper life, and we understand that they are outward and visible signs of internal growth and development. Our culture glorifies this stage of development. For hundreds of years in the West, we have celebrated the personal identity.

The identity project becomes the vehicle of the adult self-image. It functions as a "carrot" to organize our movement toward our aspirations. Our idea of who we should be is always future oriented, and we are always moving toward or away from it. Like the idea of self, the self-image is not an object. It is a highly charged and conditioned set of beliefs and attitudes with which we deeply, and mostly unconsciously, identify. It is what we sometimes refer to as "our dreams."

In adulthood, most of us organize our attempts at happiness around fulfilling our self-image, in spite of the fact that, at times, this internal picture is significantly at odds with reality. My former client, Daniel, for example, married a beautiful woman twenty years his junior with whom he had little in common, because the idea of a beautiful young woman completed his image of who he thought he should be. The longing to be happy is at the core of the human experience, and most of us will do just about anything we can to achieve this happiness. In our culture, this means that we will do just about whatever we can to manifest our idea of how we should be.

If it is at all successful, the identity project eventually develops a good deal of positive momentum. What begins as a way of overcoming the terror of no-self becomes, as Washburn says, "a way of engaging one's faculties, developing talents, learning how to meet the challenges of the world, giving expression to one's character, and in, in general, growing in effective personhood."[6] We become "pillars of the community"—physicists, lawyers, teachers, householders, parents.

And so we are very busy indeed. For a long while, perhaps even for our entire lives, we identify with the persona we create in our mind's eye, and we assume that this is who we are. The anxiety of nothingness, of emptiness, of no-self, is assuaged. We feel valued as human beings for the contributions we make as we manifest our identity and interact with the world. We feel a sense of belonging. We feel normal.

THE BONFIRE OF THE VANITIES

The meditation retreat was over, and Paula and I had walked together up to Bapuji's meditation garden, a secluded Japanese garden on a cliff overlooking the wide expanse of mansion lawn.

"So what happened to the Shadowbrook mansion, Steve? You didn't finish the story."

"Well, it was a kind of early twentieth-century *Bonfire of the Vanities.*" I told the story as I had heard it: Some have said that the mansion had a curse. Anson Phelps Stokes, the original squire of Shadowbrook, enjoyed the estate for only five years before he had a terrible riding accident. His horse stepped on a hornet's nest. It reared and plunged ahead, out of control, and finally collided with an elm tree. Stokes's right leg was crushed and had to be amputated. "Even though he regained his health, he abandoned Shadowbrook after the accident. He didn't even try to sell the property. Just kind of let the whole place go to weeds."

We walked around the perimeter of the old foundation. "Eventually, the place was sold to Andrew Carnegie." Carnegie lived out his older years at Shadowbrook, unhappy and increasingly senile, missing his castle in Scotland, where he couldn't go because of the war in Europe. He died at Shadowbrook in 1919. Mrs. Carnegie gave it to the Jesuits in 1922.

"The legend goes that as sacred land, it was never meant to be in the hands of just one wealthy family. Finally, it reverted to a place for spiritual practice."

"You said the mansion burned? How did the fire start?"

"I don't think that was ever really determined. But it was a tragic and monumental event in Berkshire County. It was a frigid night in March 1956. Everything was covered in ice. Apparently the fire trucks just couldn't get there. They say the blaze could be seen in the night sky for many miles around. Four Jesuits were killed and six other priests and brothers were injured."

We stood for a moment, pondering the enormity of that disaster. "Everything in this place seems to happen on a grand scale," Paula said.

"After the fire, the Jesuits built the new Shadowbrook building like a fortress. No wood. All brick, glass, stainless steel. Built to last two hundred years, they said."

"I guess it could never burn again, then?" Neither Paula nor I could have known, in that moment, the irony of her question.

THE TRANSMUTATION OF THE IDENTITY PROJECT

The Buddha said, "Living in this mortal body is like living in a house on fire." However solid we think our mansion is, it is already, in fact, on fire.

As a strategy for happy living, the identity project is fundamentally flawed, organized as it inevitably is around the four erroneous beliefs and the five afflictions. It cannot bring us home to our true self. In the yogic view, the identity project keeps us, like Viveka among the peasants, bound to an image of who we're not, rather than offering us an experience of who we are. In the yogic view, it is a defense against reality, against consciousness, and against our potential experience of divinity.

At some point, most of us begin to perceive that even when our goals are met over and over again, as they were for Paula, they fail to bring lasting happiness and contentment. Try heroically as we may, we cannot sustain the illusion of this solid, idealized self that we've been working so desperately to achieve.

The successful identity project, like Paula's, does not collapse in failure. Rather, it is seen through. On the night of his enlightenment, the Buddha declared, "I have seen the builder of the house!" He had seen the internal delusional structure that maintained the idea of the solid, separate self-under-its-own-power. Once seen through, it had no more power to drive his life.

Sitting in the meditation retreat I, too, had begun, in the most rudimentary fashion, to expose the "builder of the house." And when the builder of the house is exposed, we experience a new crisis of development. Just as with the earlier crises, there will be a sense of death and rebirth, and a deepening sense of authenticity—we begin to feel more like ourselves.

Albert Camus describes this moment in his final and autobiographical novel, *The First Man*. He had believed that "he had himself well in hand," as he puts it, until he stood looking at his father's grave, facing the reality of death: "In the strange dizziness of that moment, the statue every man eventually erects and that hardens in the fire of the years, into which he then creeps and there awaits its final crumbling—that statue was rapidly cracking, it was already collapsing."[7]

From the yogic point of view, the statue *must* crumble. The identity project is not a final destination for the human being, but only a transitional structure. It is only a vehicle meant to prepare us for the next step in our journey. In our culture, we have mistaken the vehicle for the destination. As a result we suffer from a kind of arrested development. At a certain point, when the self is ready to make the leap, we will long to leave the vehicle of the identity project behind. The shadow side of the self from which we retreated in early adulthood begins to reemerge. We now have the skills to face the "anxiety of nothingness" quite a bit more directly. And in order to grow into the next stage of our full aliveness, we will have to do just that.

7

THE SUFFERING

OF THE FALSE SELF

To the untrue man, the whole universe is false,—it
is impalpable,—it shrinks to nothing within his
grasp. And he himself, in so far as he shows
himself in a false light, becomes a shadow, or,
indeed, ceases to exist.

—Nathaniel Hawthorne,
The Scarlet Letter

Toward the end of my first summer of residency at Kripalu, I was
invited (as an example of a successful "graduate," I guess) to meet with
a group of thirty new trainees who had come, as I had the previous fall,
to explore a spiritual lifestyle. We were meeting in the cozy, wood-
paneled resident chapel, once a training chapel for Jesuit novices, now
adorned with pictures of yogic saints and piled high with meditation
cushions. I remembered how I had felt a year earlier—anxious, hopeful, excited, ready for an adventure. As I looked around the room, I
realized this group of seekers fell into roughly two groups: the first
were middle-aged folks like myself who had had careers, money, relationships, and all the rest, and who had found that these had not lived
up to their billing. They seemed to be driven by disappointment and by
the haunting sense that "there must be something more." The second
group were young adults in their early twenties. They were driven,
apparently, by the need to figure out who they really were in the world
of work and love. These young seekers hoped Kripalu would be the

place—the transformational space—in which they could fit together the pieces of their personal identities.

Saradananda, one of the senior teachers, noticed this division in the group as well, and he said something about it that struck me deeply: "Disappointment," he said, "is a much more fertile ground for spiritual practice than dreams."

I felt how true this was for me, how the suffering of loss, failure, and disappointment had compelled me to look deeper, to become a seeker. I took the risk of sharing some of my own story that night, and I found that many people identified with it thoroughly. One man my age quoted Paul Simon, "Don't know a dream that's not been shattered, or driven to its knees." Others had similar things to say: "I'm happy with my life in a way, but I know there's something deeper and less transient beneath it that I want to touch." "Suddenly I don't know what anything means anymore." "What's the true purpose of my life?" "Everything in my life appears to be falling apart." "I'm tired, bored, and I just can't believe that I'm really living my life fully."

Later that evening as I was writing in my journal, I remembered with a wave of sadness the meltdown of just two years before. On the night after Sean and I broke up, Mark had stayed with me all night. For a long time, he held me as I sobbed. The words that erupted from my belly over and over again surprised even me. "I tried so hard. I tried so hard." They seemed to emerge from a bottomless well of pain—a well so deep, I felt that I had tapped into an underground river. Not just *my* pain, but *the* pain. Humanity's pain. "I tried so hard!"

With Mark that night, I was experiencing the shadow side of the identity project, the dark truth from which we ordinarily flee. No matter how heroically we work at patching together our personal identities, we live always at the brink of what Buddhists call the three marks of existence—impermanence, insubstantiality, and suffering. "No matter what we do," says Buddhist psychologist Mark Epstein, "we cannot sustain the illusion of our self-sufficiency. We are all subject to decay, old age, and death, to disappointment, loss and disease. We are all engaged in a futile struggle to maintain ourselves in our own image. The crises in our lives inevitably reveal how impossible our attempts to control our destinies really are."[1]

As I thought about my time with the new trainees that night, I began to realize that my own pilgrimage had been initiated by a kind of natural meltdown of me and mine. I had tired of the Sisyphean struggle to keep the mansion of my life together, to keep stone upon stone, always resisting the pull of gravity. "I tried so hard!" What would it be like to just let go? To stop the struggle and surrender to gravity? To let the mansion crumble?

I realized, too, how much I had in common with the younger members of the group. Here at Kripalu, I felt again some of the transparency and vulnerability of adolescence. At times of self-reorganization, both in adolescence and at midlife, the sense of "I-ness" is fragile, tender, and there is a magic window through the solidity of asmita. There is a heightened sense of pain and despair, but also a magnified sense of wonder and spirituality. We are ready for an initiation into the deeper mysteries of energy and consciousness.

THE REVELATION OF THE FALSE SELF

Most people who come to Kripalu acknowledge some problems with their sense of self: they are unable to love themselves, to esteem themselves; they're tired of paddling so hard; they don't feel completely real; they don't feel that they're fully inhabiting their lives; they don't know who they are; they feel unsatisfied. Why is this, they wonder?

Interestingly enough, the yogic view and Western psychology seem to converge in their answer to this question: The ideas we have in our minds about who we should be are out of touch with reality. They may be unrealistically grandiose and inflated. They may be unrealistically devalued and deflated. Either way, we suffer. In Western psychological language, we call this the suffering of the "false self," a term coined by D. W. Winnicott.

The "false self" describes one of the major stumbling blocks of the seeker, and it must be understood if we're to comprehend the role of the second affliction, asmita, in our contemporary lives. In the yogic view, there is always some degree of false self driving the identity project, even the most seemingly successful ones.

How does this false self show up in our lives? In my work at Kripalu I regularly see three manifestations of it:

1. *The sense of self is separated from a vital connection to the body.* When I first started teaching at Kripalu, I noticed something striking. At the beginning of yoga classes, I would routinely do a brief

meditation, asking students to close their eyes for a moment and scan through their current inner experience of their body. "Become aware of sensations, aches, pains, whatever might be present," I might say. A surprisingly large number of people simply could not do this. I remember one student in particular, named Judy, whose eyes eagerly scanned the ceiling whenever I led a meditation. She couldn't locate the insides of her body. Her energy was all directed somewhere above her head. Judy couldn't bring her gaze down to the ground.

Some of us find that our ability to receive, process, tolerate, and enjoy both the pleasure and the pain of sensation and the "embodied life" is damaged. The range and depth of our awareness of our interior physical landscape is often severely diminished. This leaves us with a sense of self that is cut off from the simple pleasures of being.

In order for us to fully inhabit our bodies, we need certain kinds of responses from our environment. These include empathic holding, nurturing, mirroring, challenge, optimal frustration, and optimal disillusionment. Problems begin to happen in our developing sense of self when, as infants and children, our real emerging needs and capacities are not met with adequate mirroring, nurturing, and sustaining responses.

In the postindustrial West, the problems of the disembodied sense of self are pandemic. The reasons for this are simple: Because of the breakdown of the extended family in the latter half of this century, we depend upon the depleted resources of small nuclear families, where hardworking parents may already feel stretched and needy themselves. This nuclear family upon which we place most of our hopes is all too often an impoverished emotional environment for children. Overburdened parents feel fragmented, insecure, and in some cases terrified by the needs they feel they should be meeting but cannot. They're hungry to get their own unsatisfied needs met. Given the demands of our culture, how could it be otherwise?

Winnicott describes one particularly critical developmental moment in which needed responses are often not forthcoming. This is what he calls the "pathological feeding" process between mother and infant. Authentic feeding experiences, he points out, emerge from the baby's spontaneously arising gestures of need, which the good-enough mother meets and responds to.[2] "In pathological feeding, however," says psychologist and author Stephen Mitchell, "the infant takes its cues from impingements from the outside. The baby's own impulses and needs are not met by the mother, and the baby learns to want what the mother gives, and to become the mother's idea of who the baby is."[3]

In the crucible of the American family, children are often used to meet the needs of emotionally hungry parents. The parent may subtly—or not so subtly—manipulate the child by withdrawing love and attention when the child fails to mirror, echo, or reward the parent in a way that feels satisfying to the parent. This vulnerable parent is unable to be used by the child as what psychologist Heinz Kohut calls a "self-object," a kind of emotional home base from which the child can securely explore all sides of her experience—being merged and separate, strong and weak, limitless and vulnerable. In the absence of the safety provided by a secure self-object, the child will eventually deny her connection to her real, kinesthetic sense of her self, her needs, and her idiosyncratic energy. She will make whatever sacrifices are necessary in order to hold on to the scarce emotional supplies offered by a vulnerable parent. In order to survive, then, the child learns to become the kind of infant the parent needs rather than the kind of child she is.

This common early experience leaves us vulnerable in two ways. First of all, we do not receive a fully satisfying experience of being soothed and feeling OK. And secondly, whatever identity we find—or assume—will not be deeply grounded in our own body. Consequently, it will never feel satisfying or fully real. Inside, we will feel "brittle," as Judy did, and have a sense of living an assumed identity, one that is easily overwhelmed by external pressures and demands.

2. *Just under the surface is a deeply felt sense that "something is wrong" with the way I am.* Several years into my tenure at Kripalu, we hosted a visiting Indian *rishi* who taught a very pure form of nondualist practice. His core motto was, "There is absolutely nothing wrong with this moment." For a while, everyone in the community was walking around the halls repeating this mantra, "Everything is OK, things are already alright. Nothing to change. Nothing to improve. Just relax. Do nothing." At first this was wonderful. A huge relief. "Ah, I'm already OK."

But something unexpected began to happen. Exposure to this teacher had the interesting effect of revealing for many of us spiritual seekers just how *not* OK we felt most of the time. The rishi's mantra bumped up against a subtle sense of "notOKness" that suffused our experience and that perhaps suffused our whole spiritual path—about which more later. We found that the mantra could be incredibly irritating. It repeatedly laid bare this underlying notOKness. At a certain point some students began to reject it. It became alarmingly clear, for many of us, just how much the unconscious sense that "something is wrong" drives our behavior.

When, at any stage of development, a child's energy, needs, and particular self cannot be adequately received by her parents, her siblings, and her social environment, she may make an unconscious "script decision." She says, in effect, "The way I am is not alright. I must be another way." She becomes disconnected from her ability to savor the experience of the self just the way it is. She cannot sustain a sense of the rightness of the world. She feels, rather, the wrongness of herself. Her energy begins to focus on "how I should be" as a concept or an image, and then on manifesting that image of the self. After that, her life becomes an attempt to undo her chronic sense of wrongness.

The well-known gadfly and talk-show host Howard Stern describes this predicament poignantly:

> Maybe it was the way I was raised, or something, but I always feel like I'm garbage. . . . I think what it comes down to, and maybe this is a personality flaw again, a character flaw, but I could go to a book signing and see twenty thousand people out there and I don't feel great from that. Which is a shame. You'd think that that kind of adulation would make you feel on top of the world. And yet I don't. I don't know why.[4]

The false self is born when the environment does not welcome the self to be as it is. The resulting dissatisfaction with the nature of *being itself* colors all experience, but usually remains just out of awareness. When we are separated from our capacity to be with life the way it is, especially early in our development, our capacity to self-soothe is severely impaired. Our need for soothing and confirmation from external sources will be chronic and insatiable. Our capacity to truly hold and soothe others will also be impaired.

3. Our internal images of self become dominated by an "ego-ideal" that may be significantly at odds with reality. Early in our friendship, Paula discovered that she had a deep belief that, as she said, "It's better to look good than to feel good." We laughed about this many times, because Paula always looked good. Her clothes were simple but elegant, her hair casually stylish, and her makeup was just right. All in all a very well put together image. Paula also began to notice how important it was for her to see herself in the mirror the way she thought of herself. She worked with the mirror every morning to get it right. Her sense of herself as whole, integrated, and cohesive was dependent on her ability to actually manifest her self-concept in the world.

We laughed about her motto, and at one point, Geoff had it translated into Latin and emblazoned on one of those fake university sweatshirts. He sensed how important a breakthrough it was for her to bring her concern for appearances into awareness and to have the perspective to laugh at herself.

To some extent, most of us are unconsciously driven by our ego-ideal. The ego-ideal is simply a set of ideas in the mind about how we should show up, how we should look, feel, behave, think. This collection of ideas and mental images is created out of fragments of highly charged experiences with important love objects in our lives, and out of the messages we receive in our interactions with the world as we grow. It remains mostly out of our awareness. The blueprint for the ego-ideal is first laid down by parental injunctions about how to be, or how not to be. These highly charged messages are taken in whole. They become the foundation of our scripts for life. The ego-ideal is certainly capable of modification and change, but for most of us it's deeply hardwired into our unconscious by the time we enter early adulthood, and it matures only marginally in later life.

Under the sway of the false self, the locus of the sense of self moves away from a visceral, grounded, kinesthetic base to an abstracted and idealized base. The answer to the question "Who am I?" now becomes, as it were, "I am the one who does or does not live up to my self-concept."[5] The self-concept has now taken the place of the parental objects. We are still trying to live up to "mother's idea of who we are," except that the external mother and her injunctions have now become the internal "mother"—our ego-ideal.

Most of us have some experience of false self functioning across a wide spectrum, from the simply irritating to the crippling. I remember living through this experience of myself, especially in my twenties. During those years, when I was struggling with identity issues and didn't feel at all grounded in my sexuality, I began to notice an ongoing inner dialogue. I was constantly asking myself, "How am I doing?" In particular, I remember one day walking up Commonwealth Avenue in Boston, having just had lunch with someone reasonably famous. "OK," I heard myself saying. "You're doing great. You just had lunch with a movie star." I imagined how others back home would view this. They would perhaps envy me. And for a moment I felt assuaged. In fact, I felt euphoric. The false self, however, can never be satisfied, so within an hour I would have to reassure myself again.

The feelings we are most apt to have when living under the sway of the mental image are those very feelings of pride, euphoria, and elation that I was feeling that day on Commonwealth Avenue—when the world seemed to be confirming my self-image. The bad news is that their opposites—dysphoria, emptiness, and panic—show up when the environment does not confirm us. The feelings of elation and euphoria, which come when we momentarily meet the demands of a tyrannical false self-concept, can be exciting and energizing. Fun as they are in the moment, however, they are not deeply satisfying.[6] Those of us who have had them will know that they do not provide a satisfying experience in the body. Euphoria and elation are, in fact, as psychologist Stephen Johnson says, the "booby prizes" of life.

For those of us tyrannized by the false self, there is no true pleasure or satisfaction in accomplishment, only a desperate confirmation or nonconfirmation of our very existence. Under the sway of the false self, we cannot warmly love the self or value and esteem ourselves. We are driven to manipulate people, places, and things in the external world in order to feel alright.

A DEFENSE AGAINST THE MOTHER

The false self, though initially an effective adaptive strategy, can eventually become a learning disability. It requires us to shut down our connection with the direct feedback of our bodies, our biocomputers. In so doing, it hampers the maturing person's ability to take in information about reality. Finally, our ideas about how we should be can be so powerful that they deeply impair our capacity to see who and how we really are. Over time, the ego becomes so invested in the false self that it begins to believe in its reality. Any threat to the false self, then, or any obstacle to the manifestation of its demands, becomes a threat to life itself. We will defend, to the death, whatever we consider to be "me."

And so we sit on our meditation cushions, or at our desks, and find ourselves completely obsessed with "me" and "mine"—my furniture, my image, my career, my status in the company, my appearance. We will sacrifice the simple, direct, and real pleasures of life—just sitting, just breathing, just watching the perspiration run down my arm, just being in the sultry July day—for the hell of self-obsession. Over and over again, I have seen patients, students, friends, and myself sacrifice real, immediate life in the pursuit of the unreality of the false self. We are driven either by achievement and perfectionism, or by their flip side, worthlessness and self-loathing, to play out our ideas of how things should be rather than learning to experience directly the pain or the pleasure of how things are.

In the yogic view, the false self is understood to be a defense against energy. It is the conditioned way in which we organize our resistance to the free flow of shakti through our physical and subtle form. When the particular "mothers" in our environment cannot bring us into a full delight in our own embodiment, cannot help us to fully inhabit the phenomenal world of pain and pleasure, cannot teach us to bear the ebb and flow of sensation, we learn to close ourselves off to the universal mother. We lose touch, often at the very beginning of our lives, with the dance of the true self.

Finally, our capacity to feel the realness of ourselves and of the world is impaired. As Hawthorne says about Reverend Dimmesdale in the passage from *The Scarlet Letter* used as the epigraph to this chapter, for the false self, the world becomes "impalpable," "a shadow," and the self, eventually, "ceases to exist." Living from the false self, we experience a chronic and cloying sense of not being fully real. To the extent that we're driven by the false self, in fact, we are deeply misidentified. We're identified with only part of who we are, or with who we are not.

On some level, Paula knew that the self she was presenting to the world was not a true self. She had a nagging sense that life must be more enjoyable than she found it to be. She saw others enjoying themselves, and experiencing true pleasure, but she didn't really know how to make that happen for herself. She was becoming increasingly aware of her disconnection from her real self. The sense of not being and feeling real and grounded became more and more painful and unacceptable. She began to want desperately to feel good, to feel whole—just, in fact, to *feel*. She was experiencing the meltdown of "me" and "mine" that is the doorway to an authentic exploration of the self.

There is no telling precisely at what chronological age the self will come to one of these crossroads. One thing is certain: these times of meltdown are precious. A delicate window is opened into the very terrain explored and mastered by yogis and buddhas and seers of all kinds. In these times, the soul has a heightened potential to discover the real. There is a palpable longing for the mother, for matter, for the earth, and along with this an openness to the father, to the spirit, to consciousness.

In his commentary on the *Yogasutras,* Bhagwan S. Rajneesh identifies this meltdown of "me" and "mine" in adulthood as the entry point into yoga.

> Yoga means that now there is no hope, now there is no future, now there are no desires. One is ready to know what is. One is not interested in what can be, what should be, what ought to be. One is not interested! One is interested only in that which is, because only the real can free you, only the reality can become liberation.
>
> Total despair is needed. That despair is called dukkha by Buddha. And if you are really in misery, don't hope, because your hope will only prolong the misery. Your hope is a drug. It can help you to reach death only and nowhere else. All your hopes can lead you only to death.
>
> Become totally hopeless—no future, no hope. Difficult. Needs courage to face the real. But such a moment comes to everyone some time or other. A moment comes to every human being when he feels total hopelessness. Absolute meaninglessness happens to him. When he becomes aware that whatsoever he is doing is useless, wheresoever he is going, he is going to nowhere, all life is meaningless—suddenly hopes drop, future drops, and for the first time you are in tune with the present, for the first time you are face to face with reality. . . . When you are not moving into the future, not moving toward the past,

then you start moving within yourself—because your being is
here and now. You are present here and now. You can enter
this reality.[7]

Human beings are afflicted. But yoga asks us to look underneath our
erroneous beliefs to find the real source of our suffering. Our true
affliction is not our inability to get what we want, or our inability to get
rid of what we don't want—mostly sickness, old age, death. The true
nature of our affliction is that we are unable and unwilling to come into
our inheritance as fully alive human beings.

Life's disappointments coupled with a maturing self-observational
capacity will eventually force us to release our attachment to the false
self. Experience forces us to see under the surface of conventional
reality and to find a whole new landscape within. And as we begin to
penetrate the surface of the ideas in the ego-ideal, and subtly break our
attachment and identification with them, we begin to experience how
things really are, not how they should be. It is only when the false self
has been exposed that we are ready for the pilgrimage to the center.

8

$\mathcal{F}$ROM THE UNREAL

TO THE REAL

> We fall down and down, until we touch the
> ground, until we relate with the basic sanity of the
> earth. We become the lowest of the low, the
> smallest of the small, a grain of sand, perfectly
> simple, no expectations. . . . If you are a grain of
> sand, the rest of the universe, all the space, all the
> room is yours, because you obstruct nothing,
> overcrowd nothing, possess nothing. There
> is tremendous openness. You are the emperor of
> the universe because you are a grain of sand.
>
> —Chogyam Trungpa, Rinpoche

During my first couple of months at Kripalu one of my favorite parts
of the day was the regular evening gathering for prayers and *arati*—a
traditional Hindu ceremony of light. At about 7:15 PM all of the day's
activity ceased, as the whole community gathered in the main chapel
for satsang (literally, "in the company of truth"). There we waited ex-
pectantly on our meditation cushions, hundreds of us dressed in whites
ranging from yellowing T-shirts to elaborate silk saris, facing the great
marble altar where Yogi Desai would soon appear. Men on one side of
the chapel. Women on the other. A horde of drummers and musicians
played in the alcove, where the choir must have been when it was a
Jesuit chapel. The altar was bedecked with flowers and candles. A
klatch of orange-robed renunciates with shaved heads bobbed around
the marble steps in the flickering light.

The whole thing made a great backdrop to the drama that was about to unfold. We were gathered to hear a talk by Amrit Desai, or perhaps, in his stead, some visiting guru, Buddhist teacher, Indian politician, or the latest New Age celebrity. To begin the ceremony—and before the talk—there was half an hour or so of chanting, usually traditional Sanskrit chants, with six or eight drums beating, along with other traditional Indian instruments like little finger cymbals, perhaps a few flutes, wooden or otherwise. Before long, the huge room pounded with energy. Most of the participants were on their feet moving in some fashion—sometimes with astonishing abandon and great beauty, sometimes with just, well, abandon.

As the chanting reached its climax, it became a kind of wail. Then it slowed, abruptly, becoming solemn and quiet. Finally, utter silence. On cue, Amrit Desai glided through the door closest to the altar, adorned in a simple brown robe and perhaps a gold prayer shawl. Hair flowing. Light as a feather. The room was ready to love him.

Well, most often we were. Some days I could let myself get lost in the dancing, or in the talk, and these times could be utterly magical— truly transcendent. Other days I was bored and slightly irritated. And then, at times I just sat and wondered what in God's name I was doing there.

But it seemed that whether I felt open or skeptical on any particular day, I was almost always moved by what happened after the talk: the closing ceremony of light. A throng of saffron-clad renunciates would take over the altar, swinging dozens of little ghee-wick candles in wide arcs while the whole group chanted a beautiful Sanskrit prayer. This particular chant was so primal, its melody so haunting and inevitable, that I found myself surrendering to it. For months, I hadn't a clue what the words meant. It didn't matter. In fact, I didn't want to know. The chant itself had a mysterious effect on me, which I came to treasure. I went off to bed enraptured, soothed to the core.

Later, when I saw a translation of the prayer, I wasn't surprised.

> *May we be protected together.*
> *May we be nourished together.*
> *May we work together with great vigor.*
> *May our study be enlightening.*
> *May there be no hatred between us.*
> *Om peace, peace, peace.*

The words spoke some of the very things that the chant made me feel—a sense of connectedness to those in the room, a sense of devo-. tion to our life and work together. What ignited my interest even more, though, was the next stanza.

> *Lead us from the unreal to the real.*
> *Lead us from darkness to light.*
> *Lead us from death to immortality.*

I loved that first line. It felt like something I could stand on and could chant with all my heart. "Lead us from the unreal to the real." A heightened concern with reality was an approach to spirituality I had never found in the Christian world, but it was one that permeated my work as a psychotherapist. I wanted to know more about how it fit into the practice of yoga.

REALITY IS GOD IN DISGUISE

Right away I noticed in Desai's talks a strong thread of concern with "moving from the unreal to the real." Indeed, after a while it was clear that this notion saturated his teaching. As I began to write this book I discovered that I had highlighted many of Desai's comments about reality in my big leather-bound journal:

I honor reality. Reality is more sacred to me than my most sacred concept. Reality is the messenger of consciousness. I want to see reality; I don't want to hide from it.

Reality is God in disguise.

Acceptance of reality is what we really mean by the word "love." Love is just accepting reality. It is not necessarily an emotional experience; it is impersonal and universal.

Reality is relentless. It follows behind every denial, every avoid- ance, until it is embraced with open arms.[1]

In these teachings, Amrit was communicating perhaps the central animating principle of all yogic practice, the one stated so succinctly by Patanjali in the second book of his *Yogasutras* (II,26,28):

> The uninterrupted practice of the awareness of the Real is the means of dispersion of *avidya*.

> From the practice of the component exercises of yoga, on the destruction of impurity, arises spiritual illumination which develops into awareness of Reality.

Such a simple and powerful place to stand. The human being is transformed through the practice of the awareness of reality. As we shall see in the coming chapters, the major antidote to the five afflictions and the four erroneous beliefs is uninterrupted awareness of reality. But what is meant by "the Real," and how do yogis propose to achieve uninterrupted awareness of it?

BEHIND THE FALSE SELF

In yogic science, the project most central to the discovery of the real is the penetration into the delusion of the unreal. This is remarkably similar to the Western psychotherapeutic notion that the true self is discovered only in the process of exposing the false self. In fact, Winnicott, the originator of the term "false self," declared that our whole task is, in a sense, understanding and revealing the false self, because once freed from it everything that is left is true self. "There is but little point," he said, "in formulating a True Self idea except for the purpose of trying to understand the False Self, because it (the idea of the True Self) does no more than collect together the details of the experience of aliveness."[2]

When the man my patient Sally had been seeing called for time out in their new relationship because he felt it was moving too fast toward a commitment, she was devastated. During their few months together, she had begun to define herself in terms of her relationship with Douglas. She was, as she believed he saw her, witty, sexy, and beautiful. Now, suddenly, she was none of those things. Now she was dull, sexless, and unattractive. As we talked in therapy, she realized how much she had needed to believe in the false reflection that Douglas presented. The painful separation gave her the opportunity to say, "not that," about many of her false assumptions and to begin to ask herself who she really was beneath her hopes and his reflections.

In yoga, as well as in psychotherapy, the real is discovered within the unreal through a gradual process of discrimination. The entire practice of yoga has been described by Bhoja, one of the major commentators on the *Yogasutras*, as "an effort to separate the *atman* (the Reality) from the non-*atman* (the apparent), and to unite the individual soul with the Reality which underlies the universe."[3] This process is called *viveka*, which literally means "separating out," or discernment. Through the regular practice of discernment, says Georg Feuerstein, "the yogi develops an inner sensitivity to what is ephemeral in his nature and, as he exposes this, he comes face to face with the underlying eternal Ground of all his experiences."[4] It is not a coincidence that the hero of this book's prologue carries the name Viveka.

Chogyam Trungpa often compared the false self to a huge platform upon which we stand, supposedly for security. We work so hard on this platform of self, hammering and nailing and shoring it up as if our lives depended upon it. Perhaps we add a special roof, and an industrial-strength railing so we won't fall off our identity platform. We make it solid. We're consumed night and day with its solidity. The joke is on us, though, when we discover that these little fortresses are only a foot off the ground. We could have stepped down onto the solid ground of reality all the time, and been truly safe, without all the effort and struggle.

ONLY REALITY IS WHOLLY SAFE

Sarita and I were sitting in her office one evening after satsang, goofing on the Indian swami who had just given a talk. "Did you notice how his eyes were always going up and out, up and out?" Sarita mimicked him with side-splitting accuracy. "As if he was trying to get out of his body into some other reality. Just dying to get out of his body and off this planet! This stuff absolutely drives me insane, you know, because that's exactly what I was trying to do with drugs. I don't want any part of that kind of spirituality."

I nodded my assent.

"You know, Steve, I lived so long in the unreality of drugs and alcohol. I mean just total la-la land, for about ten years. It's a terrifying way to live. There's never any solid ground under your feet. I would lose whole chunks of my life. There are periods of weeks and months during that time that I still don't know where I was or who I was with."

Sarita believed that those people who have recovered from living in unreality become relentless in their pursuit of the real. "That's one of the main things that drew me to yoga, and in particular to Gurudev," she said. "I don't know if he always lives it, but he sure teaches it right." In the years of her recovery, in addition to yoga and Christianity, Sarita had begun working with a popular spiritual teaching called the *Course in Miracles,* from which she appropriated the motto that now was posted in large letters on the bulletin board above her desk: "Only reality is wholly safe."

One of my greatest psychotherapy mentors, Elvin Semrad, used to ask the following question about patients: "How concerned is this patient with reality?" He found that patients who don't really care about knowing "how it really is or how I really am" will never get better.

When I was working in an inpatient psychiatric hospital during graduate school, I witnessed the enormous difficulties that delusional patients have with the most ordinary functions of daily life. Some had trouble even remembering that they had bodies that needed to be fed. But according to the yogic view, we're *all* fairly out of sync with reality. As the Buddha said, "All human beings are quite deluded." The line between the staff and patients is sometimes frighteningly thin. We are all deluded. It's only a matter of degree.

The concern with reality—with "how I really am" and "who I really am"—begins with the emergence of the introspective self in adolescence. In the first decades of adulthood, most of us find out who we are by learning what we can do, what roles we can play at work and in relationship. But as the identity project matures, a new set of concerns about authenticity begins to emerge, concerns about the self as being rather than doing, concerns about the intrinsic worth, meaning, beauty, and value of the self. The emergence of these concerns signals the capacity for a new kind of relationship with reality.

Thus, the identity project finally gives way to a completely new organizing principle of the self, a developmental event that I call the reality project. As the reality project emerges, we begin to relinquish our attempts to make life the way we think it should be, and we turn our attention instead to a minute and thorough inspection of the way life really is.

At the heart of the shift to the reality project is the eagerness to investigate exactly how things are right now. The preoccupying question is no longer, "What is wrong with this moment?" or "How do I change this reality so that it conforms with my ideals?" but, rather, "What is the nature of this moment—precisely? How can I examine it more deeply?" In her recovery from life in the unreal world of addiction, Sarita found that her most important practice was not doing yoga postures, but stopping regularly throughout the day to sit down, breathe, and ask herself the question, "How is it for me right now?"

With the emergence of the reality project, the "why" questions begin to become less important, like "Why is this moment the way it is?" Why questions take us into abstractions or concepts. They retrigger the delusions of the false self. With the reality project, the "what" questions become more compelling. "What is the texture, the feel, the experience of this moment?" As Rajneesh pointed out, "One is interested only in that which *is,* because only the Real can free you, only Reality can become liberation." This is the developmental need that makes yogic practice and philosophy useful, and that made it essential for Sarita.

THE REALITY PROJECT

Sarita and I sat together in her office for several hours that night, sharing our own peculiar experiences of the emergence of the reality project. In the following weeks and months, through conversation with many other yogis, I began to formulate some of the psychological "marker events" of this developmental stage:[5]

1. A return to the body. After a recent yoga and meditation retreat, Amy, one of the retreatants, told me a story about her experience. After the second day, she actually had a visceral experience of "landing" on the meditation cushion, of arriving back in her body just as if she had been away on a long trip. "It was as if I dropped in from outer space," she said, thrilled and astonished to be home. "But I didn't even know I wasn't home until I got back!" After her experience of "landing," she had a heightened sense of smell, of sight—"colors are more vibrant!"—

and of touch. It was, for her, like discovering an entirely new subtle realm of physical reality, and she experienced it with a great deal of pleasure. "Just being in my body makes me happy. I don't have to do anything, or prove anything. What freedom!" For the first time in her adult life, Amy had tasted the possibility of a life not lived in the head—or in the abstraction of the ego-ideal—but in the very real world of current direct kinesthetic experience. Her life was changed.

Our bodies are finally our best hope to rescue us from our false selves. As Stephen Johnson says, "We are all ultimately rescued from our characterological compromises by our biological reality. . . . Only if we can be brought back to the reality of our physical existence will there be enough force to challenge and ultimately renounce the grandiose (or worthless) false self compromises which remain so seductive."[6]

Over centuries of practice, yogis discovered this truth. They discovered that we have to begin our knowing of reality with the body—the annamayakosha. There is no way around it. No spiritual bypass will work. We cannot prematurely transcend the body. We must turn toward it, not away from it.

2. *Relinquishing the attempt to dominate the body*. At the core of the false self is the experience of being dominated, and dominated in the most primitive way—in our bodies. The very real needs and demands of the child's body are forcefully rejected by powerful caretakers, and then finally suppressed by the child herself, as she attempts to embody the ideal. A true, and rather primitive example: A twenty-something yoga student of mine named Greta had been toilet trained early, not in response to her own readiness, but according to her mother's own rigid schedule. As a result, Greta did not, even as an adult, allow herself the freedom to control her own bowels without the use of laxatives.

Unconsciously incorporating the messages of our parental love objects, upon whom we have deeply depended, we learn at a very early age how to dominate our own bodies as a strategy for life. We learn how to deny and override the cues and needs of our own organism rather than how to respond to them. We begin to do to ourselves what was done to us.

While we are under the sway of the false self, and the identity project, even our attempts at creating a healthy or beautiful body may really be saturated with this subtext of domination. Even our practice of yoga may really be about "whipping our bodies into shape," as it was for Gloria, a fifty-year-old yoga student who came to yoga with the expectation that it would make her look younger. In fact, I see this every day in my yoga classes. Beginning students often ask how much weight they can expect to lose if they practice every day. Once, Gloria stopped me after class to ask how many calories I thought she had burned in *shalabasana*, a particularly vigorous posture. The single most difficult thing for yoga students to learn is precisely how to stop attempting to dominate their bodies.

But as the reality project emerges, this quality of domination begins to soften naturally. A deep level of exhaustion often surfaces, and the obsessive attempt to override the body begins to collapse of its own weight. As Gloria said with a sigh after she'd been practicing for six months, "I just don't have the energy for this 'tyranny of youth and beauty' anymore."

3. *A new quality of authenticity in caring for the self.* "I remember," said Sarita, "when I actually looked at myself in the mirror for the first time, after I'd met Amrit and begun to practice yoga. I was thirty years old, for God's sake. I just looked and looked, as though I had never seen myself before. And it was only then that I realized that I loved myself." As we begin to reexperience a visceral reconnection with the needs of our bodies, another amazing change emerges: there is a brand new capacity to warmly love the self. We experience a new quality of authenticity in our caring, which redirects our attention to our health, our diet, our energy, our time-management. This enhanced care for the self arises spontaneously, and naturally, not as a response to a "should." It feels naturally satisfying. We are able to experience an immediate and intrinsic pleasure in self-care, rather than the driven need to create a beautiful, buffed up, youthful-looking body that will meet our ego-ideal.

4. *A stand against habitual self-sacrifice.* When driven to meet our ego-ideal, we do whatever the job takes, not counting the cost to our bodies or minds. My old college buddy Joel works seventy billable hours a week for his law firm, in spite of his heart condition. My friend Jean, a terrifically busy working mother, always accedes to the demands of her selfish and demanding mother, sacrificing her own health and emotional well-being.

As the reality project emerges, there is usually a very strong stand taken against this ongoing self-sacrifice.[7] As Jean finally said to me one night, "It's just not worth it anymore. I won't do it. *I won't do it.*" This refusal can be fueled by an emerging awareness of rage at the original self-sacrifice—the self-betrayal that happened in infancy and childhood. It sometimes shows up as an awkward, and socially ungraceful, new attempt to set limits. Very often, our friends and family are not exactly thrilled by these new limits. This is understandable. It is usually precisely these family members, friends, and co-workers who have been benefiting from our willingness to sacrifice ourselves to an abstraction. Jean's newly emerging real self may adamantly refuse to pursue activities that rescue others but that torture her, refusing, perhaps for the first time in her adult life, to sacrifice health and real immediate felt needs in order to pursue perfection and achievement.

5. *An enhanced awareness of likes, dislikes, interests, curiosities:* The person who is just waking up to reality is often amazed at the extent to which he's remained completely ignorant of his own likes, dislikes, interests, and curiosities.[8] After all, the false self allows these things to be determined by others. For the first time, hobbies and other interests may be pursued not for secondary gain or external rewards, but for simple pleasure in the activity itself. This can be quite a revelation.

Karen, an accountant who had never taken an art class in her life, signed up for a course in ceramic sculpture and found, in the tactile pleasure of clay and the focus of her mind on her own creation, a new awareness of her own creative ability and a real joy in expressing that ability.

As a person's real interests emerge, they often do so with extraordinary new energy—and with an extraordinary commitment to mastery in these new and highly valued areas. The false self is, after all, not finally capable of mastering anything. There is not enough real energy in the drivenness of obligation or the hankering for the euphoria of achievement to take a pursuit to its deepest levels. True mastery can only be built upon the energy of real interest. This satisfying new connection with real interests may be accompanied by a sense of enhanced personal power—an experience of acting in alignment with the deepest self.

6. More genuine self-expression and the increased capacity to say "no." Jean's mother was furious for an entire year when Jean insisted that she limit her phone calls to one every other day. She pulled out all the stops to get her to relent: Shame: "Bad daughter!" Withdrawal: "No calls for a week!" The will: "I guess you don't need me now, so you won't need my money when I'm gone."

Jean's mother was unaccustomed to hearing the word "no" from her daughter. There was good reason why this was so. "No" is precisely what could not be said at the point of the development of the false self. We could not say, "No, don't try to dominate me like that. Let me be me!" Saying "no" to our caretakers as infants was impossible. Saying "no" as adults to our own internal critics, or to others, can be almost as difficult. It will certainly trigger the emotional impact of all of the old unconscious messages and scripts of childhood, bringing us face to face with our inability to protect ourselves as infants and children.

But when we know who we are, saying "no" is not a problem, because we know, also, who we are not. When "no" is uttered by the emerging real self, it will inevitably be voiced as a challenge to the primitive introjects and will emerge as a remarkably satisfying victory. Insignificant as it may seem to others, Jean's holding fast to her "no" with her mother was one of the great victories of her adult life.

7. The relief of being ordinary. The false self lives with a chronic sense of separation and isolation—born, simply, of trying too hard. As it begins to fall away, there can be a sense of utter relief at rejoining the human race. "Ah, I'm just like everybody else inside. I'm no better and no worse than most folks. Wow, I belong. I'm OK. So, this is the way it is with human beings." Sharon was finally able to laugh at her pretensions to being one of the "elite" of her small rural town in western Massachusetts. "Hell," she said, "who am I kidding? A town with only two bars and a general store doesn't have an elite worth belonging to." As the drivenness to earn worth through accomplishment falls away, there is a more realistic perception of the self, and a new depth to the appreciation of being an ordinary human being. There is a new lightness and a new sense of humor.

8. The preciousness of particularity and the emergence of idiosyncracy. As we experience the relief of being ordinary, we also begin to value our particular voice, our particular contribution, our particular way of doing things. Idiosyncrasy and eccentricity cannot be tolerated by the false self. But as the false self sloughs off, conformity goes with it. At this point, Sarah stopped dyeing her hair, which had been pure white since she was thirty-five. Robert, with a sigh of relief, stopped wearing pretentious three-piece suits to work at his accounting firm. Ginger, at forty-three, resumed the piano lessons she had left at age fifteen. We become, and others experience us becoming, more and more "ourselves." We experiment with a surrender to a deep, and deeply unseen, inner self that only wants to emerge and speak. And we care less about what other people think. There can be a wild new sense of freedom in this, of unpredictability, of transparency. We are no longer "other-directed." We are freed to explore our hidden selves, those parts of ourselves that feel discontinuous with the old, that may even feel startlingly in opposition to the old self. A surprising new burst of energy arises as we give ourselves permission to try on many different selves.

9. *Using relationships with important others to explore and reveal the real self.* Of all the hallmarks of the reality project, this one is perhaps the most critical: there is a pronounced shift away from using others to support our false self-compensation—our self-image—and toward using others to discover and support who we really are.

Stephen Johnson states this nicely. "In the budding of the real self there is hope. But as the real self emerges, one is fragile, vulnerable and full of feeling. The feelings may be very negative, or too much when positive, but they are undeniably real. It is this realness that one learns to cultivate and cherish. In the birth of the real self, though, there is always the profound need for others, which one has long denied or avoided. The new bud of the real self cannot exist long without the sustenance provided by a needed other."[9]

The experience of relating to important others from the core of the real self is the heart of the healing experience. Through this experience comes the proof that the newly revealed self can be borne not just by the self, but by others as well. Many of us undergoing this "waking up" experience are surprised by the enthusiasm of others for the newly discovered self within us. What a miracle to discover that we can be loved, even when there are negative emotions, even when there are emphatic new "no's," even when there is friction.

My therapy client Roger was embarrassed to tell his wife, Jenny, about the humiliation he felt at the hands of his scornful and belittling father-in-law, for whom he worked as an executive in the family paper-manufacturing business. He was ashamed of his negative feelings and was afraid she would think less of him. When he finally shared the anguish he felt, Jenny was supportive and loving. Her knowledge of his distress brought them closer, and together they formulated a plan to deal with the business and family problem.

Often as we deepen our experience of authenticity in relationships we develop a kind of "practicing" motif. At first, we may need to practice our new authenticity only with the most closely trusted others. Roger, for example, had tried out sharing his shame and rage with me before he shared it with Jenny. Then we move outward into other important relationships. The practicing is repeated over and over again, as the self gets more comfortable being in attuned relationships. Each time we successfully tolerate this kind of attunement, the false self is weakened.[10]

Nothing exposes the false self and reveals the true self like real love. This can be terrifyingly compelling. Here I think of a wonderful moment from one of my favorite films—*Moonstruck*. Loretta falls in love with a man named Ronnie, who is the brother of her fiancé, Johnny. Ronnie is the archetype of the man awake to himself—in his body, in his sexuality, in his soul. When Loretta discovers Ronnie, he has a broken heart, and he doesn't attempt to conceal his suffering in any way. Because of his own authenticity, Ronnie is able to see clearly who Loretta really is—and that she is marrying Johnny only for security. In the climactic scene, Ronnie pleads with Loretta to wake up:

> *The past and the future is a joke to me now;*
> *I see that they ain't here. I see that the only*
> *thing that's here is you.*
> *Loretta. I love you.*
> *Not like they told you love is.*
> *Love don't make things nice.*
> *It ruins everything.*
> *It breaks your heart.*
> *It makes things a mess.*
> *We aren't here to make things perfect.*
> *The snowflakes are perfect, not us. The stars are perfect.*

We are here to ruin ourselves and to break our hearts—
to love the wrong people and die.
The storybooks are bullshit.[11]

In the face of this plea, Loretta makes a courageous and fateful decision: she lets life change her. She trusts her emerging true self. She lets its energy bring her courage. And she will never be the same again.

10. An increased capacity to see previously denied aspects of reality. As the false self becomes more transparent, we will probably have some dramatic moments of realizing that the world is not what we thought it was. My friend Maria, a teacher at Kripalu, told me that it wasn't until she reached her midforties that she was able to bear seeing clearly who her father had been. Until then she had held tightly to the idealization that she had maintained throughout childhood. She believed firmly that her father had been a successful businessman and was very well respected in his work, even though she knew that he had been an inadequate father. As she began to awaken from her delusions about him, she was shocked to find how deeply she had distorted the truth. In fact, he had been fired from every job he had had, and he had committed numerous small crimes and one large one. He had systematically embezzled forty-seven thousand dollars over the course of two years from an employer who was a dear friend of the family. This employer did not prosecute him, and so the matter was settled quietly, but everyone in town knew about it. Except Maria. Why? She began to understand that the reality of it was too difficult for her to bear until she developed a stronger sense of her own self.

Maria's insight served as a kind of marker event, a dramatic outward and visible sign that she was undergoing a deep reorganization of her self. She was able to see reality more clearly. For a period of time, she was filled with a sense of wonder about this. She discovered the final gift of the reality project: however painful the truth may be, its recognition is accompanied by a visceral sense of relief. The body likes living in reality. Stepping down onto the solid ground of reality always feels better than living in delusion. It may be painful, but there is life in it, energy in it, and, like the ground, it holds us up in a way that delusion does not. "Only reality is wholly safe."

INSPECTING REALITY AT CLOSE RANGE

When the reality project emerges, the stage is set for us to deepen our practice of yoga. The ego has become strong and pliant enough to actually begin to inspect itself. We can now begin to examine our experience at a new and more subtle level. We can explore beneath the surface of the mirror of the self. The maturing consciousness begins, in Ken Wilber's words, "to learn to subtly inspect the mind's cognitive and perceptual capacities, and in so doing, has a sense of transcending them."[12] The ego actually learns to maintain what psychologist Jack Engler has called a "therapeutic split"—holding the self as both subject and object. As this development proceeds, says Wilber, "cognitive and perceptual capacities become so pluralistic and universal that they begin to reach beyond any narrowly held personal perspectives or concerns."[13] We begin to see the see-er, or, in yogic terms, the Seer.

This is the beginning of contemplative development. It is the hatching out of what is often called, in spiritual practice, "the Witness." The observing self becomes steady and resilient, able both to feel the feeling and to watch the self experiencing the reaction. What is the exact texture of the sensations, the feeling-states, the pains and pleasures of our physical selves? How does this particular mind work? What are its qualities, its patterns, its mannerisms? What is the experience of this mind thinking? There is a call, too, to touch the more subtle realms of our experience—our intuition, our precognitive knowing, our soul, our spirit.

The genius of yogic practice is that it cultivates the capacity to experience a close-range, moment-by-moment inspection of reality. In fact, yoga teaches that living fully in the moment is the only doorway into the hidden realities of the Self. Once again, in scanning my journals, I discover how beautifully Amrit Desai captured this fundamental teaching of yoga:

> If you want to experience the joyous ecstasy that life offers, there is one commitment that is absolutely fundamental: the commitment to live in the moment. With that commitment as your guiding focus, whatever you do in your daily life is part of your transformational process. Your commitment to living in the moment becomes your vehicle for spiritual growth.[14]

I also discover this warning:

> Living in the moment, however, is the most dangerous situation
> anybody ever faces in life, because everything you have ever
> avoided is revealed to you when you live in the moment. You
> get to face all the denied contents of your subconscious as they
> reappear again and again through the events of your life.[15]

As the events of the next few years would reveal, the reality project is
a game played for the highest stakes.

WHAT IS REAL?

It was after midnight, and Sarita and I were still in her office, talking.

"I have a friend who's been really close to me in my recovery process, and she's always asking me the same question, 'Sarita, are you
willing to go to any lengths to regain your sanity and your connection
with God. *Any lengths*?' " We sat quietly for a moment, letting that one
sink in.

"I find that I have to ask myself that question all the time around
here," she said. "Because no matter how much we talk about reality in
this spiritual scene, most people really don't want anything to do with
it. Like that swami tonight, they'd really rather get up and out of this
embodied human life, into some rarefied transcendent zone. This
seems like a real Indian guy thing. And, after all, this place is run by an
Indian guy. I'm always fighting this battle around here—to get people
to be real. Sometimes there's just altogether too much white, not
enough black; too much smiling, not enough rage; too much yes, not
enough no. And when I point this out, you should see what I get back.
Suddenly, I'm the Wicked Witch of the West."

I knew what Sarita was talking about. Curiously, even though
Kripalu was a hatha yoga center, there seemed to be much more emphasis on transcendence than on embodiment—on the One, rather
than on the many; on the masculine images of consciousness rather
than the feminine. As Sarita pointed out, those swamis seemed more
the rule than the exception. And yet, as I wrote in my journal the next
evening after satsang, the transcendent *is* half of the equation. Many
come to spiritual practice craving the transcendent, the spiritual, the

white, the numinous, because it is so entirely missing from most of our materialistic culture. But the transcendent is still only *half* of the equation. How do we find the right balance?

Meditating on my favorite chant, I wrote, "If we were to move from the unreal to the real, where would we be going? It seems important to understand that in the yogic view, the phenomenal world is not seen in itself as unreal. It is seen as just the tip of the iceberg. Our delusion is not that we think of the gross phenomenal world as real, but that we miss the hidden depths that underlie it. We miss its interiority. And thereby, we remain oblivious of our deep and subtle connectedness to the whole realm of mind and matter."

As Swami Prabhavananda puts it in his excellent commentary on the *Yogasutras*:

> When we say that *brahman* alone is real, we do not mean that everything else is an illusion, but rather that *brahman* alone is fundamental and omnipresent. The aspects of God, the divine incarnations, have their own relative order of reality; so do the subtle and the gross objects. The materialists—those who describe themselves as being "down to earth"—are the ones who are living in an unreal world, because they limit themselves to the level of gross sense-perception. But the perception of the illumined saint ranges over the whole scale, from gross to subtle and from subtle to absolute; and it is only he who knows what the nature of this universe actually is.[16]

As Viveka discovered on his archetypal quest, the goal of the reality project is not to disengage from the phenomenal world, but to turn to embrace it more and more deeply—to discover its hidden depths. And in order to do that, paradoxically, we do not reject the vicissitudes of the embodied life. We do not reject suffering. Rather, we turn and go through the doorway of suffering. We turn to embrace our neuroses, our conflicts, our difficult bodies and minds, and we let them be the bridge to a fuller life. Our task is not to free ourselves from the world, but to fully embrace the world—to embrace the real.

As we sat together that night, I told Sarita something I had not yet shared with another living soul. "I'm thinking of staying here. Of not going back to Boston at the end of my year's sabbatical."

"I know."

"What do you mean, you know?"

"Hello? Can we just face the facts for a minute, Steve? You love to do yoga. You're up every morning meditating for hours. You're eating up yoga psychology and philosophy with a spoon. You've been here nine months now, and you're obviously thriving. Your face looks completely different from when you arrived. It's so obvious. Why would you leave?" Sarita didn't mince words.

"Yeah. Well, this certainly has been the 'transformational space' I've needed this year. No doubt about it. Fabulous. But making a permanent lifestyle of it. That's another thing altogether, Sarita."

She shrugged. "What's your worry?"

"Well, just the stuff we've been talking about tonight. Is this place out of balance? If it's an unreal world, how am I going to find my real self?"

"Oh, come on, Steve. Every place is a little out of balance, isn't it? You still looking for the perfect place? You've got to push up against it. Test it. Challenge it. Challenge the guru. Be real yourself. You could make a contribution here, you know.

"You know, sometimes Amrit is just blowing smoke, of course. But what he said tonight about being a possibility in disguise. That stuff is true," said Sarita. "We're possibilities in disguise. And I can see your possibilities turning into realities here. Can you throw that away?"

Part Three

ENCOUNTERS WITH
THE MOTHER AND
THE SEER

9

$\mathscr{T}$HE TWIN PILLARS OF THE REALITY PROJECT

When you open your eyes to the world

You are on your own for
    the first time. No one is
even interested in saving you now.

and the world steps in
    to test the calm fluidity of your body
from moment to moment

as if it believed you could join
    its vibrant dance
of fire and calmness and final stillness.

—David Whyte,
"Revelation Must Be Terrible"

"**S**teve?"

It was Jeff on the phone. He sounded distant, disconnected, and not at all himself. "Can you come and pick me up, please?" There was a little-boy quality to his tone.

"What happened? I thought you weren't finished until Friday."

"I don't know. I kind of freaked out, I guess. I'll tell you more when you get here."

Jeff had been away at a ten-day meditation retreat, his first, and he seemed to have crashed and burned after six days. I dug my car out of the remains of the previous night's blizzard and drove the hour and a half to the meditation center. As I drove up the drive to the center, I saw Jeff waiting for me at the edge of a snowbank, wrapped up in his down jacket, looking lost and forlorn, a vacant stare on his face. There were no binoculars around his neck.

"I'm sorry."

"Sorry? You don't have to be sorry, Jeff."

He dived at me, clung to me, and began to sob. "I'm sorry. I'm sorry." Big heaving sobs. "I'm so, so sorry."

As we drove the blustery and snow-covered roads, the story spilled out. A year and a half earlier, Jeff's father had died of a heart attack while being driven to work. Jeff had not shed a single tear at the funeral. He had supported his mother, his brother, and his sisters. He had wondered about his own reaction at the time. But he had assumed that he was not grieving because he was glad that his father was dead. After all, he believed his father had hated him and had competed with him. Certainly his father had bullied and shamed him his entire life. What was to grieve?

As Jeff sat in meditation practice day after day at the retreat, the emotional reality of his relationship with his father emerged. His father had been a high-ranking officer in the navy. Straight, tight-lipped with his feelings and praise, he had enormously high expectations both for himself and for Jeff. Jeff never measured up. Finally, in his late teens, as he went off to college, Jeff had given up trying and had withdrawn from the relationship. Ten years later, when his father reached out, Jeff had rebuffed his appeals for healing their relationship.

Now, in the midst of deep meditation practice, Jeff had begun to face a very difficult truth. It wasn't just that his father had hated him. It was also that he had hated his father. He wasn't just the persecuted. He was also the persecutor. Jeff had actively rejected his father and had felt some pleasure in doing so. Just a month before his father's death, he had even used his coming to Kripalu to sadistically taunt his father. "I'm a failure, Dad. Look what I'm going to do with my life after Yale."

Now Jeff felt unbearable guilt and sadness. "I'm sorry. I'm just so sorry."

Jeff was overwhelmed by these discoveries. After six days of intensive meditation, he was exhibiting all of the signs of a personality on the brink of disorganization and fragmentation. "It's so strange, Steve. I'm on a roller coaster. Some moments things feel realer than they ever have. I see my father and myself clearly. I see my mother and what she had to live with. And other moments everything seems completely unreal. Distant. Like I'm looking the wrong way through my binocs. For the past couple of days, I've been touching myself just to see if I'm really here."

Jeff seemed to feel soothed and calmed by my presence. On the trip home, I put on some of his favorite music—the Fauré *Requiem* and Elgar's *Enigma Variations*—and we cut and dove through the snow-blown landscape. We stopped at a quiet little restaurant and had a meal of comfort food—meatloaf and mashed potatoes.

"What's happening to me?" Jeff asked after we got home to Shadow-brook. "Am I having a nervous breakdown? Last night I got terrified that I was going to end up like my cousin—in the bin, and on meds for the rest of my life."

THE TWO WINGS OF PRACTICE

Like the spiritual warrior that he was, Jeff had dived into the *vipassana* meditation technique with what the Buddha called "strong determination." Following instructions, Jeff had done sitting and walking meditation for thirteen hours a day, watching his thoughts, following his breath, paying attention to a subtle new inner landscape of sensations in his body. Not surprisingly, waves of thoughts and feelings that he ordinarily kept out of awareness began to come into view. At first this was fascinating to him. He wanted more. He stayed later at night in the meditation hall than anyone else. This was magic. Soon, however, the insights became overwhelming. Yet once he had begun to open up the process, he wasn't sure how to shut it down again. This was when he began to panic.

Jeff was not having a nervous breakdown. He was simply experiencing what happens when awareness, or clear seeing, loses its connection with the other wing of witness consciousness—equanimity. When insight moves too quickly to uncover painful aspects of mental and emotional life, the personality can become disorganized and fragmented. Under these conditions, there can be a sense of disorientation, a deterioration in cognitive functioning, and an experience of depersonalization and dissociation—as Jeff discovered.

In the yogic traditions, the simultaneous cultivation of both clear seeing and the calm abiding self are required for the emergence of the fully alive human being—the jivan mukta. In the yogic view, the major obstacle to our consciousness is our unconsciousness. We need to see more clearly, especially into areas that are blocked from our conscious awareness. But just as important, we need to cultivate our connection with a deep vital center, the source of our being, or what I like to call the calmly abiding self. This means developing a nonreactive, non-judgmental, quality of acceptance, and learning to warmly love our selves and others. These qualities are naturally cultivated when we feel safely and securely held and soothed in relationships with self, with others, and with God.

For his quest to be successful, Jeff did need to hone his awareness, to look deeply under the surface of things, as he well understood. And he would certainly survive to meditate another day. But when he returned to the meditation cushion after his traumatic experience, he would take with him a deep appreciation for both sides of the reality project—the twin pillars of clear seeing and calm abiding.

CLEAR SEEING

Since Vedic times in ancient India, yogis have been called seers. It was accepted wisdom that yogic sages could penetrate the space-time continuum with their highly developed awareness. They could "see" the subtle bodies of human beings, or the planet, and could literally peer into the unmanifest realms. When Viveka ascends the sacred mountain, he finds himself in the sphere of Shiva, the seer. Here he encounters the powerful consciousness of yogic seers, which is also the archetypal masculine—transcendent awareness merged with the formless One of Brahman.

Shiva (in the form of Rudra) instructs Viveka in the refinement of the capacities of the mind. Viveka discovers, in deep states of meditation and yoga, how the normal human capacity for attention can be developed to the limits of its extraordinary dimensions. He discovers that ordinary human attention, which is discursive, intermittent, and passive, can be trained to become active, one-pointed, and autonomous. Through honing the powers of attention, ordinary mind can be transformed, revealing completely new and astonishing powers and structures of mind. This is a mind that is capable of seeing through the kleshas and the four erroneous beliefs. This transformed mind is capable of penetrating not only the unconscious, but also the realm of realities that lie hidden behind the phenomenal world. The mind then becomes an instrument for penetrating into the essence of things, for taking possession of, or assimilating, the real. "Then the wisdom of the yogi knows all things as they are," says Vyasa in his commentary on the *Yogasutras.*

In the final stages of practice, even the mind's awareness of itself—or self-consciousness—disappears. All subject-object separation vanishes, and the subject becomes absorbed in the object. All that exists at this point is the object as illumined by and revealed to consciousness. And then, finally, all that exists is pure consciousness: chitta. In the words of the *Yogasutras,* "Then, the Seer is Seeing alone." Clearly, this is a mind that has developed capacities of which we in the West have been almost completely unaware.

CALM ABIDING

When Viveka descends the sacred mountain and enters again into the marketplace, he comes into the sphere of the Wise Woman, the energies of the archetypal feminine. During his yearlong stay with the Mother, Viveka learns to embrace the experience of embodiment, to open his heart to the energies of the phenomenal world. The Mother teaches him to see all beings as manifestations of the One (Brahman), and to see the whole world as simply the play of the divine. As Viveka is healed in relationship with the Mother, he discovers the depth of compassion in his own heart for all beings, and for himself. In the process, he refines his capacity for equanimity, for happiness in his embodied human condition.

Adepts in all the contemplative traditions discovered that clear seeing could not proceed to full maturation without the development of another skill of equal importance—the capacity for equanimity. In one passage, the *Bhagavad Gita* defines yoga as "equanimity," using the Sanskrit word *samatva,* which literally means "sameness" or "evenness."[1] This quality of evenness is essential to the practice, because it creates an instrument of knowing that is nonreactive. Yogic teaching says that we have to learn gradually to tolerate sensations and feelings in the physical body, and thoughts in the mind, without reacting to them by either holding or pushing away. Craving and aversion (raga and dvesha, the third and fourth kleshas, respectively) roil the body-mind and create a kind of white noise in the system that obscures seeing clearly. For this reason, the development of a compassionate, grounded, centered, continuous, and abiding sense of self is at the core of yogic practice.

When we deeply internalize the Mother's holding, comforting, and soothing, we develop this deep, calmly abiding self, a self that is equanimous and nonreactive, a self that is always connected with the source of the Mother. This is what the *Bhagavad Gita* refers to as "steadied wisdom" *(sthita-prajna)*: "He whose mind is not affected in sorrow and is free from desire in pleasure and who is without attachment, fear, or anger—he is called a sage of 'steadied insight' *(sthita-dhi)*." (II.56)

As Viveka discovered during his apprenticeship at the edge of the forest, the systematic creation of this calmly abiding center required not only the holding and soothing of the Mother, but also a process of purification. Before Viveka could pass through the last obstacle between him and home, he had to cultivate the health and strength of his body. This aspect of practice focused on creating the "hard wiring" for the energies of consciousness—literally strengthening the structure and the form of his instruments of perception. Through the practice of yoga, the physical structure is said to be "baked," or refined, creating a form strong enough to tolerate and hold the powerful energies of the fully alive human being without being roiled or destroyed by them. Without the creation of this hard wiring, as Viveka saw, it was simply not possible to tolerate the subtle levels of awareness into which the quest would take him. Like Viveka, without the development of a compassionate and equanimous body and mind, we literally cannot bear what the seer reveals to us.

Not surprisingly, human communities interested in generating the fully alive human being discover these two poles of practice over and over again, in every generation and in diverse parts of the globe. In Buddhist communities these two aspects of practice are often called wisdom and compassion; in the world of psychology, we sometimes identify the creative interplay between insight, bringing unconscious processes into awareness, and support, building the foundations of a cohesive, continuous, and nonfragmenting sense of self. In yoga, these two poles of practice are the twin pillars supporting the central yogic strategy for waking up: witness consciousness. The reality project cannot proceed without the equal development of both poles of practice.

LEARNING TO ACKNOWLEDGE, EXPERIENCE, AND BEAR REALITY

When I was a young graduate student in Boston, the psychoanalytic community boasted a number of teachers and mentors of enormous stature: Erik Erikson, Sofie Freud Lowenstein, Robert Coles, John Mack. But none of these, I think, was more loved and admired than Elvin Semrad. By the time I came onto the scene, Semrad was already a legend. He was a training analyst and former president of the Boston Psychoanalytic Institute, professor of psychiatry at Harvard Medical School, and, for more than twenty years, clinical director in charge of psychiatric residency training at the highly regarded Massachusetts Mental Health Center. Though he wrote no books—only a series of two hundred or so highly technical papers—he became one of the most important teachers of his generation.

Semrad seemed to embody both of the poles I have just been discussing. He was a man of ample girth—solid, grounded in reality, and remarkably plain-spoken. His very presence seemed to create a deep sense of safety in patients and young therapists alike. He exuded a sense of calm abiding. And within the big, safe space that he created, there was ample room for patients and students to explore the whole range of their emotional and mental landscapes, to look unflinchingly at who they were, and at who others were.

Semrad believed that in order to be fully alive, it was important to explore all facets of the self's experience. In the safety of his presence, patients and therapists could begin to risk freeing up their awareness and their imagination, letting them roam where they needed to. He was big enough to allow patients and trainees to use him as an emotional home base for their own investigations. "A therapist is a kind of service man," he would say. "There are so many things a patient can want to use you for, and if you can swallow your own ideas of how things should be, you can perform a real service."[2]

Semrad's formulation of the goal of psychotherapy was brilliant, concise, and complete: "Through the work of psychoanalysis, the patient must come to acknowledge, experience, and bear the reality of his life—both the painful reality and the pleasurable reality of it. Then, he can finally put into perspective the feelings that arise in the process of living."[3]

Acknowledge, experience, and bear reality—I loved Semrad's statement. First of all, I loved his devotion to reality. He always made patients feel that reality was the safest place to be. He trusted the wisdom of the unconscious completely. He wanted to reassure us that we could step down off the platform of our delusions onto the solid ground of reality.

But secondly, I loved his definition because it strikes just the right balance. It includes not just the project of seeing clearly (acknowledging), but adds an important nuance to that—the capacity to fully experience life. Seeing, as he rightly points out, has to be done with the whole self. In order to be known, reality must be experienced, with the body, the feeling life, and the life of the mind. This is entirely consistent with the yogic view.

One of the central findings of yogic experimentation into the phenomenology of the self is that reality cannot be described or defined in any satisfactory way. It must simply be realized, fully experienced in the body-mind. The single goal driving the whole teeming, colorful world of Indian spirituality was atmavidya—"knowledge of the soul." But for yogis, knowledge meant something quite different than it does for us. In the yogic worldview, the only kind of knowledge that liberates is "direct knowledge of the self"—that is to say, experiential knowledge. The reality of the field of intelligence, energy, and consciousness must be known directly, experientially, in the cells of the body-mind and in all the koshas. This is quite consistent with Semrad's view of the process of psychotherapy.

Semrad completes his formulation with a brilliant stroke. In addition to acknowledging and experiencing life, we must learn to "bear" life, with both its attendant vicissitudes and pleasures. By "bearing," Semrad means creating the capacity in the self to tolerate the experience of life. He means creating the container to hold life in such a way that we are not shattered by it. He means developing the calmly abiding center as a continuous home base from which it is possible to range freely through our entire experience. Semrad knew that without the foundations of the calmly abiding self in place, the experience of awareness can simply be shattering, fragmenting, and traumatic, as it was for Jeff.

Semrad advised that we never underestimate our capacity for delusion. "Sometimes I think the greatest sources of our suffering are the lies we tell to ourselves," he said.[4] At the same time, however, he respected the heroic effort it takes to see through this veil of delusion, and he always counseled compassion, self-love, and multifarious techniques for soothing the self and others. In his psychoanalytic work, Elvin Semrad was unknowingly aligned with the best wisdom of the Eastern traditions. Let's look more closely at the two wings of practice that he exemplified: clear seeing and calm abiding.

THE FIRST PILLAR: CLEAR SEEING

Catherine was a Presbyterian minister who was on a leave of absence from her church to spend a year at Kripalu, learning about Eastern spirituality, yoga, and meditation. When she arrived in the community, she was surprised to find that we didn't meditate and do yoga all day long. We all had jobs connected with the running of the center— anything from cutting vegetables to mowing lawns, from secretarial work to administrative work. After her first week of orientation, she was asked to take a newly vacated position of inventory manager in the Kripalu shop, where we sold books, tapes, and yoga clothing.

"Hmm," said Catherine, gazing over the top of her half glasses, and peering abstractedly through her gray bangs. I could tell she did not want to do this job. She told me later that she did have a momentary flash of intuition that said clearly, "Don't do this," but she immediately suppressed it. Catherine had a strong belief that spirituality was about surrendering, a belief she had nurtured in her work with the church, and she decided on the spot that it would be good for her to "surrender her ego" and take the position. "Of course I'll do it," she said, with her characteristic Katharine Hepburn–like determination and wholesomeness.

Three months later, Catherine had mastered the complicated computer system used to manage hundreds of thousands of dollars' worth of inventory. She was working overtime to reorganize the procedures of the department, so that it would be more efficient. "It seems," I thought, "that she really *has* surrendered to this."

Then something extraordinary happened. Catherine charged into the office one day after lunch. (She was feeling nothing, she told me later, except a certain manic kind of drivenness.) Without even thinking, she sat down at her computer screen and typed in the special code to delete the entire inventory from the data bank. This was a code that was only used once a month, after a full inventory had been taken and just before new inventory was entered. It was a complicated enough code that it couldn't have been entered accidentally. Catherine had just "accidentally on purpose" dropped a bomb into the midst of her carefully honed data. She was about to perpetrate a disaster.

In a panic, Catherine realized what she had done. She watched in horror as "DELETE, DELETE, DELETE" flashed across the screen in big letters. She tried everything she could to stop it. Nothing worked.

Catherine's mind raced. She was desperately hoping she would be able to stop this disaster and cover it up. How could she have done something so stupid, so reckless? But even more terrifying—how could she have done something so hostile, so aggressive, so angry, so, well, subversive? What would people think of her? Could she avoid telling her boss? Could she save face?

Finally, there was only one thing to do. She had to find her supervisor right away and get her help. She did. Together they called for backup from the software specialist who had written the program. There was a way to stop the process. Catherine allowed herself to be led through the procedure on the phone. The old inventory was saved. Catherine sat down, exhausted, trembling. She cried as her supervisor sat with her. "How could I have done that?" she kept asking. "Why? It wasn't me! It was like I was taken over by someone else."

Why, indeed? What was going on with Catherine? It's fairly simple. She wasn't taken over by someone else, of course. She was taken over by herself. Catherine was royally pissed about working as an inventory manager from the very beginning. She didn't want to do it. But she wanted to please. She wanted to be spiritual. She hadn't been able to say no. And so, she had not listened to the small voice of her intuition. She had shut it up. She had buried that voice so deeply, in fact, that she wasn't even aware of it. Her feelings lived, though. They lived in the basement of her awareness. Unconsciously, Catherine felt used. She seethed with resentment. She felt she was betraying her own intentions for her sabbatical. Part of her wanted to throw a bomb into the place. And she did.

Many truths were revealed in the course of this drama. But for our discussion, the most important one is this: Much of our behavior is driven by motivations—wishes and fears, hopes and dreads, loves and hates—of which we are completely unaware. Catherine was angry. Yet she remained astonishingly unaware of the depth of her anger. "Denial," as the bumper sticker says, "is not just a river in Egypt." It is a very powerful defense mechanism that allows us to keep out of awareness aspects of reality that we cannot bear, or aspects of ourselves that are not consistent with our ideas about who we are or who we should be.

Among the many brilliant insights brought into our culture in this century by psychoanalysis, this is perhaps the simplest, and the most important: Much of mental and emotional life is unconscious. It happens completely outside of our conscious awareness. Most reasonably educated Americans now give lip service to this insight. We know about slips of the tongue, dreams, accidents, and "forgetting." We know, at least theoretically, how the unconscious leaks out. We know about what Freud called "the return of the repressed." But when we actually do meet the unconscious at work in our daily dramas, as Catherine did, it can be astonishing. Most of us, most of the time, cannot bear to acknowledge that we live up to our necks in the dark waters of unconsciousness. We spend our days acting out little dramas driven from the dark recesses of the self.

We can "put away" the lunatic, raging aunts and the sex-obsessed, alcoholic uncles of our psychic life. We can lock them up in the basement of our consciousness. But the more energy we expend in securing the basement door, the more dramatic their appearance will be when they get out. To paraphrase Carl Jung, that which we hold unaware in our unconscious will eventually come to us as fate. These split-off aspects of our self will appear as strangers, as enemies, as "not us." They will appear as "the hand of God." But one thing is absolutely sure. They will eventually be in our face, and often in the unkindest and most surprising of ways.

Catherine was unconsciously committed to the projects of her "false self," the first and most obvious of which we have already discovered—proving her worth as a spiritual professional, a minister. It turned out that one of the reasons Catherine wanted to come on a yearlong retreat was that she was exhausted, worn out from overriding her feelings, from dominating her self in the service of a wildly distorted and grandiose ego-ideal. Catherine was perfectionistic, driven in her "spiritual" work, and overidentified with her successes and failures in her career in the church. Her underlying, distorted sense of worthlessness was all based on childhood experiences that still lived, completely outside of her awareness. Success in the spiritual realm had become just another hook for her false self.

But now here is the key question. Wouldn't a year of spiritual practice eventually have softened Catherine's distortions, perhaps allowing her more access to her vulnerability, her limitations, and her many-faceted emotional reality? Well, not necessarily. The problem was that Catherine's new spiritual project was caught in the same web of perfectionism and achievement orientation as the rest of her life. And the result would be the same, because as we have seen, the false self is a kind of learning disability. Catherine would still experience no true satisfaction as long as her spiritual search was unconsciously driven by the need to please others and disprove her worthlessness.

Catherine came to Kripalu because she was looking everywhere she could think of for "ways of finding out" who she really was. There was a strong drive toward self-discovery. This was right on the surface. But underneath, there was also a strong drive to remain hidden, and to use spiritual practice to manifest her unconscious projects, her grandiose ego-ideal being only the most obvious of these.

What does Catherine need? She needs to understand the particular nature of her unconscious projects. How are they in opposition to her conscious projects? What engine is driving her buried life? As Semrad once said to a group of therapists in training, "Laymen often think that the best way to deal with any difficult situation is not to deal with it—to forget it. But you and I have the experience that the only way you can forget is to remember."⁵

Freud understood that these intrusions of the unconscious into our conscious lives are enormous gifts—"letters from the unconscious," as Jung said about dreams. For all her spiritual work and practice, however, Catherine did not have a structure in place that would allow her to open these letters. The message they carried was too painful for her to look at. Within a week or so her experience with the computer seemed to vanish into the mists of her unconscious. I thought, sadly, that in spite of her best spiritual intentions, this lovely, dedicated person would almost certainly repeat these episodes again and again, until she was finally able, in Semrad's terms, to "remember herself."

PARALLEL LIVES

Psychoanalysis has a second insight to add to our understanding of the buried life: Mental processes—fears, wishes, hopes, dreads—operate in parallel. This means that we can easily desire and fear the same thing. We can want and not want the same thing, just as we can love and hate the same person. This insight mirrors the wisdom of the contemplative traditions, which see mental and emotional life as always under the sway of duality. In these traditions it is understood that there are two sides to everything human: underneath fear there is often a wish, underneath hope there is often unconscious dread, underneath love is the shadow side of hate, underneath gain is often loss. Praise and blame, fame and ill-repute. And on and on. When we look under the surface of our lives, we can see how refusal to acknowledge this parallel aspect of the buried life causes us to suffer.

A patient of mine named Cassandra once brought the following problem into therapy. She had loaned a considerable amount of money to her younger brother, Sam, so that he could send his young son to an expensive special summer camp for diabetic children. Sam's son had a great experience at the camp, and it really changed his life. Cassandra felt terrific about being able to help. As the years passed, however, things soured. Sam would not repay Cassandra's loan. He had a good job. He was a member of a fundamentalist church to which he tithed. And yet, he could not make a single payment to Cassandra. He acted lovingly toward Cassandra and her family, when he saw them. He made many promises of payment, then broke them. Cassandra felt furious and helpless. "He's supposed to be a Christian," she said, "but he's stolen my money."

What was happening? Sam loved Cassandra, and always had—of this he was aware. But at the very same time he hated her. His hate, unlike his love, lived in the basement of his consciousness. He could not let himself face it. Why did he hate this generous sister? For one thing, Cassandra had been their mother's special child. She had done extremely well in school, better than he, and had then prospered in her career. He resented her. Paradoxically, he hated her for having the money to give him. Unconsciously, he felt entitled to her money as repayment for the inequality in their lives.

As long as Sam remained unaware of this seething resentment, there was little chance of Cassandra's getting her money back. As long as he could not face his feelings toward his sister, he was destined to act them out. "What remains unconscious will come to us as fate," as Jung said.

Note that Sam was living a spiritual practice—Christian fundamentalism. Yet he was acting in a way that contravened everything he believed. He had, in effect, stolen a large amount of money, not from a stranger, but from a sister whom he loved. Yet, because his spiritual path did not help him cultivate seeing clearly into the unconscious roots of his behavior, he was incapable of living up to its requirements for ethical behavior.

Sam's church helped him to feel connected with God and others. He felt safely held and soothed in the arms of his religion. It immeasurably aided his development of equanimity, of a calmly abiding self. But without cultivating the power of clear seeing as well, his practice could not help him to avoid suffering and could not help him stop contributing to the suffering of others.

THE SECOND PILLAR: THE CALM, ABIDING SELF

When Jeff called me from the retreat center, I knew exactly what had happened to him because it had also happened to me. Several years earlier, I had undertaken a monthlong vipassana meditation retreat. For thirteen hours a day I did sitting and walking meditation, practicing a technique that is specifically designed to develop awareness. For the first couple weeks, I watched in amazement as floods of hitherto-repressed memories and experiences were brought into consciousness. Suddenly, there was my first-grade teacher, Miss Hanson; my grandmother's hand rubbing my back; my sister's face at about age two. Long-forgotten moments of childhood arose, sometimes with ineffable sweetness, sometimes with terrible pain. The experience was shocking, astonishing, and completely compelling. I was riveted. The technique just kept opening doors. I sat on my cushion and downloaded days, weeks, months, years of experience from my childhood. I felt as though I had tapped into the mother lode, a vein of gold in my unconscious.

Two weeks into the retreat I began to feel intensely anxious. I couldn't sit still. During breaks from sitting, I began to walk obses-sively—first two miles, then five, then ten miles. I was moving fast—two times around the lake for everyone else's one. At times my body was burning with energy. Too, I had uncomfortable moments, some-times hours, of feeling dissociated from my body. In fact, it seemed as though every day I had a new disconcerting mental or emotional expe-rience, many of which I recognized from the *Diagnostic and Statistical Manual of Mental Disorders*. For a couple of days, I began to feel as if I were disappearing. This was terrifying. Then, I noticed that between sitting sessions I was regularly checking in the mirror to see that I still existed. I was beginning to lose that all-important continuous sense of myself, as I knew some of my patients did. Sometimes, when I'd look in the mirror, I wasn't sure who was staring back at me.

Finally, I panicked: Is this it? Am I going crazy? I knew it, I knew I was basically unstable. I made a desperate late-night visit to one of my teachers. "Sylvia," I said. "I'm losing it." She was calm and sooth-ing. She gave me a cup of tea and sat me down on the sofa. And we talked. After listening to me for a while, she smiled and said in her most assuring voice, "Stephen. This is OK. You're not going crazy at all. In fact, you've refined your awareness to a very high degree. The only problem is that you've done too well. Your awareness has grown faster than your equanimity. You need to go back to a practice that creates equanimity. We'll focus on that for the rest of the retreat, and you'll be fine." For the rest of that retreat, my practice was to focus on building a calmly abiding center that could keep pace with the unsettling new awareness I had developed. Eventually I regained my center.

Reality is difficult to bear. There is a good reason why we keep aspects of ourselves hidden. Seeing too clearly, or too soon, can create a dangerous amount of instability in a self that is organized around a certain amount of delusion (which is of course how we're all con-structed). As I discovered in my meditation retreat, even a healthy self can come unglued when overwhelmed with too much painful truth. Clear seeing needs the calmly abiding self.

Back in my room after getting Jeff resettled, I pulled out my journal and, recalling my own terrifying experience of fragmentation and my conversation with Sylvia, I added a new schematic beneath my earlier diagram of the relationship between shiva and shakti.

AWARENESS	EQUANIMITY
Clear seeing	Calm abiding
Mind	Heart
Wisdom	Compassion
No-self	Self
Seeing through the self	Building up the self
Insight	Self-soothing
Acknowledge	Bear
The Seer	The Mother

Understanding spiritual development as a tension arc between these two poles is crucial. Unfortunately, both psychotherapeutic and spiritual practice in our time have suffered from an absence of the "second pillar," devoting themselves in an unbalanced fashion to the notion that awareness is, of itself, healing.

In psychotherapy this belief has shown up as a bias toward techniques that soften and dismantle defensive structures. The classic psychoanalytic approach to therapy focuses on revealing and resolving conflict between various aspects of the self—uncovering and working through the roots of inhibition, guilt, anxiety, obsession, and so forth. In the consulting room, this often means relentlessly uncovering impulses, drives, and feelings so that conflict can be resolved. Even in the popular imagination, there is an understanding that the real work of psychotherapy is making the unconscious conscious. This notion has filtered down to the pop psychology level where there is still a proliferation of intensive programs that are meant to "break you down," so that "you can get real"—revealing what is hidden.

Not surprisingly, this same bias shows up in our spiritual practices. We prefer to "cut to the chase," and we assume that this is accomplished through the more advanced insight-oriented techniques. Certainly this is what I was doing during that monthlong retreat. In many cases, however, we have taken these practices out of a traditional context that is really quite a bit more balanced. At our peril, we focus all of our effort on cultivating awareness, often ignoring the vast repertoire of self-building and equanimity practices that are meant to go hand in hand with insight. In fact, the preliminary practices of yoga are almost all about building the calmly abiding self.

In recent decades, psychotherapists, too, have developed a new emphasis on the cultivation of the calmly abiding center. In the work of Heinz Kohut, the founder of what is sometimes called self psychology, the focus of treatment is not so much on uncovering unconscious conflict, but on building the foundations of the self. These foundations read like a laundry list of the factors of equanimity: the capacity to self-soothe, to warmly love the self, to value and esteem the self, and to experience a satisfyingly cohesive sense of identity.[6]

Self psychologists discovered that when these foundational capacities are strong, conflict within the self is more naturally revealed and more easily worked through. Resistance to clear seeing is softened. And, in the presence of such strong foundations, all the more subtle potentials of the self naturally emerge over time.

My students often ask me to describe equanimity. I tell them I cannot do better than to tell the story of my greatest teacher of equanimity—my cat, Mr. B. Long before my immersion in yoga, I had a cat whom I had given a Sanskrit name—Bonanda, after a character on the late-night TV comedy *Mary Hartman, Mary Hartman.*

It didn't take long in the presence of Bonanda to realize that this animal was deeply spiritual, that he was, in fact, enlightened. He had clearly earned his name in an earlier life. Nothing shook Bonanda. One day, Mr. B., as I came to call him, was sitting in my front yard, calmly surveying the neighborhood like a little sphinx, all knowing, and all seeing. Head up, eyes scanning slowly up and down the street. Two doors down, something unusual happened. My neighbor's large and ferocious German shepherd, Queenie, got out of the house. She was in turn surveying the scene on the street when her eye caught sight of Mr. B. Queenie stood perfectly still for a moment, ears up. She crouched. Then she charged, like a rocket, directly at the composed little figure of Bonanda. Mr. B did not budge. Did not blink. He stared with utter nonconcern at Queenie's raging approach. A foot or two from Bonanda, Queenie, completely taken aback by the cat's unflinching ease, put her two paws out in front of her, skidded to a stop, and ran back to her own yard. Mr. B. put his head back down on his paws. That was that.

This is equanimity.

CULTIVATING EQUANIMITY

Several weeks after Jeff's meditation-meltdown, he, Paula, and I were sitting in the dining chapel at Kripalu, talking about the importance of creating equanimity in practice.

"Now I understand why my Quaker meeting for worship has become so important in my life," Paula said. "It's the place in my life where I really seem to be cultivating equanimity." She described her Sunday routine, which was always the same. She would arrive at the simple white eighteenth-century meetinghouse early and sit in a back pew, next to a big window that overlooked a little garden. As soon as she sat down her whole body seemed to calm deeply. The other fifteen or twenty worshipers entered gradually, silently.

"I've gotten used to the pattern," said Paula. She described it: First her breathing is shallow and rapid. But as she sits in the silence, she can feel her breath naturally begin to slow down into long, relaxed waves. Her mind slows, too; at a certain point it simply shifts gears into "doing nothing." In the silence and stillness, and with the support of the centuries of prayer seeping from the blue walls, deeply buried images of the past—smells, memories, visions—waft up unbidden. At times they arise hand in hand with pain that catches in her belly. At times they come with ineffable sweetness. And as she sits in her regular spot, looking out the window onto the garden, she has a profound sense of peace.

Paula mentioned other experiences, too: quiet times alone or with her family, meditation, yoga, journaling, conscious breathing. "These are the very experiences I think of as spiritual practice. These are the times I feel most connected to the source of my being, to God." Paula went on to say that in the context of certain kinds of relationships—especially in her new friendships—she felt that she could allow herself to drop down into her center.

The self can neither exist as a cohesive structure nor generate experiences of well-being apart from a contextual surround that is sustaining in this way. Paula, Jeff, and I needed this "surround" as much as we needed oxygen. We all need to have a healing experience of being safely and securely held (metaphorically speaking), and whether this happens in the context of psychotherapy or spiritual practice does not matter. It is within this sustaining, evocative, and properly responsive environment that our whole subjective, internal world can be expressed, expanded, and enriched.

Interestingly enough, Paula discovered that when she was experiencing her center, her awareness was also newly alive, capable of going both inward (as in Quaker meeting) and outward, to more fully meet sensations, feelings, and experiences. From this place of calm abiding, she felt capable of being fully present for herself and for life. She momentarily felt her deep connection with all beings. Her awareness was free to go out to meet life and to penetrate life more fully.

In yoga it is understood that the experience of the abiding self is not so much discovered as it is created, moment to moment, in a field that is properly evocative, sustaining, and responsive. Most of my students at Kripalu have not studied self psychology, but they know this experience from the inside out. They've found many of the words that describe it: "connection, permission, simplification, self-trust, inner stillness, time alone, a good friend, quiet, focus, breath, faith, continuity."

"UNCOVERING CONFLICT" OR "BUILDING UP THE SELF"?

Tom, Paula, Nina, Geoff, and I were sitting in the early October sun, having lunch in the grass by the Charles River. We'd just attended a talk given by Tom at a psychotherapy conference at Boston University. A month earlier, I had told each of them, by letter and by phone calls, that I would not be returning to practice in Boston at the end of my sabbatical year. Nina and her husband, Martin, had beat a hasty path to my door to try to convince me otherwise. She and I were still working through the bumps from that painful surprise visit.

Between bites of my chicken-salad sandwich, I was telling them the story of Viveka, his encounter with the Seer and the Mother, and the Eastern contemplative point of view on awareness and equanimity. "What fascinates me is that these traditions acknowledge the creative tension arc between these two poles—insight on the one hand, and building up the self on the other. The mind and the heart are brought together. This is a powerful combination, and I don't think it's one we've even begun to achieve in psychotherapy."

"It does seem to me we've split these two aspects of growth in our culture," Tom said, and he went on to describe his view of this predicament. Psychology and psychotherapy have become the guardians of mental processes, the experts in the process of seeing through the defensive structures of the mind. When we're ready for clear seeing beneath the surface, we seek out a therapist. Likewise, religion and spirituality have become the guardians of source, of the deepest forms of self-soothing, of compassion, of the calmly abiding self. When we're searching for source, we often seek out spiritual practice.

"Well, I certainly agree that these functions have been split," said Geoff. "In my neck of the woods, it seems that most people go to church just to get comforted, held, consoled, certainly not for what you call clear seeing. People go to church to go to sleep, not to wake up."

Paula objected. "I think maybe 'go to sleep' might be a little strong. In my Quaker meeting there's something more than consoling going on. I'm not just soothing my despair, but also making meaning of it. And also celebrating life."

"Steve's right about one thing," said Nina. "Most religions don't confront the unconscious. Don't actually try in any way to dismantle the defensive structure. If what you're saying is true, though, Steve, it sounds like the Eastern traditions do try to see through the armoring of the self." Nina chewed on her sandwich thoughtfully for a few moments. We all watched the first signs of spring on the Charles—an occasional sailboat, a big cruiser filled with bundled-up boaters.

"The issue is really balance," I said, elaborating a bit on my current thinking. "In practice, there will always be a movement back and forth between awareness and equanimity." When equanimity is weak there will be increasing fragmentation. When awareness is weak, we'll find ourselves constantly hijacked by our unconscious projects. As more abiding center is cultivated, it calls for and creates the container for more awareness. As awareness is honed, and more of the unconscious is revealed, it calls for a stronger abiding center to hold it.

Nina turned toward me with a serious look on her face. "I see what you're talking about with these two sides of the project of waking up." There was an edge in her voice. "But do you think they're both present at Kripalu? I mean, when Martin and I were out there two weeks ago, I certainly got a sense of the safety and soothing. But too much of that can produce a kind of *Magic Mountain* scene. I mean, are you really going to *face* anything there?" I could hear the fury in her voice.

"To be honest, Nina, I think I came to Kripalu for that soothing part of spirituality, connecting with source, more than I did the awareness part. I had already had a strong dose of looking clearly at hard reality."

"Yeah, exactly my point. I just don't want you hiding out," she said, " 'cause that's not going to get you anywhere. You should never have ended psychoanalysis. You know, this has to get worked out in relationship. You can't do it in an ivory tower or on a yoga mat."

I had to chuckle at this one. "Try living with more than three hundred people in your face day in and day out, eating, sleeping, working, and you'll see that it's not hiding out. You get triggered. Your stuff gets exposed. You have plenty of opportunity to work through it, believe me."

"You know, Neen," said Tom, "you're not acknowledging the huge debate that's raging about this very issue right now in the shrink world. I mean, do we uncover conflict or do we build up the self? There are strong points of view for both. You're just being a clunky Freudian."

Nina swatted Tom good-naturedly with a magazine, and we all settled back in to finishing lunch.

Uncover conflict or build up the self? I leaned back on the grass, gazing up at the clouds skimming like sails overhead. Both, I thought. Both, in a balanced spiritual practice. Both, too, in a successful psychotherapeutic process. But Nina was right about one thing. Both of these pillars of the reality project have to be developed in the context of relationship. We cannot become real in isolation.

EQUANIMITY: ON HOLDING

AND BEING HELD

Within the city of Brahman, which is the body,
there is the heart, and within the heart there is a
little house. This house has the shape of a lotus,
and within it dwells that which is to be sought
after, inquired about, and realized. Even so large
as the universe outside is the universe within the
lotus of the heart. Within it are heaven and earth,
the sun, moon, the lightning and all the stars.
Whatever is in the macrocosm is in this microcosm
also.

—*Chandogya Upanishad*

When I was about four years old, I lived "within the lotus of the heart," staying for a year with my grandparents in their big old Victorian house in the little town of Phelps, in upstate New York. For me, the house was a vast new universe unto itself, with its immense oak-paneled staircase and library, long dark hallway upstairs, ancient mysterious ancestors staring down from portraits on the wall, and cavernous attic filled with trunks of antique clothes and toys, covered with dusty sheets. I can still remember the utter and complete safety of that house—my little bed, tucked in a corner of a big room and covered with stuffed animals. Mostly, I remember the big warm lap of my grandmother, her beautiful face, her soft breasts, into which I was welcome to snuggle. I remember how she smelled. I remember her sitting on my bed at night as I went to sleep, talking with me and my stuffed animals, in a soothing voice that seemed all I could ever want. This was paradise. It was a rich, solid, old world that I imagined had always been, and would always be.

In those magical months, I had the experience of feeling safely and securely held in the arms of both my grandparents. I could walk uptown holding the hand of my Aunt Gertrude and look through the big plate-glass window of the handsome limestone town hall to see my grandfather, who was then town supervisor, always in a three-piece suit, working at his desk.

So powerful was this immersion that the experience of being held and soothed became a permanent place inside me—a place I could evoke in memory when I needed it, a place I still return to, my emotional home base. Thirty years later, when both my grandparents had died and we sold the house, my twin sister and I stood in the middle of the packing crates and sobbed. The house itself was saturated with the love of these two people. But we realized that day that that love had also saturated us. It was in our eyes, in our hearts.

THE FOUNDATIONS OF EQUANIMITY: ON BEING SAFELY HELD AND SOOTHED

In the yogic view of the world, consciousness exists as a potential in the "seed of the self," or the "egg of Brahman." Yogis believe that there is an actual subtle physical center of spiritual consciousness called "the lotus of the heart," situated in the center of the chest, and that it is "first among equals" of the centers of consciousness in the body, because it is the subtle umbilical cord that connects us with the source of the divine Mother. There is a great mystery connected with its awakening. Though it lies as a potential in all of us, it can only be called forth by another awake human heart. Just as a physical human being can only be born from the body of another human being, so, too, consciousness must give birth to consciousness. It does not come about through "practices" or postures or scripture or knowledge or purification. It happens only in the magic of relationship—and not a relationship with an impersonal Absolute (atman/brahman) but with a human embodiment of the divine. As Bapuji put it, "The key to your heart lies in the heart of another."

We awaken to our calmly abiding center through deep relationship and connectedness with others who have found their own center. We need others like this to be so close to us that they are, in fact, almost like extensions of ourselves. People who have deeply internalized the capacity to feel safely held and soothed, comforted, calmed, grounded, and centered in themselves, like my grandmother, have a unique capacity to transmit this to others.[1] When we use someone in this way, they become for us what Heinz Kohut has called self-objects. They are at one and the same time other (objects) and self. They are as important to us as oxygen and food, because they allow us to literally take them inside ourselves. We take them in viscerally, and, in effect, we borrow their calmly abiding center until the experience of centeredness is evoked inside our self.

One of our deepest needs, then, is to merge our hearts with powerful, safe, solid, and loving objects who hold us physically in their arms and who also hold us emotionally in their hearts. Kohut calls this a narcissistic need—the need for merger with idealized self-objects. My grandparents were most important self-objects for me, allowing me to relax into the stable, calm, nonanxious, powerful, and protective environment that they created with their care. Within the vast and safe container of their nurturing, I was allowed to discover my true self.

Western psychology has come to understand that the self cannot exist as a cohesive structure apart from these self-object experiences. Without them, we cannot generate an inner experience of well-being. In Western psychological terms, the very foundation of equanimity is the capacity to soothe the self. And this capacity we can only internalize through having been safely and securely held and soothed ourselves. It doesn't take perfect holding and soothing, and it doesn't take a lot. As Semrad said, "A little bit of love goes a long way." But it does take a minimum amount—what Winnicott called "good enough" soothing.

This is not only a Western psychological insight. It is central to the architecture of yoga. And yet, in their transmission to the West, many yogic practices have lost their original relational context. Many Western spiritual seekers seem to think that yoga and meditation are things that they do by and with themselves, that opening the heart comes about through repeatedly entering altered states of consciousness, dissolving the physical body into white light, and merging with the One. The truth is, however, that all the yoga postures in the world cannot create the opening of the heart. In their original context, yogic practices were completely submerged in a web of relationship—relationships to extended family, village, teachers, holy men and women. In many cases "practice" was simply opportunity for relationship to develop, and though it may not have been commented upon, it was, in fact, the relationship, often with the guru, that was the key transformational ingredient.

THE TEACHER AS MOTHER

Yogis developed an entire science of relationship, acknowledging it to be the foundation of all subsequent spiritual development. The relationship with a beloved teacher (guru) became the doorway to the most profound relationship with the beloved—God in her many guises and forms. For some seekers, indeed, the entire path may be relationship. This was so for many students at Kripalu, who used Amrit Desai as an idealized object of love and devotion.

In Indian spirituality, the teacher, his or her being, extended family, and home or ashram all become a kind of refuge for the student. The yogic scriptures are full of references to the teacher as "mother," and many scriptures refer to the process of being born out of the womb of the teacher. For example, the *Athara-Veda,* composed as early as 1000 BCE says, "Initiation takes place in that the teacher carries the pupil in himself, as it were, as the mother bears the embryo in her body."[2]

A thousand years later another scripture (the *Hevajra Tantra*) puts it, "The school is said to be the body. The monastery is called the womb. The yellow robe is the membrane. And the preceptor is one's mother."[3]

Amrit actively promoted the image of ashram as a "refuge," a "safe haven." I had heard him use this language in the talk he gave to our group on my first day—the guru's house as a kind of chrysalis for transformation. It lent an air of magical safety to the entire life of the community. We were protected by magical forces—as long as we remained in the "womb."

The teacher is seen as a manifestation of the shakti, or the divine Mother—the steady stream of power and love emanating from the heart of the universe. Even if the teacher is male, in his role as "mother" he embodies the female principle of generativity. He or she becomes a "womb" or an "exoskeleton" for the student as she develops her own capacities to self-soothe. Gradually, the student internalizes the teachings, and comes to experience the teacher as "inside" rather than outside. The river of life, of shakti, and of the divine Mother, are now flowing within. The student's connection with source has been awakened.

In contemporary Western culture, the psychotherapist often provides precisely this kind of refuge for the person seeking healing and rebirth—though the archetypal images of mother and womb are rarely invoked. The relational aspects of the contemplative traditions are just now beginning to be explored, but when they are more fully understood it will be seen that they share two fundamental premises with the world of Western psychotherapy: that which is damaged in relationship must also be healed within relationship, and character can only truly be transformed through relationship—not through solitary practice.

THE ARCHETYPE OF THE ORPHAN

The archetype of the Orphan appears over and over again in yogic lore. This is the student who remembers the "arms of the teacher," perhaps from previous lifetimes, but who is now separated from the grace of the teacher's presence. Without the real presence of the teacher, and without the return to his or her "womb," the student knows he cannot awaken the true connection with the river of life, with divine Mother. The archetypal story of the Orphan in yogic literature is usually a tale of longing, desperation, and spiritual depression. Though it often includes a suicide attempt, there is usually a happy ending, with the teacher archetype appearing at the last possible moment.

Within the yogic lineage at Kripalu, there is such a story—the story of Bapuji's spiritual depression, which I briefly sketched in chapter 2. From the depths of his despair and suicidal wish, the nineteen-year-old Bapuji cried out to the divine Mother to take him home. In the moment of his greatest anguish, as he knelt in the temple of the Mother, he was found by his guru—who turned out to be Lord Lakulish, one of the great immortal saints of India. Through his relationship with this remarkable teacher, Bapuji's suffering and despair were transmuted into a deep relationship with God. Bapuji was thus "reborn" in the womb of this mysterious saint, transformed into a *yogacharya*—a teacher and master of yoga.

The very same outlines of this archetypal tale appear in the story of one of the greatest of Hindu ecstatics and mystics, the nineteenth-century Indian saint Ramakrishna—who was widely believed to be a supremely realized Self *(paramahansa)* and an avatar (incarnation of the divine). Ramakrishna found the premature deaths of his brother and his father almost impossible to bear, and he came to the brink of suicide, calling upon the divine Mother, and losing himself in his longing for her. He later claimed that he had become "positively insane" in his longing for the Mother, and he spent most of his time "inebriated" with visions of various forms of Shakti. Finally, a middle-aged woman—a wandering renunciate named Yogesvari—arrived mysteriously and became Ramakrishna's first teacher, providing for him the real human form that he needed in order to transform his longing into a direct realization of the source within. The real presence of the Mother in his life allowed Ramakrishna to open his heart to the universal Mother, and he subsequently had many ecstatic experiences such as the one he describes in the following passage from his writings:

> Suddenly I had the wonderful vision of the Mother, and fell down unconscious. . . . In my heart of hearts, there was flowing a current of intense bliss, never experienced before and I had the immediate knowledge of the light that was Mother . . . a boundless infinite conscious sea of light . . . a continuous succession of effulgent waves.[4]

Through the safe haven created by his teacher, Ramakrishna overcame his unbearable sense of separation and transformed his destructive tendencies into what he called "the joyful play (lila) of a child in his Mother's Mansion of Mirth." Through the rest of his remarkable life, Ramakrishna always used the language of mother and child in explaining his relationship with God. As he once put it, "One must have the yearning for God of a child when his mother is away."[5]

THE TERROR OF THE ORPHAN

As a psychotherapist, I discovered what it was like for people who had never been safely and securely held and had never been soothed with warm, responsive, yielding love. These were people who, as a result, did not yet have inside themselves a visceral experience of that calmly abiding center; people who could not even evoke from memory, as I could, that deep sense of being absolutely alright, absolutely safe, reassuringly held.

I discovered that patients who did not have enough of a taste of this experience had a terrifying sense of shakiness, fragmentation, and impermanence at the core of their sense of self. Indeed, they did not have a sense of their own abidingness at all. Some, I discovered, were so without a center that they did not even know that I would recognize them from week to week. They literally did not know that they existed in a continuous way in the minds of other people. And so, they felt compelled to tell me their whole story over and over again, like Coleridge's ancient mariner.

Several very painful things happen to those of us who have not been held and soothed enough. First of all, we will have a chronic internal sense that something is profoundly wrong, that the world is not safe. We will not feel at home in our bodies. We cannot feel that everything is fundamentally OK. There is no place inside us to land, to snuggle into, to rest, to refuel. No internal safe harbor.

And second, there will be a profound sense of aloneness inside. This sense of aloneness is different from loneliness. With loneliness we can call up the memory of having been held. We can feel how even now, at a distance from the one we love, we are being abidingly held in our loved one's thoughts and heart. In separation, we'll feel sad, and we'll feel the pain of longing and yearning to be held again, but we can always evoke the sensory experience of closeness. With aloneness, however, that evocation is not possible, or it is less strong. Perhaps it is fleeting. Perhaps it comes and goes.

But when it cannot be called up at all, there is a deep sense of panic. We feel as if we are literally coming apart. We cannot connect with that abiding center, that sense of our own continuity. This is, in fact, the worst kind of anxiety. It's called annihilation anxiety. We actually feel that if we don't get connected with a source of soothing and holding, we will cease to exist.

This experience of losing our center, of falling apart, of fragmenting, can happen to all of us under stress. Several years ago I attended a professional conference on Nantucket Island. The friend I was to travel with had to cancel at the last minute. When I got to the island, it was rainy and dreary. I knew no one. I spent the day before the conference alone in my tiny guesthouse room reading a novel. But I began to feel depressed. I felt sad. I felt lonely. And the loneliness began to deepen into a kind of aloneness and anxiety that I had not felt in a long time. I couldn't get comfortable. I went for long walks. I felt more anxious.

The next day, I found a couple of other lost souls at the conference, and we adopted each other. We literally merged together into a tight-knit little foursome—a regular "enmeshed-ego-mass." We went everywhere together for a couple of days, until, through the experience of finding temporary self-objects, we all found our feet again and began to go our own ways. We all need self-objects throughout our lives, and we may adopt emergency self-objects at any time.

Patients in psychotherapy who feel intensely fragmented, and who have no capacity to find or use self-objects, however, often hold out the prospect of suicide as a kind of "sustaining fantasy." For these souls, the wish for suicide can be a wish to "lie down in the arms of the great mother earth." In death there may be the hope of being united with the ever-giving, ever-holding God, or the wished-for mother. Indeed, this was precisely the fantasy in the minds of both Bapuji and Ramakrishna as they pondered suicide. Sometimes, the fantasy of achieving this deep sense of peace is enough. Tragically, however, if the fantasy itself is not soothing enough, a patient will actually commit suicide in order to find this experience of union.

THE FORTRESS OF LOVE

The story of my grandparents' house as the archetype of the Lotus of the Heart has a kind of paradisiacal quality to it. But the truth is that the experience of being safely held can emerge under the most seemingly difficult and adverse conditions as well. John Steinbeck portrays such an experience in his novel *The Grapes of Wrath*. Through the harrowing experiences of eviction from the farm, the trip to California, the death of several family members, and the banishment of the beloved son, Tom, Ma Joad holds the center.[6] When everyone else is demoralized, there is a stream of abidingness and loving-kindness coming from her that just won't quit.

A scene from the book portrays how one human being who is connected with her own center is able to hold an entire family in the arms of her own equanimity.

Says Pa, "Funny! Woman taking over the fambly. Woman sayin', we'll do this here, an' we'll go there. An' I don' even care."

"Woman can change better'n a man," Ma said soothingly. "Woman got all her life in her arms. Man got it all in his head. Don' you mind. Maybe—well, may nex' year we can get a place."

"We got nothin', now," Pa said. . . . "Seems like our life's over an' done."

"No, it ain't," Ma smiled. "It ain't, Pa. An' that's one more thing a woman knows. I noticed that. Man, he lives in jerks—baby born an' a man dies, an' that's a jerk—gets a farm an' loses his arm, little waterfalls, but the river, it goes right on. Woman looks at it like that. We ain't gonna die out. People is goin' on—changin' a little, maybe, but goin' right on."

"How can you tell?" Uncle John demanded. "What's to keep ever'thing from stoppin'; all the folks from jus' gettin' tired an' layin' down?"

Ma considered. She rubbed the shiny back of one hand with the other, pushed the fingers of her right hand between the fingers of her left. "Hard to say," she said. "Ever'thing we do—seems to me is aimed right at goin' on. Seems that way to me. Even gettin' hungry—even bein' sick; some die, but the rest is toughter. Jus' try an' live the day, jus' the day."[7]

Even in the midst of the most grinding poverty and dislocation, Ma Joad had a realness and a solidity that allowed the whole family to feel real and solid.

My own grandmother created both an internal and external container for this nurturing. Her kitchen was an external extension of her lap. It was warm, spacious, comfortable, nurturing, and always well supplied with sugar cookies and molasses cookies baked especially for her grandchildren. She was deeply present and empathic. And her loving-kindness, like Ma Joad's, had a warmth and a sweetness that made it sink in deeper. And both women had another skill—they saw the way things were and they named them. My grandmother saw reality clearly and was willing to name it. There was a sense about her that, like Ma Joad, she could not be blown away. She was not going to be knocked over by life. And as a result of merging with her, there developed inside me a place that was not going to be knocked over, either.

Shakespeare's sonnet 116 expresses this same quality of the indestructibility of the Mother: "Love is not love / Which alters when it alteration finds, / Or bends with the remover to remove: / O, no! it is an ever-fixed mark, / That looks on tempests and is never shaken."

THE DIVINE MOTHER IS EVERYWHERE

During my first year at Kripalu, it was clear to me that the big brick fortress on the hill, with the archetypal Father-Mother in residence, had provided a special kind of transformational space for thousands of seekers. It was a safe space, where those of us who felt that we were coming apart could feel held together, and those of us who wanted to intentionally risk coming apart (in the interest of growth), could do so in relative safety. Some had found it useful as an environment for long-term restructuring of the self, others as a temporary, emergency holding environment in which they could reliably drink in a sense of cohesiveness from the outside in.

Early in my second year at Kripalu I received a visit from a friend of mine who is a distinguished psychoanalyst in Boston. After spending a few days in the community, he said to me, "Gurudev reminds me of Semrad in the kind of safety he creates for everyone here. This really is 'the peaceable kingdom,' isn't it?"

I told him my surprising discovery. While many of us had traveled great distances to find our idealized spiritual teacher—in this case, Gurudev—most of us actually had little or no real personal contact with him. But in the safety and consciousness of the community, I had discovered many friends who acted as "step-down transformers" for his presence—friends who actually had a much more reliable, direct, and sustaining role as self-objects for me. I discovered that my real spiritual teachers and gurus were all around me, invisibly submerged in the context of my daily life. Finally, it was the community that played the role of mother for me, not the guru.

For many of us, our experience with our original sources of merger, our parents, was disappointing. But none of us relies solely on our parents, or even our psychotherapists. There are so many people in the world who might love us in the way we need to be loved, who might provide for us a haven, who might lend us their center, even for a few weeks or months. We may not recognize the power of their contribution at the time, but in retrospect, when we think of our lives, these are the human beings who will shine in our memories.

Week after week, for example, I sit with Hilda, my piano teacher, and receive amazing gifts. She's a woman in her sixties who had been a musical genius as a child, making her Carnegie Hall debut at seventeen, studying for seven years with one of the greatest teachers of the twentieth century, Artur Schnabel, and concertizing in Europe. She later left her remarkable musical career to raise twelve children, and to create a farm with her husband in the Berkshires; after farming, she returned to music as a teacher. Her absolute passion for music vibrates through her, and as I sit next to her every Tuesday night on the piano bench, playing some Schubert four-hand fantasy, I receive her powerful generativity. In sharing our regular musical moments, I am invited to participate in the deep abiding center of her heart and her musical imagination. Then, miraculously, I take some of it away with me. Now it's inside.

All human beings who have developed the capacity to be an abiding presence can transfer this capacity in a kind of cellular, visceral way to others who don't have it. We all know people who have this capacity, and we know that they're not necessarily spiritual teachers or psychotherapists. They are people who are so full of the river of life that they cannot help transferring it to others. Ramakrishna used to say that people who are themselves connected to the source are like "big steamships, carrying hundreds of other Souls across the ocean of suffering."

Exposure to such human beings evokes in us that calmly abiding center that already exists in each of us in potential form. Suddenly, we discover that we ourselves are connected to the source. We've been hooked up to it through others. That calmly abiding center becomes a steady stream of energy, of light, flowing through us. Through contact with this kind of presence, we discover our lives coming alive with meaning and purpose, because we're connected again to the stream of life from whence we came.

Psychologist Erik Erikson used the word "generativity" to describe this capacity to awaken the calmly abiding center in others. Listen, for example, to another one of Semrad's students talking about what this most generative of teachers meant for her.

> His simple statements had a peculiar power, an immediate familiarity which reminded me of the experience of reclaiming repressed memories—thoughts and feelings newly available, but bearing the sense of always having been known. His plain talk often brought a pulse of recognition, a sense of shared experience. He allowed the impression that he had been there, wherever, or that he would readily go, using the man or the woman in himself, as he would say. And there he sat, in his amplitude, very often smiling mischievously, teasingly, wisely, kindly, enigmatically, diabolically, attesting to the safety of taking life on, simply—of acknowledging, bearing, and finally putting into perspective the feelings that went with the living of it. "We're just big messes trying to help bigger messes, and the only reason we can do it is that we've been through it before and have survived." He was not all and everything, but he was very much. As my teacher, he let me use him as I needed—and by example taught me to help my patients in that way.[8]

Behind the everyday forms of Hilda, Dr. Semrad, Grandpa and Grandma, Ma Joad, is the river of love. They are personal manifestations of reality—the divine Mother at work everywhere, bringing her children back to her. These are the real gurus in our lives, teachers who are really doing the heavy lifting, allowing us to merge and separate, merge and separate; connecting us, moment to moment, through their presence, with the river of love flowing from the heart of the universe. The real transmission of source consciousness happens in the simplest moments of our lives. In the yogic view, all of these human forms are simply the divine Mother at play.

THE RIVER FLOWS WITHIN US

When conditions are auspicious, human beings emerge into adulthood with the "good enough" rudiments of a calmly abiding center. Under the proper conditions, this resilient seed can be nurtured into the most magnificent qualities of the fully alive human being: generativity, compassion, gratitude, and unitive consciousness. These qualities can emerge through an intentional process such as psychotherapy or spiritual practice, or simply through the grace of life unfolding.

Once the river of life is awakened in us, we cannot help giving it away. The spirit of generosity is expressed in the ancient Buddhist archetype of the *bodhisattva*, the awakened being who dedicates his or her life to the liberation of others. In a psychological sense, the bodhisattva is called to let himself be used as a self-object for others, to safely hold and soothe, to let his heart become an abiding home base—in Ramakrishna's words, to become an ocean liner.

As Steinbeck reveals, the seed of this abiding center was so warmly planted within Tom Joad that he inevitably begins to feel his own generativity. The river is alive in him. In the midst of the most grinding of odds, what emerges naturally is the most sublime of all essentially spiritual qualities: he feels his compassion for all beings, and he feels his identification with all beings.

> Tom laughed uneasily, "Well, maybe like Casy says, a fella ain't got a soul of his own, but on'y a piece of a big one—an' then— Then it don' matter. Then I'll be all aroun' in the dark. I'll be ever'where—where you look. Wherever they's a fight so hungry people can eat, I'll be there. Wherever they's a cop beatin' up a guy, I'll be there. If Casy knowed, why I'll be in the way guys yell when they're mad an'—I'll be in the way kids laugh when they're hungry an' they know supper's ready. An' when our folks eat the food they raise an' live in the houses they build— why, I'll be there."[9]

The calmly abiding self, created by the most mundane and simple of human experiences, matures into the most noble: loving-kindness. The still point becomes a pulsing, living stream of energy, of light, emerging from the source that is beyond time, beyond place, beyond personality. It is the unmoved that is always moving. It is the center that is everywhere.

11

$\mathcal{A}$WARENESS: ON SEEING AND
BEING SEEN

"What is REAL?" asked the Rabbit one day, when he and the Skin Horse were lying side by side near the nursery fender. . . .

"Real isn't how you are made," said the Skin Horse. "It's a thing that happens to you. When a child loves you for a long, long time, not just to play with, but REALLY loves you, then you become Real."

"Does it hurt?" asked the Rabbit.

"Sometimes," said the Skin Horse, for he was always truthful.

—Margery Williams,
The Velveteen Rabbit

I looked around the circle at my colleagues as I read to them some of my favorite sections of *The Velveteen Rabbit*,[1] and I noticed that Susan was crying. This did not surprise me. For several weeks, it had been clear that Susan was not happy.

"The way you've got these books organized is all wrong," she had said to me earlier that day with a thinly disguised sneer. "Obviously the philosophy section should go over here next to the yoga books. Why don't you organize them logically?" She started to move the books around before I could respond.

I felt my belly tighten. I took a deep breath and let out a big sigh. It was going to be another one of those days. Susan was probably right. She usually was. But her attitude had such an edge to it.

Susan was a thirty-seven-year-old lawyer who had come to Kripalu on a yearlong sabbatical. She had been forced to take some time away from her big New York law firm because she had just spent five years working herself to the brink of an early grave. Two years earlier she had begun to develop serious colitis, and finally her doctor laid down the law: "You've got to take a serious break from this schedule."

Susan had been assigned to work for me in the shop, where I had been a manager for just a couple of months. It was turning into an impossible situation. Susan seemed to be one of those human beings who would rather be right than happy. She had to be right. She had to know everything. Her attitude was saturated with condescension and arrogance. Even though she had chosen to be at Kripalu for "a time of healing," she seemed to hate herself for being there. She hated the fact that she had been "weak" and gotten sick. She seemed determined to recover on sheer willpower and brute determination. Susan also hated the notion that in order to be part of the community she had to do "menial work." And it was a huge blow to her ego that she had to work for me. She let it be known that she was at Kripalu for one reason and one reason only. She wanted to be close to the guru. Working was, at best, a distraction from her real goal.

Susan had developed an intense idealization of Amrit Desai. She often referred to him as a sage, or a seer. She believed that he was one of the few fully enlightened gurus in America, and that he was, as she often said, "the real thing." In deference to "living in the guru's house," she always wore white—designer white. She went religiously to evening satsang, placing herself prominently wherever it was rumored he would appear. She deeply believed that the more contact she had with him, the sooner she would herself become enlightened. Susan was not messing around. In her career she had gone for the best—Harvard Law School. Now, she was going for the best guru she could find, and for nothing less than enlightenment. "Liberation in this lifetime—jivan mukti," was her goal.

Susan had an acute and interesting mind. She was very knowledge-able about yoga metaphysics. She talked intelligently about training her awareness to penetrate the unmanifest realms. She talked knowledge-ably about atman-brahman and the Absolute—about an intellectual kind of freedom. But to me she seemed distinctly unfree and unhappy.

I understood that there was something very distorted in how Susan saw herself, what she demanded of herself, and what she demanded of others. But I was still trying to figure out how to work with all of this when the unexpected happened. Sitting around in a circle with all her fellow workers in the shop, listening to *The Velveteen Rabbit* in one of our late-afternoon staff meetings, Susan had shown another side of herself altogether. "I just don't feel real. I feel like that damned rabbit. Stuffed with sawdust. A phony rabbit." Susan pulled herself together quickly, dabbed at her eyes with a tissue, and laughed it off. I suspected that part of her was horrified at what she had just done. But for a brief moment, she had allowed us to see the other side of her commanding presence—the fragile, brittle, empty, scared side that she usually kept tightly under wraps.

In that moment of vulnerability I felt my heart open to Susan. I understood that she got under my skin because we had so much in common. I liked to be right, too, after all. And as she began to show me more and more of her hidden sides, I came to like and admire Susan very much indeed.

ON SEEING AND BEING SEEN

The story of the Velveteen Rabbit brings us face to face with another major insight of contemporary psychoanalysis: The ideas we have in our minds about who we are, and who we should be, were formed early in our childhoods by how we were seen by important others. Psychologists now understand that mental representations of self and other are deeply formed in childhood and continue to guide our interactions with others well into adulthood. These mental representations are enduring and they play a central role in our suffering and confusion about reality.

Like the Velveteen Rabbit, in order to feel real, we all need to be recognized and affirmed. We need to be accepted, and appreciated; most important, we need to be seen with loving eyes, and reflected back with warmth and enthusiasm. Psychologists call this the narcissistic need for mirroring. It is considered a narcissistic need as important as the need for merger which we discussed in the last chapter. We need to be seen and reflected back just as much as we need oxygen and food.

Why is mirroring so important? Well, we might consider the fact that we cannot look at our complete physical selves with our own eyes. We can see parts of our bodies directly with our eyes, but not the whole thing. We look eagerly at photographs of ourselves in home videos, and we think, *That can't be me. That's not what I look like.* This is a central fact of the human existential dilemma: In order to see ourselves, we must rely on reflection. In some ultimate sense, we don't really know what we look like, or who we are, without the use of mirrors.

It is the same with our internal worlds. Some of our interior landscape we can see, but much of it must be seen by others, then reflected back to us. And the quality of the seeing is critical to how we see ourselves, and to who we become. The eyes with which we are seen become the eyes through which we see ourselves. Those eyes may be loving, or despising, or ambivalent, or cruel and rejecting. Whatever they are, one thing is certain: it is these eyes that we will inherit.

For quite a few years the Velveteen Rabbit lived in the nursery cupboard, "and nobody thought much about him." The storyteller makes it clear that outwardly, the Rabbit was beautiful, even grand: "In the beginning," she says, "the Rabbit was really splendid. He was fat and bunchy, as a rabbit should be; his coat was spotted brown and white, he had real thread whiskers, and his ears were lined with pink sateen." Beautiful as he was, however, the Rabbit knew he was stuffed only with sawdust. With all his outward splendor, he had an aching sense of being unreal.

It was not until he was discovered by the Boy, and seen with eyes interested particularly in him, that the Rabbit began to feel real. Indeed, it was only through the regular, miraculous reflection of himself in the boy's loving eyes that the Rabbit came alive. He began to experience the realness of himself, and of the world. He began to see himself as the Boy saw him.

The Boy's seeing was powerfully infused with an imagination that could believe in the realness of his stuffed bunny. And this way of seeing had immense consequences, as the story reveals. The bunny became what the eyes saw. It was just a tale. But it was an archetypal story with deep truth for those of us who haven't yet been fully seen into being. And so, Susan cried.

Unfortunately, most of us were seen, as children, with eyes that were imagining much more complex and ambivalent scenarios than those of the Boy and the Rabbit. These complex reflections of ourselves became the building blocks of our own seeing, and have exerted an important influence over the ways in which we see even now, so many years later.

Research psychologists have shown repeatedly the tenacity of the distortions in our seeing: we see not what is there, but what we've seen before, and what we therefore expect to see over and over again.

SPIRITUAL BLINDNESS

If we are interested in the path of yoga, we will eventually be compelled to explore the foundations of the human capacity to see reality clearly. Susan was in many ways correct in her understanding of this primary focus of yoga, and her longing to see reality was in alignment with all of the classical scriptures. In the final stages of practice, indeed, all that remains is pure seeing. Yogis describe highly refined states of perception in which all subject-object separation is dissolved, and, as the *Yogasutras* put it, "The Seer is Seeing alone."

In my time at Kripalu, however, I discovered an intriguing paradox. In the yogic world, an air of unreality permeates discussions about the real. This is what Sarita and I were noticing that night in her office after the swami's talk. As she had astutely pointed out, often the very eyes of these visiting swamis revealed the quality of avoidance of reality. They were always looking up. They would be talking about the third eye and looking in that direction. Up. Up. Up. Everything was up. "Seeing" came to mean something remarkably abstract and inward-turned, and it seemed to completely bypass the importance of seeing the realities of the phenomenal world in which we live in this very moment.

Susan's situation, of course, highlighted this paradox. What is the use of being able to dissolve the body into light, to lose subject-object separation in deep states of samadhi, if we cannot even bear to see our true face in the mirror? Why do we think we can, or should, penetrate the most refined aspects of the five kleshas and the four erroneous beliefs, when, in the most gross kinds of ways, we are having trouble acknowledging, experiencing, and bearing the reality of our simple daily life?

Facing delusion is extremely painful. For many of us, alas, like Susan, our spiritual projects seem to be flights away from the consequences of our daily acts of delusion—flights, indeed, away from reality more than flights toward reality. Our spiritual motto might as well be,

"Bring us from the real to the unreal." Like Susan, we may desperately wish that spiritual practice could be something we could do in the privacy of our own rooms, on our yoga mats, away from the revealing vision of others.

Susan frequently expressed a wish to "see"—to be the seer. This wish was conscious and on the surface of things. But she had a powerful unconscious wish to remain hidden—to not see, and to not be seen. This side was completely out of awareness, and over and over again it undermined her movement toward the goal of clear seeing. If we look under the surface of Susan's dilemma, we will discover the source of her unconscious commitment to not seeing and not being seen. We will discover that in order to get her most basic needs met as a child, Susan had to learn precisely how not to see certain aspects of reality, and, having learned this approach, she remained committed to not seeing as a way of coping.

Many spiritual seekers participate to some degree in this strategy. Much of spiritual practice then becomes, in fact, a flight from clear seeing and its implications, an attempt to remain somehow outside our lives, rather than in them. Harvard psychologist Jack Engler gives us a very helpful list of some of the ways in which avoidance of the real can motivate our so-called spiritual paths.[2] For some of us, "spirituality" can be unconsciously driven by:

~ *A quest for perfection and invulnerability.* We may be especially prone to the quest for perfection if we feel all too imperfect, or if we have been badly hurt and don't want to ever have to feel that vulnerable again.

~ *A fear of individuation.* We may be anxious about stepping out into the world, assuming responsibility for ourselves and our life, shrinking back from competition, comparisons, or achievement.

~ *Avoidance of commitment and accountability.* We might conveniently relabel this avoidance spiritual "detachment," or, in New Age terminology, "just going with the flow."

~ *A fear of intimacy and social involvement.* It's striking how many of us drawn to spiritual life have a history of difficulties with intimacy and closeness in relationships, or disappointments in love, and how being in a spiritual community allows us to feel a sense of belonging without resolving these underlying fears.

~ *An inability to grieve and mourn important losses.* All the spiritual teachings and practices about "letting go," "renunciation," or "detachment" can actually substitute for a genuine facing of personal grief and loss, and the painful feelings associated with it.

~ *An avoidance of feelings.* So many drawn to spiritual practice have difficulty with strong emotions like anger, sadness, and disappointment. Spiritual traditions label these as kleshas and as unwholesome, and so we might take this to mean we shouldn't feel them, and then we feel guilty or unspiritual if we do. Sometimes the experience of pleasure and sexuality seems to be even more problematic for people drawn to spiritual practice.

THE ARCHETYPE OF THE USED CHILD

Many of the avoidances on Engler's list were characteristic of Susan's flight from the real to the unreal. But how do we make sense of the paradoxes in Susan's story—the tension between being seen and being hidden? In order to understand what is driving Susan's malaise, and her retreat from a full life in the body, it is useful to understand the archetype of the Used Child, one of the major themes in the psychological and spiritual suffering of our time.[3]

Susan's family looked good on the outside. And why wouldn't they? All of their resources were devoted to looking good for the community. This was an entire family with a "false self" image. The internal experience of the family was hidden at all costs from outside eyes. It was one of emotional poverty and deprivation, competition for scarce resources, and very little real connection with and identification with a visceral experience of pleasure and satisfaction.

As we saw in chapter 7, the children in a family like Susan's are inevitably used to meet the needs of the parents. It cannot be otherwise. The parents, depleted and needy, either subtly or not so subtly manipulate the child by withdrawing love and "supplies" when the child fails to mirror, echo, and reward the parent. The parent is unable to be used by the child as that all-important emotional home-base from which the child can securely explore merging and separating, can experience both her strength and weakness, her limitlessness and vulnerability.

Susan's father idealized her, frequently referring to her as his "golden child." He clearly felt gratified by her "cuteness" as a child, and as she grew up by her obvious intelligence and competence. Susan's father felt himself to be intellectually unworthy and inferior, and her gifts became a way of compensating for his own gnawing sense of inadequacy. He basked in the glow of her achievement and her specialness.

Susan's capacity to see herself clearly was inhibited by eyes that wanted to see and bring to life only one side of her aliveness—her magnificence, her talent, her intelligence. Her limitations, vulnerabilities, and smallness remained unseen, unilluminated by love, and definitely "not OK." Later on in life, these aspects of Susan's reality became for her not just the unseen, but the unseeable. Susan, like all of us with some components of false self, became prematurely committed to one side of reality only. As we have seen, the false self is fundamentally unrealistic, because it believes itself to be more perfect, omnipotent, self-sufficient, and capable than could be true, or, in some cases, conversely, believes itself to be more imperfect, empty, unworthy, and powerless than could be true.

Susan's efforts to attract her parents' attention and love, and her competition with her younger sisters for the scarce emotional resources in the family, inevitably led her into overachieving. Her own ambitions to prove herself, and to attract attention, masked early unmet longings and a resulting chronic sense of unworthiness and emptiness. She complied with becoming who she thought her parents wanted and "needed" her to be, so she was driven to be outwardly successful.

Susan continued to "act out" this unresolved conflict through her legal career. She remained deeply attached to and identified with her successes and failures, in a way that was still driven by the unconscious need to please and to attract nurturing and emotional "supplies." Her reactions were, thus, overdetermined and unconscious, and often inordinate. She experienced the "brittleness" of a life based on the attempt to manifest the ego-ideal. She didn't feel real. She was starving for mirroring, for real feedback, for someone to see her into reality, to see through the facade of her false self. It's no wonder she connected so deeply with the Velveteen Rabbit.

To the extent that a child is used in the way Susan was—to meet the parents' needs—she is left with a sense of not being a real subject, but an object to be used by others. This leaves the Used Child with a chronic fear of being used but also, paradoxically, with an unconscious wish to repeat the experience of being used in order to complete it. In addition, children who have been used cannot help repeating the using by using others. People who worked closely with Susan, myself included, felt used.

In so many ways, the false self these experiences elicit is also supported by our culture—a culture that encourages growing up quickly, that encourages separation and individuation above needing and bonding; a culture that promotes grandiosity, encouraging achievement and perfectionism, and the objectification of others, sexually and emotionally; a culture that in fact supports the compensatory self-sacrifice that many of us make from our false selves—a self-sacrifice that might be quite valuable to others, but from which we get no real pleasure.

EMPTINESS, ISOLATION, AND TERROR

Like the Velveteen Rabbit, the Used Child is lost in plain sight. A sense of unreality perfumes the air around her. And, like the Rabbit, her legs are not real. There is no groundedness in reality. Behind the drivenness is a sense of terror; behind the perfectionism is an empty stare in the headlights; and behind the charm is a deep sense of isolation.

1. Emptiness. One of the most evocative images of the Used Child appears in the popular 1970s American movie *Fame*.[4] This film describes the story of Doris Finsecker and her classic "stage mother." When Doris's mother looked at her, she did not see anything that was peculiarly Doris. She saw only an extension of herself, her own hopes and dreams. When, after much *Sturm und Drang*, Doris is finally accepted as a student at a prestigious high school for the performing arts in New York City, her mother receives the call and yells out excitedly across the room, "Doris—we're in!" In her mind's eye, Doris and she are one.

This kind of "seeing" (or not-seeing) gives Doris the implicit message, "Without me, you're nothing." And Doris feels like nothing. What's being seen into aliveness is her mother's image of who she should be—the prototype for the "false self"—and Doris clings to this image. And why would she not? This is all that's being nurtured into being. But it is not enough to make Doris feel real. The "false self" always creates this feeling of emptiness and worthlessness at the core. And as Susan discovered, this emptiness may drive any number of projects meant to disprove and undo it.

2. *Isolation.* Though Susan could not articulate it at the time, she arrived at Kripalu desperate to be seen. The false self in its fortress of achievement always lives in isolation from intimate relationships. This is inevitably so, because grandiosity and perfectionism cannot survive true intimacy.

Susan had been isolated from relationship because she found, as she did in her brief encounter with me, that whenever she got to know someone well, they were disappointing. They were not good enough. Limitation, vulnerability, imperfection, and ordinariness were precisely what Susan could not tolerate in herself, and as a result, she certainly could not tolerate them in others.

When Susan got too close, what she saw reflected back in the mirror was too painful to look at. "Loser!" She discovered that it was best not to get too close to mirrors. All of the conflicts that existed inside her would inevitably be revealed in her experience of being close to others. She knew unconsciously that living alone she might be clever enough to circumvent intense scrutiny, but she could not escape it in close and authentic relationship. And so, she avoided this authenticity as much as she could.

3. *Terror.* In Samuel Beckett's play *Waiting for Godot,* Estragon and Vladimir are waiting for the elusive Godot to come to them. Periodically, "the boy," a messenger from the mysterious Godot, arrives to inform them that Godot's arrival has been postponed again. In spite of the fact that the same boy returns to them over and over again, the boy does not recognize Estragon and Vladimir. At first, this is simply a bit unnerving. Finally, the simple "drip, drip, drip" of not being seen or recognized becomes positively life-threatening. Vladimir and Estragon become desperate to be seen. The whole environment becomes infused with an unbearable lack of reality. When the boy asks, "What am I to tell Mr. Godot, sir?" Vladimir says, "Tell him . . . tell him you saw me and that . . . that you saw me! (With sudden violence) You

did see me! You're sure you saw me, you won't come and tell me tomorrow that you never saw me!"[5]

In the absence of appropriate mirroring, even the person with a well-established sense of self will begin to have this experience of the terror of annihilation. Imagine how much more vulnerable we are to this terror when, like Susan, we have not yet established a strong sense of self.[6]

BEWARE THE GURU ON THE GOLDEN THRONE

The Used Child among us looks constantly for the all-knowing self-object who will reflect her back the way she wishes to see herself. She seeks to participate in the "glow" of these larger-than-life beings, wanting so much to be a part of the halo of specialness and omnipotence that often surrounds them. Susan believed that in Amrit Desai she had found such an all-powerful man who would not let her down. He was, after all, in her opinion, a fully enlightened human being. At last, her quest was to be fulfilled.

Susan used to "get a glow on" around the guru. She and Amrit beamed at each other. He beamed as well, of course, because he was getting reflected glory from her, the Harvard lawyer, just as she was from him. To be affirmed, recognized, admired, and even adored—this was what she seemed to hunger for most. Because she was not really in a relationship with him (she saw him only on more or less formal occasions) she could maintain her idealizing transference. She remained at a safe distance and maintained what she believed was a mutually loving, admiring relationship. She refused to hear anything negative about him. Unreality hovered around this "relationship" like bees around honey.

Mirroring of this highly idealized sort involves using others primarily for the purposes of acknowledging and aggrandizing the false self. We want to be prized, special, and we want our specialness echoed. We relate to special others not as they are, but as we think we need them to be. They are objects for us, just as we were objects for our parents.

For the first few months of her residency, those of us who were working in the trenches with Susan on a daily basis got to see only the shadow side of her projections. She had to keep her own sense of worthlessness and inadequacy out of awareness, and she did this by projecting it onto those of us who were ordinary schleppers. In her mind, the worthlessness did not exist in her—it was in us.

The first crack in Susan's idealization of the guru appeared several months after she arrived. She discovered one day that she had been rebuffed and virtually ignored by the guru, when she was intentionally excluded from an important meeting. She went into a tailspin. How could he do this to her? In one very powerful evening of sharing with her roommate, Sandy, Susan allowed herself a torrent of tears and risked exposing her sense of worthlessness. Sandy sat with Susan for hours, helping her to come to grips with reality. "The guru doesn't really even know who I am," she discovered. She had made up the relationship out of her own powerful wishes and longings. But Sandy was able to hold her through this profound disillusionment.

Over the coming months, Susan began to see more clearly how focused she was on this one powerful character, and how distorted that was. She saw how it had promoted her avoidance of the many real relationships that the community offered her. She was shocked to see how needy she was for the guru's approval. The discovery of her pain, and the fact that it was alright to feel it with normal human beings, was a "marker event" for her, a dramatic and visible outward sign of an inward change. The encounter with real feelings and the discovery of the depth of these feelings in the presence of someone who really cared about her—Sandy—helped to begin a process of transformation. Susan began to be more connected with a sense of real self—real suffering as well as real pleasure.

Over the course of time, Susan saw through her idealization. She saw Amrit more realistically, and this was liberating for her. She saw, too, that those of us with whom she was in real relationship were her true gurus.

This is not just an American yoga story. It is, in fact, the archetypal story of the guru in Indian scripture. The true guru is a requirement for the practice of yoga, because he or she initiates the seeker into the realm of truth, through relationship. The true guru—the *sadguru*, or "teacher of the real"—is capable of initiating the spiritual seeker into knowledge of the Absolute, Brahman. So often in the archetypal stories, this guru is not a glorified, triumphal being, but is disguised. Yogic lore is full of cautionary tales about true gurus and false gurus, and the gem of wisdom in most of these tales is just this: The true guru is not the one sitting on the golden throne.

> Many are the gurus who rob the disciple of his wealth, but rare is the guru who removes the afflictions of his disciple.[7]

> There are many gurus, like lamps in house after house, but hard to find, O Devi, is the guru who lights up all like the sun.[8]

In Western psychological language, it is most likely that the "guru on the golden throne" has himself (or herself) become lost in the all-too-powerful hopes and wishes of students and seekers. As Jack Engler reminds us, "When students see the teacher as perfect or realized or enlightened, the teacher may come to see him or herself that way. . . . Idealization can unconsciously reinforce the teacher's residual narcissistic needs to be admired and powerful. They can also create a climate of unreality around the teacher."[9]

The true guru has eschewed any outward and visible signs of power. It must be so, because when we understand the guru's real role, we will see that a major part of it is to lead the seeker through the birth canal of optimal disillusionment. With our true gurus there is a glow, to be sure, but the glow is inward, secret, subtle, and must be detected by the student. So many of the greatest masters of yoga have been eccentric, elusive, shabby, and completely uninterested in external omnipotence and charm. Ramakrishna, for example, perhaps the greatest yogic avatar of the last century, wore a shabby, old "wearing cloth" that was perpetually falling off. The same was true of the great Neem Karoli Baba, Ram Dass's guru. These teachers had no sense of themselves as being "special." As Ramana Maharshi put it about these true gurus:

> The Guru is one who at all times abides in the profound depths of the Self. He never sees any difference between himself and others and is quite free from the idea that he is the Enlightened or the Liberated One, while those around him are in bondage or the darkness of ignorance. . . . There is no difference between God, Guru, and the Self.[10]

The true seers of ancient yogic lore, like most of the great Western saints, are thoroughly human, and though they may have some extraordinary powers, they still most often seem eccentric in some ways, and completely ordinary in others. Real gurus are, like the Skin Horse, invisible to the ordinary naked eye. Their own inner magnificence and splendor can only be seen by the eye of the true seeker, who is capable of peering beneath the surface of gross apparent reality. The outward polish has long since been worn off, but the inward glow of truth is real and abiding.

By the time Susan left the shop after her year's internship, she had begun to acknowledge who her true teachers were. It takes time to adjust to a radically new way of experiencing life, the self, and others. But for Susan there was great power in her understanding that she had been initiated into the Real by those of us in the community who cared about her and loved her for her vulnerabilities as well as her strengths. She discovered that true seers are almost always hiding out in ordinary circumstances.

THE COMMUNITY AS GURU

Though Amrit often seemed to believe the powerfully idealized transferences and projections onto him, he nonetheless had a clear and consistent point of view about the importance of other human beings in the ongoing creation of the self. He understood that only other human beings can initiate us into the Real. One of his most useful proverbs was this: "Company is more powerful than willpower."

This was a classic Amrit Desai insight—simple, concise, elegant. He understood that effort and will do not create consciousness. Consciousness is transmitted in relationships. We seek friends, lovers, communities, who can see us, hold us, bear us. Frank Lloyd Wright said, "We create our buildings and then they create us." Likewise, we construct our circle of friends and our communities and then they construct us—precisely by how they see us into being. Company is more powerful than willpower.

In the healing of the false self, the importance of creating community cannot be overemphasized.[11] For the real self to emerge, we urgently need a social network of appropriate self-objects who love, support, challenge, and sustain us. Such communities help us to accept and embrace all sides of our human nature. They do not continue to call up and reinforce our delusion of superiority (or inferiority). Rather, they help us to name it, and thereby to expose it, as Sandy did for Susan.

In the archetypal story of the narcissist, it is always the encounter with the truth-teller that turns the situation around. In *Fame*, the story turns around when Doris moves into the new environment of the school, and suddenly she's being seen with eyes that are interested in who she really is. Her teachers are particularly interested in seeing her gifts as they really are. Doris comes alive. She has the added advantage of being seen not by just one new pair of eyes, but by an entire new community of them—eyes, for the most part, committed to seeing the life, the creativity, the magic in others. In the reflection of these new mirrors, she recognizes a self she has always intuited but had never really seen before. Being seen in this way literally evokes Doris's genius, her talent, her aliveness. She has the exhilarating experience that it's all right there, just waiting to be called forth. Throughout the rest of the film, Doris becomes real. She still has her mother's eyes, but she also has a whole new repertoire of seeing, which finally begins to evoke a new sense of authenticity.

A caring community can help us create a safe domain in which personal experiences can be expressed, expanded, and enriched. And in this safety we can have a brand-new experience of authentic, deeply personal experience.[12] In these safe new reflective surfaces we can—like Doris—try on new aspects of the self. We can discover how flexible we are, and how much more there is to us than we thought. We have multiple selves, variable and changing selves—and to claim these new versions of ourselves feels like liberation.

People like Doris and Susan, who have kept others at bay with their false and incomplete selves, are usually surprised by the welcome they receive when they share their vulnerabilities and insecurities.[13] As Susan was able to break out of her isolation and let people see who she really was, she was astonished to find how much people liked her. As she began to feel safer showing her vulnerabilities, she began to share some of her writing projects—poetry and short stories. This was a hidden self she had not dared show, and the more she showed it, the more it grew. She began to learn the value of expression versus suppression, the value of intimacy versus isolation. She discovered, as

Doris did, that huge amounts of energy were freed up as she claimed the whole of her life.

THE MATURE OBSERVING SELF: WISDOM, INTUITION, AND INTERDEPENDENCE

Later in the archetypal tale of the Velveteen Rabbit, both the Rabbit's initial grandiosity and his later worthlessness are worn away. He grows very shabby. "But," the storyteller instructs us,

> the Boy loved him just as much. He loved him so hard that he loved all his whiskers off, and the pink lining to his ears turned grey, and his brown spots faded. He even began to lose his shape, and he scarcely looked like a rabbit any more, except to the Boy. To him he was always beautiful, and that was all that the little Rabbit cared about. He didn't mind how he looked to other people, because the nursery magic had made him Real, and when you are Real shabbiness doesn't matter.[14]

By this point in the tale, the Rabbit has had an experience of transcendence of his obsession with self, with "me" and "mine," with "am I Real?" He knows he is real, and that is the end of it. The Skin Horse points out to the Velveteen Rabbit that "once you are Real, you can't become Unreal again. It lasts for always." The structures of our consciousness are profoundly altered by the experience of becoming Real.

On the base of this emerging real self will arise the ability to see clearly—to perceive reality. The self can now see its own nature, can see through the false-self construct, and finally perceive itself to be what it always was—born divine, nonseparate, connected with the whole field of mind and matter. Transcendence is simply the normal maturation of the self. As our most basic needs and longings are met by the environment we create for ourselves, transformation happens.

The highest capacities of the human being to see reality clearly are rooted in the simple experiences of being seen. We cannot see without having first been seen. We cannot wake up without interacting with a consciousness that is awake. Spiritual practice in the contemplative traditions works with the rudiments of the capacity to see clearly, and then it builds them into all of the extraordinary potentials always present in the seed of the human being.

The deepest structures of the mind are evoked in this process of seeing clearly—the intuitive awakened mind, *buddhi*. This is a mind, an awareness, a consciousness, that can move anywhere, that is not separate from anything in the whole field of mind and matter, that is not restricted by fear, clinging, holding on. This is the mind that can acknowledge, experience, and bear all of life. This is the mind and body that can be fully in the dance and, at the same time, be fully in the calmly abiding center.

Susan had come to Kripalu longing for enlightenment. Instead, she got liberation. She awakened from the dream of separation in which she'd lived. She knew irrevocably now that her real self existed in a network of interdependence. She awakened from the painful isolation, emptiness, and terror in which she had lived, and found that she could step down onto the solid ground of earth, to live with the rest of us extraordinarily ordinary human beings.

As she left, I believed that she knew how to find and build community around her and, that she would find the mirrors she would continue to need. That she would continue to thrive as she created a deep sense of mutual belonging with her surround of loved ones, mentors, and co-workers. She went back to a new law firm in Manhattan—smaller, more realistic for her energy levels, with a schedule that allowed her to work on her writing and poetry.

When Susan left the shop and Kripalu Center to go back to Manhattan, she gave the staff a wonderful gift—an engraving of a rabbit, with the following words inscribed beneath it: "Once you become Real, you can't become Unreal again. It lasts for always!"

12

AWAKENING THE WITNESS

> When will you learn, O mind,
> to sleep in perfect comfort
> between the captivating lovers,
> holiness and defilement?
> Only when you can keep
> these two consorts peaceful
> beneath a single roof
> will you truly encounter
> the brilliance of the Goddess.
>
> —Ramakrishna,
> Translated by Lex Hixon

"**K**eep pushing," said Douglas in a frantic whisper. "And for God's sake keep your voice down. You're going to wake somebody up."

Jon grunted his assent. He was pushing as hard as he could, leaning into the car at the driver's side with the door open, trying to steer the silent vehicle down the dark lane. Small beads of sweat were forming on his forehead. The sky was clear, the night dry and sultry, the stars brilliant, but there was almost no moon.

Their hearts were beating fast. "What do you suppose they'll do to us if we get caught?" asked Jon.

"Just keep pushing," said Douglas. "We're not going to get caught."

It was well past ten, half an hour after lights out, and the ashram was silent. Jon and Douglas heard only the sounds of their own heavy breathing and the steady chorus of crickets in the July evening. The rich smell of newly cut hay wafted up from the field on the right side of the road.

Finally, the car reached the end of the long drive. Douglas, who had been pushing from behind, was drenched in sweat. Jon had stubbed his toe on a concealed rock and was swearing quietly under his breath. As the car rolled silently onto the highway, it began to pick up speed. They both hopped in. The headlights were on now. The engine turned over. Jon stepped on the gas, and in a few moments the ashram buildings had receded into the dark distance. The "bros" were on their way to town!

Jon turned on the radio full blast. Freedom. The windows were open. The air was cool on their faces. "Wow," said Douglas. "Just like *Cool Hand Luke.* We escaped. We did it." They gave each other a high five. Their bodies moved in rhythm with the music. It was good to be alive.

Ten miles up the road, the car entered the outskirts of a small town and there, just at the edge of town, was the bros' covert and dangerous destination: an old-fashioned ice-cream parlor. Jon and Douglas got out of the car and stood for a few moments surveying the territory. They looked at the list of ice-cream flavors. They smiled at the girl behind the service window. "Chocolate?" said Douglas, with his eyebrows raised. Jon smiled.

They sat in the car savoring the moment. The radio was still on. They both held the largest possible paper dishes full of ice cream—four scoops. Jon had hot fudge added to his, and whipped cream. This was heaven.

Suddenly a police car drove up and parked next to them. Jon saw the alarm on Douglas's face, and without so much as another breath, they both instinctively jammed their ice creams under the seat.

Douglas and Jon's ice-cream crime cleverly avoided the detection of law enforcement officials, but in the next moment, as they looked wide-eyed at each other, they each realized what had just been revealed in that moment of intense guilt, and they howled with laughter and surprise. "Oh my God," Douglas said. "Do you believe we just did that?"

Jon looked back incredulously. "What the hell is going on here?"

What indeed? How had something as lovely and innocuous as ice cream become so highly charged a substance that it had to be hidden from the police? How had an innocent evening's drive to the ice-cream parlor become so supercharged with the notions of the profane, the evil, the hidden? One assumes that this is not exactly the fruit of yogic practice that Bapuji had in mind. Here were craving, impulsivity, guilt, self-rejection, and fear writ large. Here was restraint transformed into indulgence, self-control morphed into hedonism, moderation become lust. This was decidedly not a moment of yogic "coolness" but an intense moment of the heat of opposites. What did it mean?

In the early years of the Kripalu community, the purificatory practices of yoga were taken very seriously. The practices of the purification of the body (bhutashuddhi) included not just a highly structured practice of celibacy (brahmacharya), but strict moderation in diet (mitahar) and in all other forms of entertaining the senses, as well. At different periods, such as the one that Douglas and Jon were living through, the entire community ate an ascetic macrobiotic diet—rice, vegetables, some fruit, beans, and nuts. Brothers and sisters were often separated so as not to arouse sexual passions. Everyone lived a vow of poverty, chastity, and, to some extent, obedience. The emphasis was everywhere on renunciation as the path to God, on transcendence of the body's various hungers. The conservation of sacred energy, restraint, chastity, purity, light: these were the watchwords.

Jon and Douglas had come to the ashram seeking God, seeking enlightenment, seeking freedom. Yet in that one electric moment at the ice-cream parlor, they saw that something about their strategy was fundamentally flawed. They did not feel more free. Was there a yogic explanation for this?[1]

THE PLAY OF THE PAIRS OF OPPOSITES

Central to the yogic view of the world is the observation that all phenomena in the conditioned world manifest as polarities, or "pairs of opposites" (dvandva). "Pain and pleasure," as Amrit liked to say, "come as twins—as two ends of the same stick." Where pleasure is, there pain will be. Where attraction is, there aversion will be. And love and hate; hope and dread; wish and fear; gain and loss; praise and blame; fame and ill-repute.

This is simply the way it is in the relative world of time and space. What we think of as the opposites of life are actually as connected as mountain and valley, back and front, light and shadow. Though appearing as opposites, they are really one single, indivisible whole. One of the great spiritual laws of yoga is, "The One Thing," or brahman, "is always present as two." This unity of polarities begins with the most fundamental aspects of life—matter and spirit, self and not-self, human and divine. Though appearing as two, they are really "the One without a second."

Western psychologies, too, have wrestled with the problem of opposites. Carl Jung believed that the movement of all psychic processes relied upon what he called "the principle of opposites." The very energy of mental and psychic life itself, in this view, depends upon polarities and "contending forces" in the inner and outer world. Jung believed that the "trip to the center," or the full maturation of the human being, required bringing all aspects of opposites into consciousness.

Yogic scriptures everywhere acknowledge that the polarization of life's energies is one of humans' central problems. Patanjali, as we have seen, lists raga and dvesha as the third and fourth afflictions. These two important opposites, attraction and aversion, stand as representatives, in his simplified form, of all of the polarities of the embodied life.

In itself, the apparently dualistic nature of our phenomenal world is not a problem. We can live with hot and cold, love and hate, gain and loss, light and shadow, sacred and profane. The problem is that we human beings inevitably tend to choose for one side of the polarity and against the other side, artificially attempting to split life down the middle. We choose only the mountaintop and eschew the valley. We cling desperately to pleasure and attempt to banish pain. We chase frantically after gain and run from loss. Or perhaps we do it the other way around, choosing the "dark side" of the polarity—hate over love, fear over wish, dread over hope, loss over gain.

Whichever way we attempt to split the polarities of life, one thing is certain: we will suffer when we do. Life lived from only one side of a polarity is extremely difficult, as we have seen. It takes an enormous amount of energy to continually push away the denied aspect of the polarity. For what we deny inexorably intrudes into our convenient organization of life. Whatever aspect of reality we split off from awareness will continually be presented to us by life. And more often than not, it will come to us, as Jung said, as fate—an unwanted and feared intruder. The more energy we have used to suppress it, the more powerful will be its reemergence in our lives.

This book so far is full of examples of people who have experienced difficulty precisely because they've tried to artificially split the polarities of life. Catherine (in chapter 9) attempted to banish her natural assertiveness, only to find that her resulting rage threatened to blot out the entire inventory of the shop. Sam (also in chapter 9) was able to bear his feelings of love for Cassandra but not his equally powerful feelings of hate, and so he was destined to "act out" that hate by refusing to repay her loan. And, of course, Douglas and Jon at some point chose tofu and rice over ice cream, the "spiritual" world over the sensory world, only to find ice cream haunting their dreams and dark nights.

Most religious and spiritual systems attempt to work with the poles of opposites by suppressing one side, using the sledgehammer of will-power, morality, and "the law." Yogic philosophy and practice, how-ever, offer a way to work directly with the daily visceral experiences of opposites, harnessing the energies of "both ends of the stick" for the creation of the fully alive human being. The primary yogic strategy for working with opposites is called witness consciousness. We'll now turn to an exploration of some of the central principles of this remarkable technique.

A SECRET LIFE

By the time I arrived at Kripalu, much of the rigidity of earlier years had softened. There was no longer any need to push silent cars down the driveway at night to get ice cream. And yet, there were still several enormous, brooding cultural polarities—most notably, it seemed to me, the split between sexuality and spirituality. In the Kripalu tradition, the conservation of sexual energy was understood to be the single most important pillar of kundalini yoga, and so, in the early years of my tenure, yogic celibacy was still being strictly practiced. Attempts to conserve sexual energy led to a whole host of heroic efforts, sometimes comic, sometimes tragic, to suppress and "rechannel" the power of sexuality: brothers retaining their semen for months and even years on end; manic physical activity and exercise, to sublimate the energy of sexuality; willful withdrawal from the slightest forms of sexual stimula-tion, including dietary practices that forbade the eating of garlic, on-ions, and caffeine. For years, the community lived with the delusion that the sexuality of healthy young Americans could be somehow suc-cessfully split off and suppressed, and the energy rerouted up the "cen-tral channel" as awakened kundalini. As we shall see, this was a delusion central to the conflagration that would later engulf the community. Long before this final drama, however, it was clearly affecting individual lives. None more so, I think, than my friend Connie's.

Connie was a beautiful, thirty-two-year-old Colombian woman, the daughter of a high-ranking diplomat. She had silky brown hair, worn in the style of Jackie O., whom she quite resembled; she had large almond-shaped brown eyes and a slight olive hue to her skin. Connie's clothes were always understated, but elegant. Her small, slender frame lent her a quality of vulnerability. This fragility, however, was belied by a certain smart toughness in her presence. She had been a successful television producer in Los Angeles, and was known in TV circles to be capable of holding her own with even the most powerful media personalities.

Connie and I had become close friends in what was for both of us the first year of our residency at Kripalu. We worked side by side prepping veggies for some time, cutting carrots and singing songs I had learned during my college year abroad, when I had hitchhiked through the tiny villages of remote Colombia.

One October evening after dinner, as I was sauntering up the road from the main building to an outbuilding on the campus where I was then living, Connie came running along behind me.

"Steve," she called breathlessly, "wait up."

When Connie reached me, she opened her arms, threw them around my neck, and began to sob uncontrollably. I held her. "That's OK, just let it go, Connie." The flood of tears continued, preventing her from telling me what was wrong. Finally, we walked over to a bench by the edge of the mansion lawn, and she began to breathe more normally. Eventually the story emerged.

Connie had a secret life. She told me that five months earlier she'd begun to leave campus late at night to hang out in a bar and pick up men. She would dress up in her trashiest L.A. outfits, put on enough makeup so that her look screamed "easy," and sneak out the back way, unseen. Connie then hopped into her car and made her way to a local dance bar where there was known to be a lot of cruising. This didn't happen regularly, she explained, but came in waves. For weeks on end, she said, she would be "fine." But some weeks she would go several times, occasionally sleeping with several different men in the course of as many days. During what she called her "binges," she was "obsessed with sex," she said. "Haunted." She found herself particularly partial to truckers, bikers, and cops—tough guys who seemed to be her opposites.

Connie was completely mortified to be telling me her secret. And yet, her hand had been forced. Something had gone wrong. One of the biker-types had begun calling her. He wouldn't let go, and she felt she was on the brink of being stalked. What should she do?

As more of the story spilled out, it became clear to me that Connie had come to the ashram on a kind of geographical cure, trying to leave behind this driven sexualizing, which had developed during her eight years in Los Angeles. For the first seven months, Connie said, she was completely free of the compulsion to go cruising. Her dream had come true. She had left this part of her nature behind in L.A. The fresh air, the mountains, the yoga, the spiritual lifestyle: all of this had "completed" her so that she did not need to look for sex. But when the fantasies and behaviors started to reappear in the spring, she was crushed. She described to me the trigger for her first experience. She had had a difficult confrontation with her supervisor, and afterward Connie had felt enraged. Without even thinking about it, Connie marched right up to her room, got out her outfit, drove to the bar, and ended up picking up a married man and spending the night with him in a motel.

"I feel like a monster," Connie said, "like this part is not really me." She told me that she felt that while "the spiritual part" of her was her true self, this was a lower self she needed to exile once again. It came into her harmonious spiritual life as an intruder, and she did not want it. She worried that she might be a multiple personality. "Steve, this thing just takes me over. I'm powerless. Am I, I don't know, like, schizophrenic, or something?"

As it turned out, of course, Connie had neither a multiple personality disorder nor schizophrenia. In fact, she was much more normal than she imagined. Upon further investigation, Connie found some useful approaches to her dilemma within yogic philosophy and practice. And over the coming several years, she would cobble together a fascinating synthesis of both yogic and Western psychological wisdom in order to heal the split between her sexual life and her spiritual life.

CHOICELESS AWARENESS

The problem of how to integrate the poles of opposites became, early on, one of the central concerns of yogic sages. They arrived at a simple, elegant, and practical solution to the dilemma.

First of all, yogis identified a profound paradox at the root of the problem: Although embodiment is central to our nature as human beings, nonetheless, we remain largely at war with the embodied state. The fact is that by our very nature we live immersed in a phenomenal world, and we experience that world directly through the medium of sensation in our bodies. In every second of life, our bodies are responding to stimuli, both internal stimuli coming from the mind and body, and external stimuli coming through "the five sense doors"—taste, touch, smell, hearing, sight. Indeed, being human is just one big light show, sound show, smell show, a constantly exploding touch, feel, and thought extravaganza. And yet, though our very nature is sensation, ironically we have enormous difficulty directly acknowledging, experiencing, and bearing the raw sensations of life. Anyone who has ever attempted to sit in meditation for just ten or fifteen minutes to observe the internal whirlwind of sensations in the body will know this is so. On a moment-by-moment basis, we recoil from the sensations of life.

Contrary to conventional wisdom, this inability to tolerate sensation is just as true of pleasurable sensations as it is of painful ones. We cannot bear feelings of craving, wanting, and attraction any more successfully than we can bear feelings of aversion, hatred, and repulsion. Indeed, Jon and Douglas went to the trouble of pushing the car halfway to town that night precisely because they could not bear the sensations of wanting and craving, longing and desire. As they ate, they could not bear their feelings of guilt. They couldn't just feel them. They had to act on them, in order to "eliminate" them. We could hardly overstate how difficult it is for us to learn to acknowledge, experience, and bear the moment-to-moment life in our bodies—pleasurable life, painful life, sexual life, the life of our desires, just plain human life.

Our attempts to choose strongly for and against experience are usually a strategy to control or avoid feelings and sensations that we cannot bear. We move toward what we like so that it will continue; we move away from what we dislike so that it will end. We try to hold on to the ebb and flow of sensation, to control the light and sound show. But this strategy is seriously flawed. Indeed, it increases our suffering. The show, alas, is out of our control. First of all, as we have already seen, choosing one side against another severely diminishes our capacity to see clearly, setting us up for all kinds of unwise courses of action. Secondly, the choice sets us in opposition to reality, by trying to artificially separate what is absolutely and inextricably joined. And, thirdly, it increases our reactivity to the experience of sensation, rather than decreasing it. It diminishes our equanimity.

But is there any other way to live? Isn't this "yo-yo effect" just in the nature of being human? Well, sensation, yes, yo-yo maybe not. Yogis discovered a third way, a path that does not split the world into pain and pleasure, right and wrong, good and bad, sacred and profane. They discovered a path that does not require us to suppress the energy of desire, but allows us to fully experience it. Patanjali writes of this third way (I.33) as the development of a kind of "impartiality in spheres of pleasure and pain, virtue and vice." The fifteenth-century scripture called the *Vedantasara* (The Essence of the Doctrines of Vedanta)[2] describes the practice of *titiksa,* a cultivation of an attitude of impartiality, patience, and endurance toward the pairs of opposites, a practice this scripture honors as one of the six treasures of life.

This impartiality and neutrality toward polarities is referred to by some modern yogis, including those in the Kripalu tradition, as "choiceless awareness." Choiceless awareness is a third way because when we're practicing it, we do not push away any sensation. We do not believe the pairs of opposites can be separated. Rather, we develop our capacity to experience the way things are, to live each moment fully, to receive the whole light and sound show. In a sense, we do not choose against any experience—we choose for all of it.

THE WITNESS: BREAKING THE CHAIN
OF CONDITIONING

Putting choiceless awareness into practice requires that we not tune out our experience of attraction and aversion but tune them in even more deeply. Yogis discovered that if we can learn to train our awareness enough to acknowledge sensations as they arise, to experience them fully and to bear them, then we can no longer be bound to the wheel of opposites. We are no longer whipped around by our conditioned responses to pleasure and pain. We can no longer be compelled to act unconsciously on the sensations.

Desire is not the problem. Attraction is not the problem. Aversion is not the problem. The problem is learning to live with the "bare reality" of the phenomenal world. The skillful means used in yogic practice to explore this bare reality is called witness consciousness. If craving and aversion are the central afflictions in the yogic view, witness consciousness is the primary skillful means for freeing us from our bondage to them. There are six primary characteristics of the witness:

1. *The witness does not choose for or against any aspect of reality.* The witness does not split life into good and bad, right and wrong, high and low, or spiritual and not-spiritual. The witness does not take sides, but experiences a kind of "choiceless awareness."

2. *The witness does not censor life.* The witness allows all thoughts, feelings, and sensations to receive the light of awareness, without discriminating. There is absolutely nothing that the witness cannot see, feel, and experience. There is no shadow, no shame, no repression that is not capable of being penetrated by witnessing. The witness is not judgmental in any way, but practices self-observation without judgment.

3. *Witnessing is a whole-body experience.* Witnessing is not an intellectual exercise. Quite the contrary. We actually witness our experience with our whole body, allowing ourselves to feel the reverberations of sensations throughout the whole physical-emotional organism. Indeed, when the witness is finely honed, we can sometimes feel the reverberation of experience throughout all of the five sheaths.

4. *Witness consciousness is always present at least in its potential form in every human being at every moment.* The witness is the essence of our divine, awake, already enlightened nature. We don't have to create the witness. This quality of consciousness needs only to be recognized, evoked, claimed, and cultivated.

5. *The witness is the part of already awake mind that is capable of standing completely still, even in the center of the whirlwind of sensations, thoughts, feelings, fantasies—even in serious mental and*

physical illness. From the witness, we can stand back and objectively observe our experience even as we're having that experience. Even as the witness stands as the still point at the center of the storm, though, this part of our consciousness can fully "dance" with life, directly experiencing all sensation, all activity in the mind, the heart, the body. It moves with experience, even as it remains completely still, anchored and grounded.

6. *The witness goes everywhere.* The witness is connected to the whole quantum field of mind and matter. Witness consciousness stands outside time and space, living in the eternal now of the unmanifest realms, while also penetrating time and space. Witness consciousness is the quality of the self-aware universe. It is the intelligence, the "sight without a seer," that saturates the whole quantum field of mind and matter.

BORROWING A WITNESS

Surprisingly, contemporary Western psychology has developed a notion of witness consciousness that is in many ways similar to the yogic view. Psychologists believe that "the witness"—sometimes called the "observing ego"—is a capacity that naturally emerges in the developing human being, once we have established a "good enough" separate physical and emotional sense of self. When the supporting structures of the self are sufficiently in place, we can mentally stand back and observe, evaluate, and find perspective on our own experience, even as we're in the midst of having it. Psychologists, like yogis, believe that if this "seer" is insufficiently developed, we will suffer, becoming over-identified with thoughts and feelings, fusing the internal world and the external world. Without the still point of the witness, we feel fragmented, fragile, not cohesive. Indeed, psychosis is, precisely, the loss of the witness—a condition in which we become lost within our own autistic, symbiotic orbit, completely merged with primitive drives, thoughts, and fantasies. Much of psychological treatment is undertaken in order to strengthen the "observing ego"—the still point at the center of our whirling lives.

From early on in his work with patients, the goal of Freud's treatment was to bring observing ego to bear on what he called "id," which

contains the unconscious drives. This was stated in Freud's classic formulation, "Where id was, there ego shall be." Indeed, the entire point
of Freud's technique of free association was to develop a "therapeutic
split in the ego" in which the self becomes both observer and observed.
Freud believed that when the patient was truly capable of free association, observing and speaking all aspects of the internal life without
choosing for or against any one side, following the associative flow of
thoughts without blocking or censoring in any fashion, she was cured.

Through his psychoanalytic work with patients, however, Freud soon
discovered the fundamental obstacle to the healing power of witness
consciousness. He found that all patients had aspects of their inner life
that seemed completely and irrevocably hidden from view. As he explored treatment with these patients, he found that it was almost impossible to overestimate the power of the strategies they used to keep
parts of themselves defended against the light of the witness. Quite to
his surprise, he discovered that patients hid not just their pain, but
their pleasure as well. The sly smile on the face of a patient describing
an act of sadism with his wife revealed the pleasure and satisfaction he
felt in a physical act of abuse, a pleasure that he vehemently denied
and that revealed itself only unconsciously.

Freud's most brilliant work was in discovering how to bring observing ego to these areas of unconsciousness. Over the course of his career, he explored three different strategies to accomplish this.[3] His first
strategy was to work directly with memories of traumatic events that
had been "forgotten" or repressed. He understood these "forgotten"
areas to be pivotal to curing neurotic symptoms. Freud found that he
could, to some extent, open these areas of repression through the use
of hypnosis, which bypassed the ordinary defenses and brought the
repressed material into awareness. This dramatic early psychoanalytic
work of Freud is still locked into our contemporary cultural imagination, through a whole host of novels and films. Many of us still think of
psychotherapy as the process of searching for that one crucial memory
that will unlock the puzzle of our lives. In fact, Freud's thinking
evolved far beyond this stereotype.

Freud soon found that the defensive structure of the self offered a
formidable amount of resistance to his direct probing, and he moved
on to explore other techniques for penetrating the unconscious. His
next explorations were with the use of free association, dreams, and
slips of the tongue, working with the very language through which the

unconscious communicates. Instead of assaulting the defenses directly, through hypnosis, he found that he could wait for the unconscious to reveal itself. This strategy proved to be extremely effective. It also, however, proved to have its limitations.

Freud was moving closer to his most brilliant insight—his understanding of "acting out" and the "repetition compulsion." He discovered that the most difficult aspects of our experience are forgotten and repressed so deeply that they cannot be seen directly. There is, however, one way of discovering this deeply repressed material. In his work with long-term analytic patients, Freud discovered that eventually we reproduce this material not as a memory, but as an action. In order to hold this material in the unconscious, we are driven to repeat it over and over again—"acting it out" without understanding its original source or motivation. Freud called this the repetition compulsion.

One of Freud's crowning achievements was his discovery that this repeated, unconscious material always showed up in the therapeutic relationship sooner or later. In the context of a relationship in which the patient feels safely held and soothed, the patient will eventually bring the unconscious material into the room through his actions, thereby exposing it to the observing ego of first the therapist, and then, as the therapist points it out, hopefully to himself. In this way, the therapist loans the patient her observing ego, or, from a yogic point of view, we might say that the therapist loans the patient her witness consciousness.

There are certain aspects of our experience, then—usually the most painful and conflicted—that can only be seen within the field of relationship. Indeed, they don't exist only within us, but within the relational fields we create. When we carry a heavy load of repressed, hidden, and unintegrated experience, we are constantly seeking out relationships that will help us hold this experience, to reveal it in the actual dramas of our lives, and, hopefully, eventually to bring it to a more successful conclusion—to heal it. Much of our maneuvering in and out of relationships is driven by these very needs—strivings for wholeness and completion that are for the most part completely out of our awareness.

Freud unwittingly made an important contribution to our contemporary understanding of witness consciousness. He saw that consciousness is sometimes a "third force," the creative product of two individual awarenesses working together to understand and integrate experience.

Matthew Arnold makes precisely the same point in his poem *The Buried Life,* in which he attempts to wrestle with precisely those "hidden," incognito aspects of the self. In Arnold's rendering, the voices of the "buried life" only reveal themselves with utmost clarity when opened to the consciousness of a loved other.

> *Only—but this is rare—*
> *When a beloved hand is laid in ours,*
> *When, jaded with the rush and glare*
> *Of the interminable hours,*
> *Our eyes can in another's eyes read clear,*
> *When our world-deafen'd ear*
> *Is by the tones of a loved voice caress'd—*
> *A bolt is shot back somewhere in our breast,*
> *And a lost pulse of feeling stirs again.*
> *The eye sinks inward, and the heart lies plain,*
> *And what we mean, we say, and what we would, we know.*[4]

It is a point that mariners and explorers of all kinds have discovered: Reality must be, in a sense, triangulated. It takes two sets of eyes, not just one, to accurately locate the third point in space. The "third" becomes a powerful still point, constructed out of the interaction of two minds and hearts.

DISCOVERING THE THIRD WAY

Connie had two motivations for her sabbatical at Kripalu. One was entirely conscious. The other was entirely unconscious. Her deepest conscious hope—which was conflicted enough that she shared it with no one until that evening on the mansion lawn—was that her time in the safe haven of spiritual community would help her to leave the demons of her sexual drivenness behind her. Her unconscious wish, of which she was completely unaware, was just the opposite: Unconsciously, she wanted to find a safe environment and relational field, in which she could expose and explore her compulsive sexual life so that she could understand it and integrate it. She was searching for the other consciousness with which she could join in order to create "the third force"—a witness powerful enough to contain, see through, and remember her split self.

The fundamental premise of the yogic worldview is that the human being has an innate capacity and drive to mature to full aliveness. However unlikely full aliveness may seem as a goal to our conscious mind, our unconscious is always urging us to face and welcome home our demons. Connie's trip to Kripalu was actually going to be just the opposite of what she thought it would be. Much to her surprise, she discovered that the doorway into her healing was through the very parts of herself that she had wished to disavow.

Connie was now facing a seemingly intractable problem: Her secret sexual life was an area in which she experienced no discernible witness consciousness. When she went off on a sexual binge, she experienced herself as being taken over by an outside force, almost as if against her will. For hours, or sometimes days, she felt lost in the fog of compulsive sexuality. In these times she envisioned herself as a primitive huntress, the goddess Diana seeking her prey. Connie became completely identified with this archetypal hunter. And when she was lost in the hunt she felt relief, she felt unburdened, she felt free, she felt full of life and creativity. Whenever she tried to shine the light of the witness, or her observing ego, on these activities, she found a harsh, judgmental, outraged, and punitive voice—one that, at least in those protected moments, she needed to exile. It was, indeed, from this very voice that she needed asylum.

As Connie and I talked through her dilemma, one thing was clear: her strategies for managing her secret sexual life were not working. The geographical cure had failed. Her sexual compulsions had accompanied her on the flight from L.A. And, of course, the continued pursuit of the secret life was self-defeating: when she returned from the hunt, she felt guilt and self-loathing. She would sometimes bring other serious problems back with her—sexually transmitted diseases, or the odd man who turned out to be unstable. Connie had understood, intellectually, that the yogic approach offers a "third way"—a choice beyond either repression, on the one hand, or "acting out" on the other. She had studied witness consciousness in her yogic training program. But she could not access it alone.

Our evening talk on the bench was an enormous breakthrough for Connie. In allowing me into her suffering, she discovered the power of sharing the witness. She was amazed that I was not judgmental or censorious of her behavior. She was astonished that I could see this problem not as a sign of sickness, but as a doorway into a fuller life. And, she was completely amazed to hear that she had not failed in her spiritual quest: that the working through of this issue was her spiritual path—it was not a detour, or a distraction from her spirituality.

It was clear to me that Connie needed a special kind of help, more than the kind of help that I, as a friend, could give her. She needed someone skilled at helping her to methodically create witness consciousness around this area of her life, to help her open the door into her behavior, to understand, acknowledge, experience, and bear its reality and meaning, and finally to gain perspective on it. She needed to be with someone who would not encourage her to override her feelings, to attempt to transcend them, or to judge them in any way, but, rather, to help her explore them. With this kind of partnership, I felt sure that she could eventually hear the deeper message in her compulsive behavior. I referred Connie to an excellent psychoanalyst in nearby Stockbridge, and she began seeing her therapist the following week. After years of hiding, Connie was relieved that her secret life could at last be joined with her "other life."

SELF-OBSERVATION WITHOUT JUDGMENT

After Bapuji arrived at Kripalu for a four-year stay, he commented frequently on the depths of self-loathing and self-rejection he found among his Western students. Many Eastern teachers are astonished at the extent of negative self-feelings they find in the West—powerful feelings of shame and self-hatred that they apparently do not find among students in their traditional cultures (cultures that have not been twisted by "the Puritan damage"). As Bapuji wrestled with the meaning of these feelings, his heart was very moved. "My beloved child," he said at one important occasion, "break your heart no longer. Each time you judge yourself you break your own heart."

Bapuji came to believe that students could make no progress in the development of witness consciousness without first intentionally softening this judgmental voice. He spoke over and over again about self-compassion, and at one point he threw up his hands and said it was to be the sole practice of his students.

Early on in my stay, I discovered that Kripalu, Bapuji's name, means "compassion." The most persistent image I have of this intrepid kundalini yogi is not of his relentless determination for liberation— toward which end he spent twenty years in silence *(mauna)* and ten to twelve hours a day in intensive yoga and meditation practice—but of his compassion and unconditional acceptance of all things human. He was, indeed, the gentle grandfather. And the gentle grand*mother* as well, for in a lineage of male teachers, he embodied the Mother in many ways.

Bapuji could not seem to emphasize enough his conviction that the path of the witness requires compassionate self-acceptance at every step. The first law of the witness is that without self-acceptance there can be no accurate self-observation. The seer requires the Mother. She is not optional. When we're judging or criticizing our experience, we cannot fully be in it. In order to witness we have to be able to interact with what is, without needing to fight against it. Nothing has to get rejected or closed down. No part of me is any more right than any other part. I am not more invested in one than in the other. I am curious. Accepting. Allowing. Interested. Watching. This is an amazingly free place to stand. "There is absolutely nothing wrong with this moment."

There is an essential corollary to the first law of the witness, however. It goes like this: Eventually, we will react, we will judge, we will censor. But this is not a problem either! When we do react, judge, or censor, we can simply take that reaction as the object of the witness's attention. All of yogic practice is about getting under the moment of reactivity, the moment when, in order to remain comfortable, we choose for or against one side or the other of the pairs of opposites. When the reactivity happens, as it surely will, we simply examine it in the light of the witness. Reactivity is not a problem. Every level of reactivity just becomes the new object of witness. Over time, the nonreactive awareness that we've built begins to deconstruct and dismantle the elaborate superstructure of drives, impulses, pushes and pulls, light and dark, mountain and valley.

WHAT THE WITNESS SAW

Connie spent the next three years in psychotherapy. She took this work on as her spiritual practice. She was still Diana, the hunter. But now she was hunting for something different: consciousness. Connie was astonished at what she discovered. As she explored beneath the surface of her life, she found that nothing was what it had appeared. She was not a sexual lunatic. In fact, her sexual acting out was not really about sex at all. She found, to her surprise, that she was actually quite prudish about and terrified of her own true sexuality.

Connie was the daughter of a narcissistic father who felt extremely competitive with his competent and pretty young daughter. He competed with her both for the attention of his wife, and for the attention of the world at large. When he could not co-opt her many accomplishments, even in her childhood, he attempted to dominate her so that he could win what he imagined to be a competition. He argued with her, minimized her achievements, publicly humiliated her, and several times threatened to exile her from his home when she refused to be submissive. Throughout her adolescence, Connie's ongoing war with her father had a highly sexual edge to it, although there was never any overt sexual behavior.

When Connie finished college and officially left home, she worked hard to please others, and to find the approbation in the world she could not find with her father. She just wanted to leave him behind, moving as far away from him as she could go. Yet, she carried him with her in her sexual fantasy life, which was saturated with themes of dominating men and being dominated by them. In her midtwenties, in Los Angeles, with her career established, she began to act out these fantasies with real men.

The reality of her sexual fantasies and behaviors was so covered over by shame that it took more than two years before Connie was able to share them with her therapist. Together, she and her therapist painstakingly built trust, and they built the framework of observing ego to hold and penetrate Connie's inner world. As they did this, Connie's need to act out her fantasies diminished. Eventually, she discovered underneath her behaviors the hidden ghost of her father and his sadistic domination of her. Connie discovered that she was, in effect, keeping her traumatic relationship with her father alive in her reenactment of it: a classic repetition compulsion. The unconscious wish, of course, was to finally resolve the feelings around the trauma, to bring them to a successful conclusion, and to integrate them. As long as Connie was acting them out, though, this was impossible, because the acting out was actually a defense against the primitive feelings of rage, emptiness, and grief that she had never been able to acknowledge, experience, and bear.

As treatment progressed, Connie was shocked to discover that, underneath all of her dramatic sexual acting out, she had practically no real relationship with her own sexuality. Her final piece of work in therapy was to uncover her own terror and judgment of her true sexual feelings. It was only through the repeated exploration of her sexual fantasies and feelings in the context of relationship with her therapist— who was relentlessly accepting and nonjudgmental—that she was able to "grow" a witness with those qualities of gentleness about which Bapuji spoke.

Connie discovered that she did not have to banish the energy, creativity, and life force of "the monster." Instead, the monster's energy was transmuted into normal and acceptable animal instincts, passion, hunger, and desire. As Connie allowed these instincts into the light of her newly developing witness, she found delight in sex. And when she did, finally, enter into an ongoing sexual relationship, she confessed to me, happily, that she was "an animal" and that she could love that part of herself. Sexuality and spirituality came together for Connie. The dark side and the light were reunited, and Connie experienced a new kind of freedom and energy in her life, of which she had never even dreamed.

FREEDOM

Psychologists Dan Brown and Jack Engler did a fascinating study of yogis at advanced stages of meditation practice. It revealed that, contrary to our mistaken Western assumptions about "enlightenment" experiences, even very advanced practitioners continue to experience conflict, fear, anxiety, depression, addictive cravings, interpersonal dependency struggles, and so forth. But this is not quite the bad news it seems. Their report continued:

> What changes is not so much the amount or nature of conflict,
> but awareness of and reactivity to it. . . . [With practice] there
> is greater awareness of and openness to conflict but paradoxi-
> cally less reaction at the same time in an impulsive, identifi-
> catory and therefore painful way. . . . [The practitioner] may

note the intense desire until it passes, like every other transient mental state; or he/she may act on it, but with full awareness. . . . Mindfulness is said to automatically intervene between impulse or thought and action in such cases. This mechanism of reality, combined with clear and impartial observation, allows a new freedom from drive and a new freedom for well-considered and appropriate action.[5]

As we Westerners become more experienced with yoga and meditation, we will begin to become more realistic about their outcomes. A mere reduction in reactivity may seem a disappointment to those of us still engaging in magical thinking about Eastern enlightenment experiences. The increase of awareness and neutrality toward experience may be a bitter pill for those of us who were hoping for immersion in permanent oceanic bliss. But, actually, "a new freedom for well-considered and appropriate action" is a very wonderful thing. It means that we have increased freedom to choose. As Connie discovered, we become free to renounce actions that might undermine our most awake experiences of ourselves. And we become free to claim actions that express who we really are.

For the witness, everything is workable. Nothing needs to be pushed away. To the contrary: our seemingly most intractable neuroses become the doorway into full life. What emerges when we open this door is a happiness that is not the opposite of sadness, a self-love that is not the opposite of self-hate. It is, rather, a happiness that embraces sadness, and a love that embraces hate. Witness consciousness cultivates a place behind dark and light, behind good and evil—behind even personality, behind even the mind.

The path, from the very first step, is self-acceptance. The goal is self-acceptance. The fruit of this practice is self-love. Compassion for the self and compassion for others radiates naturally from every moment of practice. As we practice allowing and accepting, we open our hearts and embrace that part of ourselves, or that part of another, that has been pushed away. By cherishing, honoring, allowing all our energies, we move into that place inside that says "yes" to all experience. Yes! Through "yes" we have stepped into the plane of consciousness of the fully alive human being—the jivan mukta.

As Rumi says, "Out beyond ideas of wrongdoing and rightdoing there is a field. Meet me there."[6]

Part Four

THE SPONTANEOUS
WISDOM OF THE BODY

RIDING THE WAVE

OF BREATH

Inside and outside her head, a billion, trillion stars,
beyond count, circled and exploded. A million
frogs croaked, trees fell in forests echoing down
valleys; children cried. The flux of everything
throbbed on and on. Songs were heard in spheres
within spheres, electric, crackle, sharp. She heard
nothing. How could she, when not once had she
even heard the sound of her own breathing?

—Duane Michaels,
"Inside and Outside"

In my heady early years at Kripalu, I had the sense of unimaginable riches about to open before me through the practice of hatha yoga. Along with many other members of the community, I did between two and three hours of yoga a day. Desai and other senior residents promoted the notion that, as a result of this intensive practice, we were all on the edge of a mystical new consciousness; and they continually urged more discipline, more practice. Some, including my friends Yoganand and Gitanand, were exploring advanced and esoteric forms of kundalini yoga. Others, like myself, undertook intensive training to become certified Kripalu yoga teachers. And many of us, beginner and advanced alike, privately aspired to "the divine body" of light talked of by the great yogic saints.

By the time I began teaching daily classes, at the end of my second year of residency, I had begun to become more realistic about the goals of practice. I saw, through direct experience, that its secrets and mysteries unfold only over time—sometimes long stretches of time. Yes, dramatic change was possible. I could feel it in myself, and I saw it in fellow students—even some whom I would have diagnosed as severely troubled when they arrived. Many of us became visibly healthier, steadier, more aware. But the truly transformative moments of practice were often subtle and unexpected. They could not be willed, and they seemed to emerge from some wordless source deep within the body.

For the next several years, my own development—both personally and as a member of the community—would unfold in relationship to my practice and teaching of Kripalu hatha yoga. I became fascinated, particularly, with the psychological healing promoted by the physical practices of yoga, and, too, with the slow emergence into consciousness of the "subtle bodies" to which I alluded in chapter 5. In the three yoga stories that follow—of my student Garth, my old friend Bonnie, and my "practice buddy" Tony—I try to convey the real possibilities of regular long-term practice of hatha yoga—its idiosyncratic rhythms and breakthroughs. Woven into these three stories are mysteries I have seen time and time again—the real, everyday magic of yoga that is not much written about, but that all serious students know.

GARTH

Garth came to my yoga classes three times a week for seven years. From the first day, he stood out from the other students. Unlike most folks, who showed up for class in sweats or leotards, Garth wore old jeans and a flannel shirt. He was tall, lean, and long-limbed. Midtwenties, I thought. With his gaunt body, narrow face, slightly stooped posture, and wild explosion of curly brown hair, he reminded me of a young Ichabod Crane. Garth apparently didn't have a yoga mat or blanket or yoga ties, props or eyebags or any yoga accoutrements whatsoever. He just plopped himself down on the floor.

It was clear from the beginning that the 4:15 moderate yoga class was important to him. Neither sleet, nor snow, nor dark of night could keep Garth away. He arrived early, went to the same far corner in the rear of the room, lay down on his back and did fifteen minutes of relaxation before class. It was clear that he felt safe in that spot. When it wasn't available he was visibly displeased.

Garth seemed to be curiously split off from his body. Often, what he was doing with his body didn't look even remotely like the posture the rest of us were doing. His long arms and legs would flail as if each of them were following separate instructions. Occasionally, with his permission, I would touch him, to support him in a posture, or to help him bring his attention back from wherever it was wandering. I noticed that there was a cool quality to his body. In spite of his youth, his joints felt stiff, and his skin had a strange gray pallor. He didn't seem to be at all present in his body or his breath.

Though Garth's apparently dissociated state was rather dramatic, he was in fact only different by degree from many students who just aren't home in their bodies as they practice. Most striking, though, in Garth's case, was a visible split between his head and the rest of him. Indeed, the unique life form that was Garth seemed to be headquartered somewhere between his ears. He always arrived in class with a little notebook and pen, and many times throughout the class he would light up like a Christmas tree, pick up his pen, and jot down a thought.

Garth had a brilliant mind. A graduate of MIT, he'd gone on to write his own ticket in the software industry. At twenty-six he was unattached and, after a spectacular four years working as a programmer for a major corporation, had settled near Kripalu, where, it turned out, he was at work on a book on some arcane aspect of quantum mechanics. He told me later, he had some of his best insights for the book in my class. Garth had been spinning out quantum equations while in the "downward dog"!

For the first year of our acquaintance, Garth said barely two words to me. Sometimes, when I approached him to talk, he appeared like a deer, frozen in the glare of oncoming headlights, a kind of terror in his eyes. At some point in the middle of the second year, however, he began to smile and say hello as he came in. Eventually, he began to eat dinner in the Kripalu dining hall, after class. I frequently sat down with him, and we struck up a more or less regular conversation.

Garth's social skills were a lot like his yoga. He was, as we might say at Kripalu, "up in his head." He had a rich intellectual life, but he seemed hyperrational, disconnected from feeling or imagination.

Garth thought of himself as "a spiritual person." He always wore his *mala* beads, which had been duly blessed by the appropriate yogic luminaries. He was, if anything, overly nice and accommodating, as though playing out his notion of how a spiritual person should act. But as I got to know Garth, he began to drop his spiritual persona. I discovered that behind his shy and awkward exterior was a warm, lively, and very, very funny man.

One of the most dramatic things I noticed about Garth, early on in our friendship, was his shallow breathing. Indeed, when I sat with him at meals, I noticed that if I wasn't paying attention, I would begin to stop breathing myself. Garth's breath seemed restricted, as if he couldn't bear to penetrate down into his body, into his lungs, or—God forbid—down into his hips and pelvis. So he took little short, rapid breaths that punctuated his learned discourses at dinner.

Garth had his own unique posture in life, his own energy imprint. I recognized "the posture of Garth" as I would recognize a face—how he held his body and how it felt to sit next to him at the table; his gestures, his expressions, his tone of voice. And I was sure that Garth was, for the most part, entirely unaware of his unique postural signature.

THE POSTURES OF LIFE

In infancy and childhood, we all develop certain deeply unconscious physical postures, just as Garth did. These are neuromuscular and energetic postures that arise inevitably as embodiments of our feelings and chronic mental states—fear, joy, rage, happiness, grief, satisfaction, hunger. We each have a unique postural signature. It is one of the chief ways in which we are known by others—our gait, mannerisms, and body language.

A significant proportion of our own idiosyncratic postural signature is an embodiment of our attempts to inhibit feelings that have been too difficult for us to bear. These are the postures of the false self. They are characterized by twisting away from life, by rigidity, constriction, brittleness, and held breath.

The most astonishing thing about our complex idiosyncratic postures, especially the postures of the false self, is that most of the time they remain almost entirely outside our awareness. The first law of mental processes—of which we spoke in chapter 9—applies to our body's postures just as much as it does to our thoughts: Much of our physical life is unconscious. Many of the physical processes of our life—sensations, feelings, gestures, movements, contractions, releases, expansion—operate completely outside our awareness.

Even though we are unaware of our unique postures most of the time, others can see them clearly. We can all think of friends or acquaintances who have fairly dramatic unconscious postures. I think immediately of a patient I once had named Jack, who grew up in a notoriously tough neighborhood of Boston. A mental image of Jack is not hard for us to conjure up. We all know him. He has a certain "attitude" in his posture—jutting chin, puffed-up chest, swagger in his gait, fists ready to clench at the drop of a dime. Jack is a fight waiting to happen. His posture had initially, of course, been a reaction to real danger. But it had gradually become Jack's way of being in the world. Remarkable as this seemed to his friends, he was completely unaware of it.

The second law of unconscious processes (chapter 9 again) also applies to our physical posture: That which remains unconscious will come to us as fate. Those aspects of our physical, visceral lives that we relegate to the dark basement of our unconscious will inexorably undermine the conscious and well-intended projects on the surface of our lives. When Freud said, "Anatomy is destiny," he was, of course, referring to gender. But we now understand that anatomy is destiny in many more ways than that. Paraphrasing Freud, we might rightfully say, too, that "posture is destiny."

Jack was a dramatic example of the way in which "posture is destiny." Needless to say, his posture attracted hostility and aggression wherever he went. He was completely bewildered by this and thought that the world was out to get him. What Jack experienced as "fate" was simply the voice of his body's unconscious, trying over and over again to be heard—and finally drawing to him what he kept repressed and split off. For Jack, anatomy was destiny because he was anatomically dragging his past into his present. And as a result, he kept creating the same future, over and over again.

And so it was for Garth. His shallow breathing and tight belly, his frozen eyes and joints, the deadness and lack of life force in his body— all of these habitual and "locked-in" reponses to fear chronically perpetuated the original mental states that had long ago evoked them. They kept Garth deeply separated from life. They insured that he continued to drag the past into the present and the future. To paraphrase the epigraph to this chapter, the flux of everything throbbed on and on, but Garth heard nothing. How could he, when not once had he even heard the sound of his own breathing?

Even when there was nothing to fear, Garth's underlying mental state was awash with fear and contraction, because his body's posture mechanically and biochemically elicited it. Terror, rage, and grief were the unacknowledged waters he swam in. Fear was how the world looked to him. He was somehow deeply split off from life, from the life of his body, from the life of his breath. I did not yet know Garth well enough to know exactly how, but I was sure that his unconscious posture was creating his destiny over and over again, and that he had come to yoga as a way of breaking through a cycle that had left him feeling trapped.

Try as we might to "transcend" the voice of the body through intellect, sheer willpower, or, in Garth's case, spirituality, the subterranean power of our unconscious postures will always hold sway. The deep patterning of the body will undermine our most elaborate rationalizations, ideas, hopes, and fantasies. The entire superstructure of our adult lives is underlain by the primal language of our postures.

The primary genius of yoga lies precisely in its recognition of the critical role of the body in the development and transformation of character. Most spiritual paths begin with what yogis call the "mental bodies"—thoughts and feelings—moving us directly to meditation, contemplation, scriptural study, or prayer. Yogis took a radical step in moving the entry point of spiritual practice right to the body. The yogic traditions therefore bring our attention directly to the annamayakosha (the physical body)—understanding it to be the doorway to the more subtle interior worlds.

BELONGING TO THE HUMAN RACE

One evening I risked asking Garth a question that had long been on my mind. "Why is yoga so important to you? I mean, what does it do for you?" For a split second I saw the deer in the headlights again. Then, he nodded, staring up at the ceiling. "I'll have to think about that."

I didn't get the answer that evening. But about a week later, Garth handed me a piece of paper. He had written an essay about yoga, and what it meant to him. Garth had written:

When I was a kid, I used to secretly believe that I came from some mysterious tribe that lived on another planet. I was not a real human being like my friends or my stepsister. I had this fantasy that someday I would find my real tribe. I used to pretend that in my real world I was a prince. And when I returned home, there would be rejoicing. There would be a crown. I would be adored. I would belong.

It's the strangest thing. I don't really believe this anymore, obviously. But one day I discovered that I was thinking of my yoga spot—you know, that spot in the Forest Room where I always do my yoga—as the link that connected me with my tribe again. Like, I could be beamed up from this particular spot on the carpet. That it was auspicious somehow. That my tribe recognized the connection. So, I guess telling you this story is just a way of saying that I feel deeply attached to my yoga practice. I feel good after yoga. I have my best thoughts. I eat better. I sleep better. I calm down in yoga. Yoga is my medicine.

Through the course of the next several years, I got to know Garth well, and I learned a lot about the particular posture that he embodied. I began to see less dramatic versions of this same postural signature in others, in my work with yoga both on and off the mat. Eventually, I understood that Garth's posture in life is an archetypal human pose: it is the posture of the hated child.[1]

THE POSTURE OF THE HATED CHILD

Garth had been born into an upwardly mobile Chicago banking family. Garth's father had been divorced from his first wife and had married a much younger woman. In many ways a child herself, his new wife had desperately wanted a baby. But, as it turned out, she had wanted only her idealized image of a baby. The real experience of a cesarean birth and of the baby itself—messy, smelly, needy, demanding, completely dependent—was another thing altogether. After several painful and hysterical months of wrestling with the newborn, she had relegated Garth's care to a series of nannies and nurses. Garth grew up believing that he had been produced simply to give his father an heir to the family name. He felt hated and resented for being needy and for actually "disfiguring" his mother, as she would later say to him.

The child who enters this kind of environment takes in a very difficult message with his mother's milk: I have no right to exist. I should not be taking up space in the world. He lives with a profound, but often unconscious, sense that he does not belong in the world.

The hated child introjects, or takes in whole, the rejection of his own life force and self-expression. In an attempt to work out a solution with his caregivers that allows him to get what he can, he must take a tragic position vis-à-vis his own life force: He begins to stop living in order to preserve his life.[2] In order to shut down his apparently offensive "neediness," he learns early on to disconnect from the most basic of life processes—the body, feelings, intimacy, food, and nature itself. For the hated child the world is not a safe place. He cannot trust others, himself, the community, or life itself.

Garth told me one evening about an enduring memory from childhood. He is sitting alone and perfectly still in a large, beautifully furnished room, on an elegant and fragile Victorian chair. He is trying not to breathe, trying not to take up any space in the room, trying to be good. He remembers wondering to himself, "How small can I get?"

Physically, the hated child will do his best not to take up space in the world. This results in very much the kind of picture that I saw with Garth: The life force is blocked, restricted, and mechanical. The breath is restricted. There is often a split between thinking and feeling, which shows up as chronic tension in the neck and at the base of the skull. The eyes will be disconnected and unresponsive, as the child attempts not to see. Joints are frozen, and there is often a deep twisting away from the visceral experience of life.

The hated child believes that he will be annihilated by feelings if he lets them move through him. The false self created in order to survive the ordeal of being hated is a brittle and fragile compromise. It is deeply threatened by alive, spontaneous self-expression. The child locked in this compromise allows himself very little positive or negative feeling. Anger and rage, grief and depression must be denied at all costs, for they threaten the entire structure. The hated child must turn away from life and avoid, at all costs, meeting it head on.

So where will the hated child live? Where is there any modicum of safety? The hated child may learn, as Garth did, to live entirely in his head—in a world of rationality that is walled off from disturbing feelings. As an adult, he may find that he can withdraw into activities that offer worldly accomplishment while avoiding intimacy, feelings, and the complicated emotional lives of others.

Because his very right to exist is always in question, the hated child cannot be bad, cannot risk being obnoxious, cannot be big. Ah, but he can be spiritual. Being spiritual may offer the perfect cover, indeed, for it may involve being transparent, not taking up space, and being not just good, but especially good. Because the hated child may feel especially bad, he may need to appear especially good—the all-giving, perfectly responsive child without any offending sharp edges.

The hated child may, more than any other version of the false self, begin to feel and appear as he should appear. He may become the ultimate "as if" child, denying his angry feelings, his grief, his terror, becoming an idealized version of himself. His false self may be built around being accepting and understanding of others. Because he has dissociated feelings and thoughts, he can live in a brittle kind of way with his spiritual false self. And in his few forays into intimacy, he always attempts to offer to others what he did not get for himself. Unfortunately, this is precisely what he cannot give.

RECONNECTING WITH THE LIFE FORCE

Although he never would have put it in these terms, with the help of yoga, Garth was methodically creating the precise qualities of transformational space he would need in order to recover and to reunite with his authentic "tribe"—which was, of course, the human race.

The first need of the hated child is safety, and so it was with Garth. He had been scared out of the body. He had developed an overweening concern with security, which showed up as highly charged concern over safety in the environment. Garth's house, which held his admittedly valuable computer equipment, was a veritable fortress of high-tech security. He didn't need locks, however, as much as he needed an environment in which he felt safely held and soothed. To his great credit, he had found this. He had found his own little corner of the yoga class, where he was surrounded by safe and caring others.

The next issue for the hated child is trust—trusting himself, others, the community, and, finally, trusting life itself. Over his first two years of involvement with yoga, and with our community, it was clear that

Garth had begun to feel safe enough to risk little experiments in trust, both on the yoga mat and off. He had begun to develop some tentative friendships. He was, for the first time in his life, having a sense of belonging.

One evening Garth showed up for yoga class with a brand-new outfit—sweatpants, and a sweatshirt that said "Plays Well with Others." When I met his eyes, he showed a momentary shy smile and then went seriously back into his posture. He knew that he had arrived someplace new. He belonged. He was savoring his belongingness.

All of this was beginning to appear in Garth's yoga postures. I had noticed for months that Garth was particularly enjoying the standing postures—especially the mountain, the warrior, the triangle, and the standing bow. He told me that he liked the sense of feeling his feet in firm connection with the ground. For the first time in his life, he said, his whole body "felt strong." He could breathe deeply at moments. His arms and legs began to have energy in them, and there was even a sense of energy emanating out of his core.

Garth began to calm down. He was more and more present in his spot. At one point I noticed that he wasn't bringing his notebook to class anymore. His whole body would now light up in certain postures. And I noticed that he held them longer than anyone else.

One evening at dinner, Garth told me about a "strange phenomenon" that had happened to him that afternoon in class, while he was in a long holding of the warrior. He had begun to feel very dizzy. His heart began to race and his chest felt "full of heat and energy." He felt, he said, as though he was going to pass out. Finally, he stopped doing the posture and lay down. As we talked about what had happened, it was clear that Garth had experienced a wave of intense feelings— perhaps sadness, perhaps rage. His breathing had become very ragged, and he had attempted to choke back these overwhelming feelings that he didn't even recognize.

This was the outward and visible sign of a major shift in Garth's practice. Garth was daring to reconnect with feelings—with the subterranean life of his energy body. "This is actually good news," I said. "After all, yoga is really about learning to be present for these kinds of feelings and sensations. You know you can trust your body, you can trust the wisdom of this energy that's moving in you."

For years, Garth had heard me talking about the energy body, life force, and prana. But until this point in his practice, prana had been just a word, a concept. He was now beginning to experience it.

PRANA AND THE ENERGY BODY

Prana is life force—the stuff of those million, zillion stars circling and exploding. Human beings receive it directly into the body through the air. We take it in in other ways as well—through live foods such as fresh fruits and vegetables, through fresh water, through living, breathing trees and vegetation, and, if we're open, through the love of other people and other creatures. We probably take it in in more mysterious ways, too, I think—through music, and the sound of inspiring words, and perhaps through beautiful sights.

Yogis discovered beneath the physical structures of the body an interpenetrating and underlying subtle sphere of reality, which they called the energy body or the pranamayakosha (literally, the sheath of vital airs). The very nature of this subtle structure is movement, flow, change. Over the centuries, and particularly after the advent of hatha yoga in medieval India, adepts developed a precise anatomy of this energy body.

Yogis found the pranamayakosha to be replete with thousands of invisible channels, or *nadis*, through which prana flows, energizing and sustaining all parts of the physical and energy structure. Most of the fascinating yogic diagrams of the energy body make the nadi system look much like our circulatory system, or nervous system, but much more dense. While Western science has mapped out about six thousand nerves in the nervous system, yogis generally agree that the prana body contains at least seventy-two thousand nadis. This astonishingly detailed description of the nadis was apparently mapped out in deep states of meditation and was confirmed over and over again by hatha yogis. (Some ancient texts go even further, and supply us with maps of 350,000 nadis.)

Of the seventy-two thousand energy channels widely agreed upon, there are fourteen major nadis, and just three with which we need to be concerned. All three of these major nadis originate at the base of the spine and move upward through the body. Two of them, the *ida* and *pingala*, crisscross back and forth as they ascend along the area of the spinal column and find their end points in the left nostril (*ida*) and the right nostril (*pingala*) respectively. The third, the shushumna nadi (or central channel) moves up from the base of the spine and then divides at the level of the larynx into an anterior and posterior portion at the *brahmarandra* (or cavity of *brahman*), which corresponds to the ventricular cavity in the physical body.[3]

Many Western students of energy are now loosely familiar with the term chakra, or energy wheel. According to hatha yogis' maps of the subtle body it is precisely the junctions of the major nadis—ida, pingala, and shushumna—with the spinal column that give rise to these chakras, or particularly powerful energy vortices. As the spokes of a wheel radiate outward from the central hub, so the nadis are said to radiate outward from these central chakra hubs to other parts of the body.

Not surprisingly, perhaps, the location of the chakras correlates directly with major centers of activity in the anatomy of the physical body, occurring at precisely the locations of major nerve plexuses, or clusters. The sacral nerve plexus, for example, corresponds with the first chakra, the hypogastric plexus with the second, and then the solar plexus, cardiac plexus, and pharyngeal plexus, and so forth continue up the spinal column. Since yogis did not use dissection, they didn't know about the anatomy of the nervous system, but only about the energy system that underlies it. As it turns out, their observations were physiologically accurate.

Interestingly, too, the energy centers and pathways discovered in the yogic tradition correspond remarkably well with similar energy pathways described in other cultures—as widely varied as the Chinese in their system of acupuncture and the Hopi Indians in North America, as well as current energy research by some Western scientists.[4]

Yogis believe that this energy body is deeply intelligent, possessing what Chogyam Trungpa Rinpoche called "basic intelligence." In prana inheres the intelligence of life itself. Much of yoga practice is about learning to develop awareness of and trust in the wisdom of the energy body.

As yogis learned to experience the energy body directly and to map the flow of its major currents, they made another fascinating discovery: the breath has an immediate impact on the flow of prana through the nadis. More than anything else, it is breathing that builds and regulates the flow of prana in the human body. On the gross level, the breath physically sustains and supports the metabolic processes of all parts of the body. The very life of the body's tissues is created by, and is dependent on, the process of breath. But the breath has a more subtle function. Breathing regulates, balances, opens, controls, and channels the flow of prana in the subtle body. The major receptor sites for prana in human beings are in the nostrils. The rate, depth, balance, and regularity of the breath directly determines the quality of energy flow in the prana body. The flow of breath directly shapes the pattern of energy flow that underlies and sustains the physical body.

THE EMOTIONAL BODY: AN ASPECT OF PRANAMAYAKOSHA

The aspect of the energy body with which most of us have direct, daily experience is the "emotional body." Janet is sitting in traffic, and suddenly realizes that it's slowed to barely a crawl. Traffic is backed up for miles. She's going to be late for her important ten o'clock meeting. Suddenly feelings begin to wash over her. Energy moves. Adrenaline pumps. Within seconds she's breathing hard. Her mind is racing.

While we know that feelings are in some sense just physical, biochemical events in the body, we experience them as more than that— as energy experiences that are "interior to" the physical body. Yogic technology confirms this experience. A feeling, in the yogic view, lies midway between the physical body and the mental body. It is an energy phenomenon that interfaces with both. The nature of feelings very much partakes of the qualities of the prana body. They are constantly flowing, constantly in motion, and we often experience them as wavelike or pulselike in nature.

In considering the emotional body, it might help to conjure up the image of a small child—an infant, or even a toddler who has not been inhibited in her self-expression, or terrified or abused in any way. In the child, we can see directly the close connection between the emotional-energy body and the physical body. The physical body, not yet fully formed, is remarkably transparent, and the energy body shows right through, like one of those clear plastic anatomical bodies from tenth-grade science class. With the infant, especially, the energy body is amazingly transparent.

Emotions that move through the child are fluid and labile. The colors and volume of feelings are constantly changing. The child holds on to nothing—she experiences anger, hurt, joy, exuberance, and back to anger again, within minutes. The child does not yet know how to suppress, repress, control, or focus this flow of emotional energy, so it just moves through unblocked. We watch this display and it connects with something deep in our own experience. Our faces contort and our eyes open wide as we attempt to connect with this little energy creature, this little reflection of our own energy experience. Suddenly we're making sounds and flowing and "ga-ga-gooing" and entering into a moment of unfettered energy expression with the child. Then we remember ourselves and look around to see who is watching us.

Let's go back to Janet in the traffic jam—a more adult energy experience. In the yogic model, rather than beginning to work directly with the restless and racing mind that arises in Janet's stressful situation, we might suggest that she begin by working directly with her energy body—through the breath. Janet's breath is the "switching station" between her inside and outside, and if she works skillfully with it she can begin to integrate the waves of energy roiling through her body as she sits in her car. As her energy body is calmed, her restless mind, too, will quiet. The key for Janet in this situation is breath.

PRANA AND THE WAVE OF BREATH

Yogis describe the breath as lying precisely at the boundary between the body and the mind. Breath is seen as the bridge to the energy body and to the emotional body, which is an aspect of it. This is hardly surprising. We all have experienced the breath as a direct link to some aspect of our inner world. Most of us have experienced the shallow breath of terror, or the long deep sighs of melancholy. We will have experienced the attempt to control our breath in order to choke back tears and sobs. Or perhaps we've noticed the tender attunement of our breath with a lover as we sleep.

The body's breathing apparatus is the only physiological function that is both voluntary and involuntary. It lies at the boundary between the conscious and the unconscious. Breath connects the inside of the body with the outside world—taking the outside world in and expelling the inside world out.

The breath's position as a kind of "switching station" between the physical body and the energy body is exemplified by the role of the diaphragm, the primary muscle of respiration. The muscles of the body are of two primary types—skeletal muscles, which are striated and under voluntary control, and smooth muscles, which make up our internal organs, not usually thought to be under our conscious control. The diaphragm, unlike any other muscle in the body, is a semistriated muscle and, as such, it partakes of both the conscious and unconscious functioning of the body.

When the breath is fully open, relaxed, and free, and when all of the breathing apparatuses—lungs, diaphragm, muscles of the rib cage and chest—are unconstricted in their movements, we have full access to our internal emotional experience. This pattern of breathing is called "abdominal-diaphragmatic breath" because the wave of breath moves unobstructed through the lower abdomen, the midlung, and the top of the lung. It is characterized by a slow, rhythmic rate of respiration, with a large "tidal volume" of air. Yogis call this the "full yogic breath." It is, essentially, the normal human breath—the breath with which the healthy infant breathes.

Because the breath is so intimately connected with the emotional body, any attempt to inhibit awareness of feelings, sensations, and thoughts is immediately reflected in the breath. All defensive maneuvers involving false-self functioning inevitably involve some suppression of the breath, because they require dissociation from the emotional body. Garth's childhood wish to disappear was profoundly reflected in his breathing. He could not bear to let the wave of breath move naturally through his body, and so his breath was chronically held, shallow, restricted.

There are a multitude of ways in which full breathing can be restricted, and Garth was using all of them. The most common is called "chest breathing" or "thoracic breathing"—which is the body's automatic response to fight or flight and to all sorts of overwhelming stress. In traumatic situations, as we all have experienced, the diaphragm is constricted, and we breathe only partway down into the lungs. The lower lobes of the lungs are then split off from the breath, and there is an uneasy sense of the breath not being fully satisfying. The rate of breath is somewhat more rapid and irregular, and there is a much lower "tidal volume" of air than in normal breathing. "Chest breathing" may be accompanied by raised shoulders and contraction of the chest. Shallow breathing can also affect the voice, by narrowing the throat and thereby heightening the choke response.

Inhibition of full abdominal-diaphragmatic breath immediately cuts us off from feelings. But it also cuts us off from prana—and deeply depletes the life force in the body. An increased reliance on chest breathing to supply the body's oxygen requirements produces chronic muscle tension in the chest and abdomen, but that's only the beginning. It also increases cardiopulmonary stress, increases blood sugar and lactate levels, increases our perception of pain, decreases oxygen to the heart and brain, inhibits transfer of oxygen from hemoglobin to tissues, and increases our sense of fatigue.

The differences between deep diaphragmatic breathing and chest breathing are significant, both to the physical body and to the energy body. Abdominal breathing can increase the amount of air we take into the lungs by 600 percent—and this makes a huge difference in the oxygenation of tissues throughout the entire body. While humans can live for long periods without food or water, tissues begin to die almost immediately when deprived of oxygen.

The impact on the nervous system is similarly powerful. While chest breathing stimulates the production of shorter, more "restless" beta waves in the brain, full diaphragmatic breath stimulates the longer, slower alpha waves associated with relaxation and calm mind states. The slow, even, and deep quality of full abdominal-diaphragmatic breath leads to relaxation of the chest muscles and creates a calm and relaxed state of mind.

Yogis understood that even in the absence of any immediate stressors, "disturbed breathing," or thoracic breath, all by itself could perpetuate or recreate a state of sympathetic nervous system arousal, causing anxiety states, panic, and fear reactions. Because respiratory movements by the chest are biologically and instinctually tied up with the emergency responses of fight or flight, they automatically tend to stir up these feelings.

"Yoga postures done with conscious breathing," said Bapuji, "are ten times more powerful than they otherwise might be." Because the breath is the switch that integrates the emotional-prana body with the physical body, postures done with conscious breathing open parts of the body that may have long been shut off from the life force. And when the wave of breath moves into these exiled areas, the results can sometimes be instantly dramatic. The wave of breath opens our emotional body and through it we can experience a deep reintegration of exiled sensations, feelings, thoughts, and memories. This is precisely what was happening to Garth in the warrior pose. The breath, in its role as switching station, had opened Garth to his energy body and to a world of feelings long denied.

THE PRACTICE OF BEING PRESENT FOR EXPERIENCE

Garth and I were sitting at dinner one evening after class. He had just had another catharsis in the yoga class. A wave of energy had arisen for him in the bow pose. He felt the muscles of his chest ripple and dramatically open. Feelings began to overwhelm him. For a moment he felt dizzy, but he let himself stay present with it. He stopped doing the posture and lay for a moment on his belly. The rippling deep in the musculature of his chest turned into raw feeling. It was sadness. It was grief. Just for a moment, he stopped himself from choking it back. He let himself sob quietly. Afterward he lay still. He felt much better—quiet, present, soft.

As we talked together, it was clear that Garth understood what a triumph he had just experienced. He was present that evening, not nearly so much in his head as usual. He was beginning to penetrate the real secret of yoga—the practice of being present for experience.

Through yoga, Garth had found an orderly, safe, contained technique for making controlled forays into his emotional world, into the prana body, into his insides. To the extent that we were scared out of our bodies, we, like Garth, will have difficulty trusting the wisdom of the prana body—trusting life itself. The first task, in that case, is to learn to have a full experience of feelings in the body, and to learn to tolerate the depth, range, and realness of this life force moving in us.

Yogis discovered that human beings experience prana in the form of a wave—a wave of energy, sensation, feelings. In order to learn to attune to the wisdom of the prana body, we need to learn how to "ride the wave," how to be present for the wavelike movement of energy—acknowledging, experiencing, and bearing the inner world of sensation.

In my second year at Kripalu, I had learned a simple but reliably effective technique to unlock the wisdom of the energy body. I took the opportunity of our talk that evening to teach Garth this yogic-based practice designed to use the breath to help integrate physical, emotional, and energy experience. It is a five-part technique that cultivates the witness consciousness of the body and helps us remain present for the experience of the wisdom of the prana body. It very neatly integrates all of the major aspects of the witness—choiceless awareness, equanimity, and transcending opposites.

"It's so simple, Garth," I said. "But amazingly effective. There are five simple steps: breathe, relax, feel, watch, allow.[5] So, for example, when you hit that wave of energy in your bow pose this evening, here's how you might use it. As the wave of energy arises, begin to breathe consciously—full yogic breath. Intentionally relax your muscles as much as you can, then begin to actively feel, and explore the sensations and feelings that are arising. Watch—shift to the witness, to choiceless awareness, not choosing for or against anything. And finally, just allow the waves of energy to flow, to move, to breathe. Let it all move through you without pushing it away or trying to control it in any way."

"OK," said Garth, writing it all down. "Breathe, relax, feel, watch, allow."

"I'll tell you a story about one of the first times I used it," I said, "just to show you how it can go."

RIDING THE WAVE WITH MARK

Not long after I learned the technique, I told Garth, I went to the hospital to visit my friend Mark, who was dying of AIDS. I hadn't seen Mark for quite a few months, but I wasn't prepared for how different he would look. After many months of wasting, and a second bout of pneumonia, he looked more than anything like a corpse—just barely breathing. He was asleep as I entered the room, and I felt a wave of sadness erupt from deep down in my belly. Almost in the same instant that I felt the wave of feeling begin to emerge, I could feel myself choking it back. Could I let him see this? I decided to take some time to be with this feeling before encountering Mark, because I wasn't sure how it would be for him to have me "riding that wave" in his presence. He hadn't seen me; I could still leave without being noticed. I really didn't want to have to choke this back. I know that as soon as I start choking back feelings, I begin to feel less real. I sensed that Mark needed me to be real. I needed to be real for myself, too. I walked down through the lobby and out into an adjacent park, where I found a bench.

I began to soften my belly, and to take long, slow, deep diaphragmatic breaths. The breath touched into a well of sadness, whose intensity surprised me. Mark and I had been lifelong friends, roommates at Amherst, best buddies since. I loved him deeply, and the vastness of my grief scared me a little. I could feel the temptation to "get off this wave." Part of me didn't want to feel this, and I considered for a moment getting back up and going upstairs.

I began to coach myself in the five-step practice of riding the wave. "OK, breathe. Relax. Feel. Watch. Allow." As I breathed down, it felt dark, desolate, empty, and very, very old, somehow, like some ancient cave I had entered. As I consciously relaxed the muscles of my belly and chest, the wave of feeling began to increase, and I coached myself: "Just let it wash through you. Feel it." I moved my awareness into the well of feeling. It was way down deep in my belly. There was a tight band around my diaphragm, which seemed to be holding it back, and another around my brow. I decided to allow that to be there, rather than to struggle with it. I just moved toward it all with my awareness.

And then at a certain moment, as I simply breathed and allowed it to be there, I fell headlong into a well of feeling. "Allow. Allow. Allow," I repeated to myself. At a certain point I let go. The band around the diaphragm burst, and I began to sob. Long, deep, body-racking sobs. This went on for some time. The experience of relief was profound. Every cell in my body was experiencing it. And as I sobbed, images came to me of all the friends I had lost in recent years, mostly to AIDS. I thought of Mark's family, who had befriended me in college, I thought of my friend Karen, at the same time dying of cancer in another city. I thought of my grandmother, whom I had seen in a hospital bed ten years earlier looking much the same way Mark did today.

As the sensations and waves of sobbing began to ebb, there was a deep emotional connection to my friends, to Mark, to my grandmother, to Karen, to the suffering of all beings. My heart was glowing. It felt so good to feel my heart, to feel connected with these beings whom I loved so much. I ran through them one by one in my mind, and my heart's connection to each one felt very alive. I felt gratitude for their being, for their love, and for being human beings together, painful as it is.

As I sat on the bench with the warm afternoon sun on my face, I felt extremely peaceful. Transformed in some way, cleansed and released. I felt esteem and warm love for myself, too, and in a real way finally ready to be with Mark. In retrospect, I think it would have been quite alright with Mark if I'd "ridden the wave" in his presence, but I'm not sure I could have done it. My body wanted to choke it all back, not to be so vulnerable in this glassed-in room with nurses about. So, I did it the way I best could.

I sat with Mark most of the afternoon. We talked about halcyon school days at Amherst, the triumphs and tragedies of our lives since, and we acknowledged that we each held part of each other's life that no one else could hold. We cried together about his impending death. I saw Mark only once after that, and he was too sick to really talk. This, then, had been our leave-taking of one another.

RIDING THE WAVE: THE TECHNIQUE

Suddenly, I realized that what had begun as a teaching story for Garth had unwittingly turned into a deep, personal sharing. But as I looked up, I could tell that he had stayed right with me. We sat together quietly for a few moments, our shared silence highlighting the intimacy of the moment.

I took a couple of deep breaths, and eventually, we returned to our examination of "riding the wave." I noticed that Garth had written down the five stages of the technique in his notebook, so I went back to them, one at a time, and gave him a little more detail.

1. Breathe. The first step in the process of connecting with the wisdom of prana is conscious breathing—using the full yogic breath, or diaphragmatic breathing. The breath immediately penetrates the frozen structure of the false self. Says the poet Lao Tsu:

> *The softest of stuff in the world*
> *Penetrates quickly the hardest.*
> *Insubstantial, it enters*
> *Where no room is.*[6]

Anything that brings us back to the switching station of breath has the potential to loosen our identification with the gross body and to heighten our connection with the prana body. What happens when we redirect our attention to breath is that we immediately enter the world of energy, of movement, of arising and passing away, of constant change. There is no distance to travel to this world. We are right there. The technique of riding the wave both evokes this level of experience and helps us to be with it more and more fully.

Since the breath is the switch that integrates the emotional-prana body with the physical body, conscious breathing opens parts of the body that may have long been shut off from the life force. And when the wave of breath moves into these exiled areas, the results can sometimes be instantly dramatic, as they were, for example, in Garth's cathartic experiences in postures. The wave of breath opened his emotional body and he experienced a deep reintegration—sobbing, release, insight, relaxation.

2. Relax. Muscular tension in the body can help to inhibit the flow of energy, sensation, and feeling, keeping areas of the body defended against the wave of energy. While intentionally riding the wave it is usually best to find a comfortable posture that allows full, deep breathing and an open chest and heart, a posture into which the body can relax and keep relaxing.

The most effective area to begin relaxing is usually the belly. I have found it helpful to repeat as a mantra, "Soft belly." It's so simple. In the midst of the waves of life just soften the belly. This is a brilliant device, because when we think "soft belly," we immediately soften our breathing, and take deep, diaphragmatic breaths. This automatically shifts our entire energy experience, cutting through obsession. It grounds us. We can feel energy flowing all the way down to the lower part of the body, to our feet and legs. Suddenly, what appear to be dense and solid thoughts and feelings become permeable to the wave of energy. They're broken up. They become transparent. They move. We feel alive again.

Full yogic breath will itself help the muscles relax and will automatically cut through any fight-or-flight response. Areas of the body that continue to hold tension and constriction—like my diaphragm in the example with Mark—and unconscious visceral attempts to choke back intense sensation and feelings will begin to become obvious. We can move our awareness directly there, to explore, and to consciously relax as much as possible.

As the wave of breath and energy builds in intensity, we will surely want to get off the wave, and we may repeatedly tense up in order to defend against it. We must remember that the tension of the false self is chronic and unconscious, and that it constantly works against the spontaneous energy of prana. We must, therefore, consciously remember to relax and to keep relaxing, in order to stay with the wave.

3. Feel. Feeling in this technique is an active state. It does not mean just "having feelings," it means moving actively toward the sensations, the energy, the emotions, and into them. We "breathe into them," as if we could send breath right into their epicenter. We develop the acuity of our awareness so that we can begin to feel the whole range of sensations—their color, their texture, their intensity, their mood.

Actively feeling means turning our attention minutely toward our moment-by-moment experience—dropping what we think about what is happening, our evaluations and judgments about it, and becoming fully absorbed at the level of sensation, feeling, and energy. Learning to focus deeply on sensation in this way develops our capacity to be with sensation and feeling. We develop curiosity, so that we're interested in the exact topography of the feeling. "Where in the body is the feeling most intense? What is the exact texture of the sensation? Are there any patterns of movement?"

This kind of proactive feeling reveals one of the central laws of the energy body: Energy follows awareness. As we bring more awareness to exiled aspects of our energy body, we also open these previously unconscious areas to the flow of prana. Consciousness and energy are deeply linked. More consciousness results in more wave of life.

4. Watch. There can now be a profound and natural shift to witness consciousness, to the zone of neutrality, where we're not choosing for or against any kind of experience, but just being with experience exactly as it is. As we become absorbed in the witness, we're free both to participate in and to stand apart from our experience. We no longer fight with what is. As we drop into witness consciousness, we may experience some intuition arising from deep within our cells—a knowing that cannot be experienced through the mind alone. "Watching" is a special place we can stand vis-à-vis our experience, where we just let life be the way it is. In the zone of the witness, our attention is focused on "how is it?" rather than "why is it?" or "do I like it?"

It is important to remember that the watcher, or observer, is also the coach of the entire experience, the part of us that remains unidentified with the "problem" and remains able to coach us to stay on the wave of energy. It is the abiding voice that is constantly repeating the mantra "breathe, relax, feel, watch, allow." It is the still point at the center of the storm of energy, and it is the seat of our trusting in the wisdom of energy.

5. *Allow.* When we don't try to control our energy experience, we're free to surrender to the wave of sensation, of feeling, and of energy. In these remarkable moments of freedom, we can let life as it is touch us, because at our core we know that "everything is already OK." We know that the energy moving in the prana body is intelligent. We know that it is moving in just the right way for healing and full integration to happen. We relinquish our resistance. We let the whole, natural process happen to us. Somehow, we trust that all we need to do is to support the process in these simple ways, and it moves itself to full integration. The key to the fifth step is this: We don't have to make the wave of life happen. We can just let it happen. As we learn this kind of trust in the process, our capacity to ride the waves of life increases dramatically.

An essential aspect of the fifth step is this: we must allow the process to happen without necessarily understanding it. Insight may come later, but it will come always simply as a by-product of being present for experience. In this final step, there is a quality of surrender, of "falling into the gap" where life can change us. There can be an exhilarating sense of freedom when this happens, a deep letting go of our "grip" on life. This kind of surrender requires a willingness to be changed. It involves, too, a willingness to trust life, to keep the focus of our awareness on energy in motion instead of on trying to understand what is happening. Prana is intelligent, after all.

GARTH: LEARNING TO BELONG IN
THE PHENOMENAL WORLD

For months after our talk about being present for experience, I watched Garth's little corner of the room as he practiced riding the wave. At times I could practically see him mouthing the words "breathe, relax, feel, watch, allow." There were days when his spot came alive with energy and focus. His notebook was a thing of the past. Quantum equations were happening in his body, not only in his mind. Then, of course, there were other days when the old Garth was back. Lifeless. No prana. Arms and legs flailing.

The simple technique of "riding the wave" became for Garth a transitional object—just as *The Cloud of Unknowing* had been for Marti, my friend from seminary days (about whom I spoke in chapter 2). It became the bridge that Garth used to cross over from isolation and separation to relationship with the phenomenal world—the world of the senses, of nature, of the heart and the body. It became a mantra, the boat that Garth rowed as he traversed the river of feelings.

The first step in Garth's healing process was to begin to learn to identify himself as his body, his feelings, and the life within—rather than just his mind, his achievements, and his spirituality. He had to learn that his life force did not threaten his life. It was his life.

Garth's false self, his hyperintellectualized and hyperspiritualized self, defended him in every way against the spontaneous flow of prana. Recall that the false self is primarily a defense against energy, a strategy for keeping prana from threatening the fragile structure of the alienated self. For Garth, this defense manifested on the yoga mat as rigidity, inflexibility, and lifelessness.

One of the most significant early "marker events" in Garth's healing was his spontaneous development of the witness: He began to notice when he was not "at home," when he had "checked out," as he put it. I encouraged him to notice without judgment, to let it be OK that he had checked out. It was important that Garth's defenses be respected, not assaulted. If he needed to check out because a feeling state had become too intense, that was OK. Increasingly, Garth began to identify with his own defensive structure. Rather than a stranger, and an intruder, it became his friend.

For Garth, the river of feelings inside was a raging one. Integrating it would not be a quick process. The hated child, after all, takes in whole the rejection of his own life force and self-expression. The primitive rage at this self-betrayal and the terror that arises around the whole inner world of feeling and energy are both denied and avoided. Garth, for years, had only allowed himself to see his "good," "spiritual" nature, keeping his rage, anger, and the "infant beast" hidden deeply in the basement of his unconscious.

It was particularly challenging for Garth to let the wave of breath, prana, and awareness descend into his belly, and further down into the pelvis. He found that these areas were opened deeply when he was exploring standing postures—the warrior, the triangle, the mountain. These postures became alternately exhilarating and terrifying. Here he discovered sexual and aggressive feelings, rage, and feelings of power. He began to discover the root chakra, the energy vortex in the prana body from which core strength emanates.

Garth's ego-ideal—the highly spiritual, good, special man, who had no "evil" feelings and wishes—was deeply challenged by the raging river of feelings he began to encounter at his core. He had to learn to trust that he wouldn't be taken over by these inner demons, that, in fact, they weren't demons at all. They were just energy, just life force, just him. Then, he had to learn that this energy was not just OK, but that it was utterly intelligent, awake, divine.

The deepest suffering of the hated child is the failure of attachment—the loss of the life-giving bond with parents and other loved ones. Garth was beginning to allow himself to feel his attachment, his love—for me, for the community, for his friends. He bought himself a Labrador retriever puppy. He began to take better care of himself and his appearance.

Another visible sign of an inward change was Garth's clearly decreasing sense of specialness and perfectionism. He began to make fun of his own spiritual self-image. He had rejoined the human race. And, in particular, he had joined our community.

Most important, Garth began to be able to trust in the wisdom of life itself. He could let himself sink into the waves of energy, emotion, sensation, prana, in his body. He could open the door through the body with conscious breathing, and let the breath penetrate the tightly held structure of his joints, his neck. There was energy again in his eyes, and life in his body. He no longer twisted so much away from life, but was learning to confront it head on. Garth discovered, in his years of yoga, that to live fully is to live inside his body and to communicate from his deep, warm center.

It is through the awareness of breath and prana that we cross the bridge from separation and isolation to belonging and union. As we ride the wave, we know ourselves to be a river of intelligent energy and life—completely spontaneous and vital. As we get a taste for this vitality, we enter "the wave" again and again, learning how to tolerate being with the reality of life moment to moment. We can learn to live on the magnificent edge where anything can happen, where nothing stays the same, where our solid boundaries melt, where we experience the whole field of mind and matter as connected together in one great web of energy. Inside and outside are the same. The flux of everything throbs on and on, and we are part of the throbbing life of the universe.

14

$\mathcal{L}$ISTENING TO THE VOICE
OF THE BODY

Crying only a little bit
is no use. You must cry
until your pillow is soaked!
Then you can get up and laugh,
Then you can jump in the shower
and splash-splash-splash!
Then you can throw open your
window and "Ha ha! Ha ha!"
And if people say, "Hey,
What's going on up there?"
"Ha ha!" sing back, "Happiness
was hiding in the last tear!
I wept it! Ha ha."

—Galway Kinnell,
"Crying"

I was reading in my office, late one evening, when I heard a knock. The door opened, and Bonnie poked her head in.

"Mind if I come in?"

Bonnie, an old friend from Boston, was just finishing up her first weeklong yoga retreat. Her blue eyes beamed prana, and I thought she looked about ten years younger than her forty-three years. She'd brought us each a cup of tea, and we sat for a few moments chatting.

"I'm not the same person I was a week ago," she said. "What did this yoga stuff do to me, Mr. Cope? You guys've bewitched me."

"I don't know what we did to you, but for somebody who had to be dragged kicking and screaming to the yoga mat, you look pretty good."

Bonnie's brother, Michael, also a friend of mine, had paid for this week, as a way to help his sister get a handle on the stress that seemed to be overwhelming her life. Bonnie had received the gift good-naturedly. She had taken a week's leave from her job as an R.N. on a large psychiatric inpatient unit, had arranged for one of her sisters to stay with her teenage son and daughter, and had bought herself some proper yoga togs. She made it known from the beginning, however, that she was a dyed-in-the-wool skeptic. On the evening before the program began, Michael had brought her out from Boston, and after the three of us had dinner together she proceeded to get down on the floor and do the most hilarious parody of yoga postures I've ever seen. Her week had obviously made a dent in her skepticism.

"So tell me about the bewitching part, Ms. Bonnieananda."

Bonnie was eager to tell me about an epiphany she'd had toward the end of the week, after she had learned some basic yoga postures and had had several days to practice entering and holding the very postures she had so convincingly parodied—the mountain, the tree, the cobra, the dog, the boat, and the cat. In the first several days, Bonnie had discovered that she loved all the postures that allowed her to round forward—the rag doll, yoga mudra, the forward bend. She found that her body especially loved to contract into the fetal position. She felt relaxed and soothed—safe. This was a surprise to her.

"So this afternoon, in the final session, the teacher said we could really just listen to our body for a few moments, then go into any posture that was really calling to us. That was easy. I love this thing called the child pose. I just went right into it. Boom. And there I stayed. Couldn't move."

Once she got into the posture—a kind of kneeling, forward-bending fetal position—Bonnie didn't want to leave it. Her breathing slowed down. She dropped into a delicious altered state. For a moment in the posture, she allowed herself to feel how much she wanted to be held and nurtured. As a nurse, she was always holding others. She didn't realize how much she also longed to be held. She could feel herself "crying inside." After holding the posture for a while, Bonnie could feel a shift occur—her belly let go, and she began sobbing quietly, relaxing even more deeply into the posture. When one of the teachers came and rested her hand between Bonnie's shoulder blades, she felt a wave of even deeper grief and longing. Her heart leaped toward that hand. Her sobs deepened. Finally she rolled out of the posture, and allowed herself to be held by the teacher. She cried for what felt like forever, losing herself in vivid body memories of being held in the warm, safe lap of her grandmother.

Bonnie had discovered the archetypal posture of the child. It's no wonder she had a catharsis in it: the posture itself had allowed her access to the neediness she'd spent most of a lifetime pushing away. In the posture, she allowed herself to feel her "skin hunger," her deep longing to be touched, held, and soothed; she felt her longing to be small—to just for once not have to be the big, responsible adult, the nurse, the single parent, always facing life and being responsible for others. As Bonnie surrendered to the child pose, she became aware of all the other people she had been carrying on her back. At the suggestion of the teacher, she let them roll off. It was terrifying to let them go, but she did it for a few seconds.

Out of the subterranean depths of Bonnie's cells, viscera, and muscles came the clearest possible voice, a voice she heard that day as if for the first time. Bonnie believed she would never be the same, because, as she put it, she now knew that she could "trust my body." It was no longer the enemy, holding dangerous longings and vulnerabilities that she had to resist. Bonnie experienced how much her body wanted to wake up, to tell its secrets, to unwind, and to share its suffering. "I know now that my body has a wisdom I don't have in my mind. If I could just learn to trust it more."

She paused for a moment to sip some tea. "I can't even believe I'm talking like this. It's such a cliché. And I'm terrified it'll just wear off when I get home. Will it last? Is it real?"

Good questions. Had Bonnie just experienced a week of peak experiences, altered states that would finally have little impact on her life? Bonnie had mastered no postures. Indeed, she could barely get into many of them. She was a complete neophyte—yet, in some ways, she had received the full benefits of the practice of yoga. What would it mean for her future?

"My God," she said, "what would happen if I let myself practice this stuff all the time? Frightening to even imagine."

As it turned out, Bonnie did begin to "practice this stuff all the time," and eight years later I can write the astonishing story of her love affair with yoga, her transformation, and her fearless reclamation of her true self.

THE DILEMMA OF THE ABANDONED CHILD

Bonnie was an abandoned child.[1] Nothing so dramatic as being left in a cardboard box on somebody's stoop. Rather, Bonnie had been emotionally left by her mother before she was ready. Her body had not drunk deeply enough of the experience of being safely and securely held and soothed. Her skin had not had enough touch. She had not locked eyes with her mother enough, nor been rocked, read to, or cooed at sufficiently. Unlike Garth, Bonnie had been a wanted child, but the emotional merger with her mother had been prematurely interrupted when her mother was hospitalized with depression. The "paradise" of being safely held and soothed was lost. And Bonnie was left still hungry, grieving, bewildered, and, underneath, enraged. In order to survive, she'd stifled much of the natural neediness of infancy and childhood, and she grew up fast. She created a "false self" in which she was highly competent at taking care of others but remained deeply disconnected from her own real visceral sense of need.

At least one out of three students I teach has some deep identification with this form of false self. And how could this not be so in a culture in which parents are so often overwhelmed by divorce, addiction, single parenting, and, most important, their own immaturity and inability to self-soothe? Bonnie was her mother's fifth child in eight years. At the time of her birth, the family had just moved for the fourth time in ten years and its emotional resources were stretched thin. Bonnie's father was an active alcoholic, and though he held down a good job, the family lived in terror of his drinking bouts.

What was it like for Bonnie to be deprived of a complete symbiosis with her mother? And how did she survive the loss? Developmental psychologist John Bowlby demonstrated in his research on attachment that for a while after the emotional loss of the mother, the infant protests and demonstrates her rage and grief. But those feelings themselves are very painful and cannot be sustained for long. Eventually, the infant begins to inhibit the needing response itself. The hunger sensations themselves become the source of the pain. There is a deep withdrawal from those sensations of need. Rather than reaching out to get needs met, the infant contracts inward. Need itself becomes the enemy.[2]

As an infant and toddler, Bonnie had been in a tragic bind. In order to preserve her own life she was forced to shut it down. Her only viable option was to choose depression over expression. Finally this meant a limitation of her life force—limiting her visceral emotional output, or expression, as well as the input, or the reaching out and taking in of emotional nourishment. This kind of shutdown required many different kinds of physical and emotional contractions, which eventually became Bonnie's core unconscious postures. No matter how well Bonnie functioned as an adult, her emotional reality reflected a depleted life force and a state of perpetual mourning and unconscious rage.

THE FALSE-SELF COMPENSATION

In order to survive the bind of the abandoned child, Bonnie had to learn to deny her own needs and neediness. She had to construct a false self that would allow her to function until the process of growth could be started again—until her true self could be properly supported, sustained, evoked, and challenged.

This false-self compromise began to play itself out during Bonnie's childhood, when, in the face of her mother's obvious inability to cope, she took on a caretaking and nurturing role with her three younger sisters. Having denied her own sense of need, Bonnie projected it outward onto others. She identified with need when she saw it outside herself. As a result, she could feel others' needs intensely—or what she imagined were others' needs—and could find some satisfaction in taking care of their needs without facing her own. As an adult, Bonnie became famous for taking care of others. Not only had she constructed a whole professional nursing career around this defensive structure, but she had also become widely known in the extended family and community as a caretaker. Unconsciously, however, Bonnie felt enraged about it. But for obvious reasons, it was a role her family did not want her to change. Like her mother, she could only get her own needs met by the back-door strategies of breaking down under stress, becoming ill, or "putting out her back."

Bonnie also occasionally displaced her emotional hunger onto food, things, substances, and the attention she received for taking care of others. As a result, she felt her life was often out of control as she responded to the strange power of food, alcohol, and drugs. By the time she was in her late twenties, Bonnie had developed a secret eating habit, of which she was quite ashamed. She was at least fifty pounds overweight most of the time. But her bingeing was completely incomprehensible to her. She saw it as a strange and alien symptom that took her over from the outside.

Like all false-self compromises, Bonnie's was unstable and prone to breakdown. The needier she felt, the harder she worked at taking care of others. This intensified her own unconscious rage, and she would begin to binge, then inevitably get sick—walking pneumonia, a disabling back spasm, a flu that lasted all winter. Also, her particular compensation attracted men who wanted to be taken care of. She obliged, and under her care they became less and less functional, until, finally, she could bear it no more, and she had to throw them out. She found support from an entire lineage of women who were using the same strategy—her mother, her sisters. It was only her brother Michael who dared to challenge the strategy over and over again.

THE BODY'S INHIBITION OF NEED

When Bonnie finally landed on the yoga mat, she was aware only that her body was a problem—it hurt much of the time, and it made unreasonable demands on her. When she paid attention, which was infrequently, she sensed that her body was tight, constricted, dense. She sometimes felt unable to breathe. Bonnie was vaguely aware that she had lost her fluidity, her responsiveness, the aliveness she remembered as a child. Years of holding on to a precariously constructed self-image, years of holding on to old pain, years of holding on to her ideas about who she should be had left her in despair. She was known as a savvy, street-smart clinician on the inpatient unit. But as everyone who worked with her knew, she could also be flip, glib, overly tough, and sometimes defensive. Underneath, Bonnie was living with a quiet sense of desperation. She secretly hoped she could live more fully, but she silently assumed she could not, that what she was feeling was just the natural baggage of aging, of loss, and of disappointment.

We now know that the development of character, including the drama of inhibition and adjustment that I have just described, is played out first on the stage of the human body. The false-self compromises literally become structured into the neuromuscular, visceral, even cellular life of the body. They are "the water in which we swim"—quite unavailable to conscious perception. Here are some of the physical markers of Bonnie's shaky compromise with the false self.

~ *Suppression of breath.* Though Bonnie's posture was outwardly good, she was a shallow breather, with a constricted diaphragm. It was clear that the wave of breath was tightly under control. The fundamental expression of all living things is seen in the pulsatory movement of expansion and contraction— taking in and expelling, opening and closing. In humans, the breath is the most basic pulsatory movement. It is impossible to inhibit feelings without interfering with the normal rhythms of the breath. This is often accomplished by hunching the muscles of the shoulders forward, and constricting and shrinking the chest.

~ *Abdominal inhibition.* Inhibition of breathing actually begins at the core of the body, in the belly. Contraction of the big abdominal muscles pulls the upper part of the rib cage forward and down, and pulls the pubic bone forward and up, which draws the entire trunk into the fetal posture. This "withdrawal reflex" is the most primitive human response to danger. It automatically inhibits breathing and effectively stops grieving and crying. (Sobbing happens deep in the belly.) It has another important effect as well. By tightening the pelvic muscles between the pubic bone and the coccyx, it puts immense pressure on all of the muscles and organs of the viscera, causing spasm and contraction. In the process, blood flow to the pelvis is inhibited, with the result that life force, sexuality, and a sense of "core strength" in the center of the body are all diminished.[3]

~ *Weak legs.* When the life force in the belly is shut down, this will inevitably be reflected in the hips and legs. Bonnie had lots of problems with her legs—circulation problems, knee problems, and hip problems. When she walked, it was easy to see that she led with her head. Her feet and legs were not solidly connected with the ground.

~ *Tightness in the upper back.* In a very early, unconscious attempt to inhibit the impulse to reach out, Bonnie had developed constriction and deep muscle tension in the upper back, especially between the shoulder blades. This same holding pattern also inhibited the natural aggression, anger, and rage that might be expressed in striking out through the hands, arms, and shoulders.

~ *Locked jaw.* Another common unconscious maneuver to inhibit breathing, as well as grief and fear, is to constrict the jaw muscles and the muscles at the base of the skull. Bonnie's tight jaw was not just a cultural artifact of her Boston upbringing. It was an unconscious bodily defense against the wave of breath, feelings, and life force.

~ *Needy eyes.* Bonnie's eyes betrayed the need that she desperately sought to hide. They were searching, responsive, hopeful, easily hurt. The reaching out that had been inhibited in the rest of her musculature was present in her eyes.

As Bonnie and I sat talking that final evening of her retreat, I was astonished at how quickly yoga had begun to soften the rigid structures of the false self. In her very first week of yoga practice, Bonnie had an experience of cutting through decades of holding on. She reconnected, if only briefly, with the natural, pulsatory wave of life and breath. All she needed was this taste. Like the proverbial horse that smells the barn, she was off and running.

CLEAR SEEING: PENETRATING THE BODY'S UNCONSCIOUS

Soon after her week at Kripalu, Bonnie found a yoga teacher in Boston near the hospital where she worked, and she began to attend class three or four days a week. Over the first six months of practice, her mat gradually became a familiar place, an anchor. She felt safe there— grounded, quiet. Some days she would just take her yoga mat out at home and lie down on it. No postures, just deep relaxation. Her kids knew: "Don't bother Mom when she's on her yoga mat. You'll die!"

Bonnie's commitment to practice represented an extraordinary piece of recovery for a woman healing from the pain of emotional abandonment. First of all, it was time set aside specifically for self-care and self-nurturing. For the first time in her adult life, Bonnie had found a place where she didn't have to override her felt needs and vulnerabilities; on her mat she had moments when she believed that the adult in her could nurture the child. Until now, Bonnie's life had been devoted to denying her early abandonment by attempting to prevent further abandonment at any cost—usually, as it turned out, at great cost to herself. She tried to be good, to do good, to care for others, to be lovable. None of this, finally, really worked to keep the experience of abandonment at bay. Her real work was to acknowledge that the abandonment had already taken place, to grieve this loss, and then to stop abandoning herself.[4] Yoga became one arena in which she could methodically practice not abandoning herself.

Bonnie began to learn some of the rhythms of long-term practice. She found, for example, that she could usually depend on postures to be a clear mirror of her mental state on any given day. Though the postures remained the same, her experience of them was different every time. One day, the camel would be almost a religious experience. She would enter it and find that the muscles between her shoulder blades would relax and melt like butter. Her chest would stretch open, and she could feel her heart. Her body would begin to vibrate and tingle, and her mind would be relaxed and happy. On those days, she was amazed to discover how much of her seemingly physical limitations to stretching and opening were actually in her mind rather than in her body. The next day, she might not even be able to get into the camel. Perhaps her mind would scream "no!" or her body would feel too tight, too grumpy and unwilling.

In the first year or so of her practice, Bonnie sometimes found herself doing postures the way she did life, denying her own real needs, trying to please, focusing on her friends in the class as a way of ignoring herself, playing the clown. After a while, though, she discovered that nobody in the class really needed her to take care of them. Her instructor actually cared about how she was feeling inside, about how the postures felt inside her, and she redirected Bonnie over and over again to her internal world. The class itself became a supportive, sustaining surround of human beings who cared about her and respected her, but who were not overly involved in her life and were not receiving caretaking from her. The class, too, was always there. Every Monday, Wednesday, and Friday. All she needed to do was, as she put it, "suit up and show up."

As Bonnie dropped the need to make her experience be the way she thought it should be, her intuitive mind opened up. She had what she called "aha! experiences." When she stopped trying to do the postures properly, she began to learn how to stop trying to do life so properly, as well. As she forgot her struggle with life and just dropped into the body, she found that answers sometimes revealed themselves. There were little releases, little insights almost every day. She began to feel, on the mat, that she was more and more connected to the beginnings of a real inner life.

Bonnie was discovering that the more she practiced listening to her body, the more clearly her body would speak to her. After decades of learning to override her body's messages, this was a revelation. She found that her attitude was the key: when her body knew she was listening—respectfully, with real curiosity and trust—it would generously reveal its secrets.

Bonnie discovered, too, that her body would speak more clearly as she stopped trying to dominate it. When she practiced postures with no thought of comparing, achieving, proving, or improving, her body would respond. After a while, she decided it was OK to let herself enjoy the postures she felt drawn to—the forward bends, the child pose, all of the postures in which she got to hold herself. She learned to identify with (rather than judge and reject) the defenses in her body, and to appreciate that those physical impulses had in some sense saved her life.

LEARNING AND UNLEARNING

A great deal of the practice of yoga on the mat is about learning and unlearning—exposing and unlearning old habits of perception, and learning to hone the human perceptual potential in altogether new ways. Over the course of long-term practice, this happens in three important ways: developing the instruments of proprioception (body awareness), restoring conscious control to the most refined centers of the brain, and penetrating the deep internal body.

1. Developing the instruments of proprioception. At the beginning of
most yoga classes, I have students simply stand for a moment with their
eyes closed, and I ask them to intentionally scan their body with their
awareness: soles of the feet, ankles, knees, hips, belly, chest, arms,
neck, head, face, crown. Almost everyone who does this finds, usually
to their astonishment, that there are areas of their bodies that are
completely "numb"—that exist completely outside their conscious
awareness. Students often have the unsettling sense that somehow the
"circuits have not been hooked up" to one or another part of the body.
"When I close my eyes, I just can't even seem to find any sensation in
the area of my hips," says one student. Indeed, the circuitry is weak.
In the process of relegating these areas of the body to the unconscious,
the neuropathways into sensation have been underused. The
neuropathways are there as potential, but the brain's skill in intentionally using them has been underdeveloped.

The good news is that our restriction of awareness is learned behavior. It can be unlearned. Yogis have proven that we can learn how to
redirect our awareness into every aspect of our physical life—not just
the musculature and the surface of the body, but the viscera and even
deeper structures of the body as well. And the best news is that in the
process of "hooking up the circuitry" again, we will naturally begin to
remember what the body has forgotten. The intentional practice of
yoga postures has the effect of "re-membering" us—reuniting us with
the lost parts of our self, our experience, and our history.

The science of physiology has coined the term "proprioception" for
the act of receiving and interpreting messages from our own bodies.
Proprioception literally means "our own reception"—and through it we
are able to feel the warmth in our hands as we sit quietly, or the
beating of our hearts, or the burning in a group of muscles that are
chronically in spasm. Through proprioception we are able to discriminate subtle shades of feeling and sensation—to both perceive and in-
terpret stimuli from the field of our own visceral reality. It is the
capacity for proprioception, indeed, that helps us to feel real and
grounded on the earth. When people lose their proprioceptive capacities through diseases of the neuromuscular systems, they often describe
a feeling that they've lost something central to their humanness.

The practice of yoga postures is intentionally designed to develop
our proprioceptive capacities to a level of supernormal refinement.

There is no magic in this. It is simply a matter of training attention. A well-balanced series of postures will systematically open up every area of the body for exploration, giving us a methodical way of scanning the body, and training our attention to penetrate every aspect of it.

When we begin practicing postures, we may notice that our attunement to sensations even on the surface of the body is quite gross. But as we take different areas of the body as objects of our concentration, our capacity to focus attention grows. We rediscover those neuropathways into sensation only through trial and error, but as we discover them we can eventually learn how to use them and bring them under our conscious control. Finally, our perception becomes so refined that we begin to penetrate the surface of the body, the armor of the musculature, and at later stages of the practice the subtlest functioning of the internal organs.

As we train our attention in this way, we'll also begin to notice our postures throughout the day, not just on the yoga mat: Oh, I'm standing here, and I can feel my shoulders hunching forward, pulling me in. What am I feeling? What am I reacting to? Something old? Something in the moment?

Postures have, in themselves, no magic power. Even the most seemingly "advanced" practice, if it is driven by fear, aggression, perfectionism, and unconsciousness, will not automatically create transformation. Postures simply provide a methodical way of training attention, so that movements and areas previously relegated to the "basement" of the primitive brain can be brought into consciousness.

2. *Restoring conscious control to the higher centers of the brain.* Because yoga asanas are not so much about exercise as they are about learning and unlearning, it is not the movement itself, but the quality of attention we bring to the movement that makes postures qualify as yoga. Yoga actually begins to change the body by reeducating the brain. There is a particular way of moving, characteristic of classical posture practice, that heightens our brain's capacity to draw areas of the body's unconscious up into consciousness. Slow, deliberate movement anchors the mind in sensation and allows a deep relearning to happen. Western science has now discovered why this is so. When muscles are moved slowly and consciously, the movement is brought under the control of the most refined aspect of the brain, the neocortex.

We now understand that human beings possess not just one brain, but three brains working in coordination—each brain having evolved out of the earlier, more primitive level. The first level controls essential functions like heart regulation, blood circulation, respiration, locomotion, and reproduction. The second brain layer refines the essential functions of the first, organizing them into greater movement coordination, with more attention to aggressive and defensive actions. The second layer also organizes the whole field of primitive emotions—fear, anger, and sexual desire.[5] When we're acting in involuntary and unconscious ways, the behavior is often being regulated by the lower brains—driven by primal needs and patterns of hunger, greed, and aggression.

The triumph of human functioning, however, is the third layer of the brain, the neocortex, which is the seat of voluntary learning and the source of conscious actions. As human beings mature, more and more control of the sensorimotor system is taken over by the neocortex. Behavior, movement, and adaptation become voluntary and conscious, and less and less driven by regression to involuntary reaction and "override" by the primitive brains.[6]

The refinement of our proprioceptive capacities requires moving the locus of control over the area of concern—the musculature, initially, and later the nervous system, organs, fluids, and subtle body—to the most refined centers of learning in the neocortex. From there, control moves to the seat of witness consciousness, or *buddhi*, a structure in the mind that has not been identified by Western science, but that has been described in detail by several millennia of yogic practitioners.

There are certain ways of practicing on the mat that ensure that this will be so. Interestingly, Patanjali nailed the most important of these almost two thousand years ago: "The posture is steady and comfortable." When the body moves beyond the point of comfortable toleration of sensation, we lose our equanimity—we lose the balance of the mind. When this happens, deeper levels of awareness are no longer possible. The mind becomes restless and dissociated. We move away from experience rather than toward it.

As Bonnie discovered early on, certain components of practice are essential to promote optimal learning and unlearning.[7] These are:

~   *Creating an environment in which concentration is supported.*
    A quiet, uninterrupted space without distractions of any kind,

even music, can be important, especially when concentration is weak.

~ *Moving slowly and deliberately.* When we're untying a complicated knot, we know enough to look carefully first, then gently undo the tangle. A hard yank on the cord will just make the knot tighter.[8] So, too, with the body's knots. Slow, intentional movement creates a kind of absorption in the mind that allows precise internal sensations to be tracked very consciously. This kind of movement keeps awareness centered in the neocortex and works against the body being hijacked by the primitive brains.

~ *Keeping awareness focused on the internal sensations and feelings.* We are interested in the internal experience of the posture, not in trying to recreate some picture from a book. While alignment is important, too much preoccupation with the external experience triggers the false-self complex, which is located in the more primitive unconscious brain. In order to keep attention focused, expectations for achievement and external success must be minimized.

~ *Moving gently without strain.* Straining is extremely counterproductive. It only creates tons of sensory feedback that is really irrelevant to what we're trying to bring under conscious control. It is important to minimize white noise in the system as we're focusing deeply. Therefore, it is best always to keep it simple—to do less rather than more. Part of internal safety comes from monitoring the feeling of the posture in the body. There must be plenty of permission and encouragement to watch and get to know where one's own individual edge is, learning to honor that and not forcing a posture beyond those limits. Forcing will not help the muscles relax. Quite the contrary: if we attempt to voluntarily force a muscle that is involuntarily contracted it will contract even more tightly, finally to the point of spasm.[9]

~ *Cultivating persistence and patience.* In order to relearn deeply wired-in patterns, there must be plenty of repetition, done with consciousness. Effort is brought to bear, in the real practice of yoga, not in forcing complicated and difficult postures, but in doing postures consciously, slowly, and deliberately. This requires the cultivation of patience and strong determination—

but not force. Force and aggression simply override the consciousness that we're trying to create.

3. *Penetrating the deep inner body.* As proprioception becomes refined, awareness begins to penetrate not just the musculature, but the organs, glands, the fluids, and even the bones. This seems odd and unlikely to us Westerners. Our Western medical model is suffused with a split in awareness between the outside of the body and the inside. The outside of the body—the skin, the muscles—is seen as available to awareness and volition. The inside of the body, however, is seen as automatic, reflexive, dark, unfathomable, and primitive—even, for some, unclean.[10] Not only is it repulsive and irrational, but it is outside our volition, and hence outside our responsibility, as well. This attitude allows us to maintain a split—the "outside" as conscious, the "inside" as unconscious. The result is that we can banish feelings we don't want to face to the inside of the body, where they manifest as disease or malaise. Then we are apt to disavow responsibility for them, seeing them as alien invaders.

When Western scientists began to study the feats of yogis, they were, for a time, obsessed with charting and describing the supernormal feats of internal bodily control, control of so-called "involuntary processes." In a famous experiment at the Menninger Clinic, for example, it was documented that Swami Rama was able to slow his heart almost to a stop for significant periods of time and to bring it under conscious control.[11] Such feats are a direct assault on our worldview. Yet, yogis have shown for millennia that our blindness to the insides of the body is just another one of what Deepak Chopra calls our "premature cognitive commitments." Awareness can naturally penetrate even the so-called involuntary organs—the digestive tract, the heart, the lungs—raising their functioning into the control of the higher centers of the brain, and making them conscious and voluntary.

Surprisingly, Swami Rama's feats are not that far beyond the scope of many Westerners' practice. In my own experience, I've found that it is not unheard of for us to develop a level of witness consciousness of the body that is capable of penetrating organ systems. In fact it's quite common with Western yogis who are afflicted with some chronic internal imbalance.

In more advanced practice, awareness of organs becomes an anchor for the mind. When we're involved in any kind of fight or flight reaction, blood, energy, and awareness are diverted from the organ systems to the musculoskeletal systems so we can act quickly and effectively. When we sense and feel our organs, however, the body and breath calm down, anchoring our awareness deep inside. Simply bringing awareness to the soft tissues of the organs counteracts the tension of stress reactions.[12]

REMEMBERING THE FORGOTTEN BODY

Several years into her practice, Bonnie had an extraordinary experience. She happened upon a period of three months one summer when she could practice postures almost every day, in a studio with a small class of other students. After fourteen years on her nursing unit, she had earned a three-month sabbatical, and she decided to take it so she could focus on her yoga practice. That summer, as her attention became increasingly sharp with daily practice, she discovered a tight little ball of energy just behind her right sitz bone, tucked somewhere deep in the middle of her gluteus muscle. Always, when she attuned to her body, she could feel it—tight, throbbing, and aching. It was relentless. For weeks she pushed it away, reacted to it, felt her aversion to it, hated it. Finally, she decided to try another approach. She allowed it to be there. She spoke to it. She explored the whole area around it with her awareness, as she moved through postures. She made friends with this inscrutable voice from her body. She asked it questions: Who are you? What do you want? What do you have to say to me?

One day as she was working in this way, she felt a new layer of unconscious reality emerge into her awareness. Just below the surface, she could feel a deep and involuntary twisting in her body. She "saw" this twist as if she had suddenly developed X-ray vision. She could see how it pulled her entire right side into contraction, pulling her head down, tightening her right shoulder and pulling it back, and pulling her right hip up and in. Her belly seemed to be twisted into a permanent knot, and she could feel how her lower rib cage was being pulled down toward her pubic bone. She felt as if her belly was in a vise. How could she possibly have been unaware of this!

A few classes later, when she looked in the mirror, she could see the twist in her body with her own eyes. Why hadn't anyone seen it before?

A doctor, a physical therapist, a massage therapist? It was so obvious to her. And then she saw something even more amazing. The whole body was pulling toward that "energy cyst" in her right hip. She also noticed for the first time a deep ache in the area of her right kidney. Suddenly it felt as though someone had kicked her there.

As Bonnie worked with this twist over the next several weeks, she discovered that the real center of the twist seemed to be in the area of the right kidney. On days when she was "going deep," as she put it, the energy cyst in her hip magically dissolved, and the throbbing intensified in the kidney area. As the kidney opened, the throbbing took on vivid new emotional colors. Day in and day out it throbbed. It ached. It felt like lead. Dense. Impenetrable. It felt like an ancient trapped scream, or perhaps a black hole of grief. Then one day, as Bonnie continued to make room for it, it shifted and softened, and a huge wave of terror poured through her. The dread and fear literally took her breath away. The first time she experienced this, she stopped doing postures and sat down.

Gradually, over the course of several weeks, Bonnie learned to bear the fear when it surfaced, and as she did, the fear that had initially taken her breath away deepened into grief—a black heaviness. Every few days a new wave of this grief surfaced. Deep sobbing would rack Bonnie's body, penetrating the thick, leaden sadness. Then would come a euphoric sense of release, and she would be fine for a few days.

The energy cyst in the kidney area took on a central role in the drama. It throbbed and poured forth images, feelings, and sensations: red rage, black grief. Along with the physical releases came memories that felt as though they were emerging from her cells. Among them, Bonnie had primitive images of her life at the time of the birth of a younger sister, Tracey, when she was two years old. For the first time, she understood this to be the occasion of her mother's final abandonment of her. Rage erupted toward her sister and toward her mother. She had no idea she had these feelings of rage toward Tracey, even though she had always felt uncomfortable with her.

As all of this arose, Bonnie found that she needed not to be alone in this again—not to repeat the earlier abandonment that she seemed to be reliving. She discovered a psychotherapist who was also trained in yoga therapy and she began, over the last weeks of the summer and fall, to work with her twice a week. The therapist helped Bonnie contain what was coming up, supported her in staying with the work, and provided the witness when Bonnie lost her own equanimity. The most important role of the yoga therapist in this case was simply to be present. Bonnie knew how to "do the work." But she couldn't do it unless she had what she hadn't had before—the reliable experience of being safely held and soothed.

During the course of that remarkable summer, Bonnie began to understand that her entire physical structure had literally been twisted into a knot around the painful issue of her mother's emotional abandonment. The knot had penetrated deeply into her body and her energy body, so deeply that remnants of it would almost surely remain for the rest of her life. Nonetheless, as Bonnie honed her proprioceptive skills through yoga, she could keep the impulse to twist away from her own deeply felt sense of need above the threshold of consciousness; she found this in itself to be remarkably freeing. When she was aware of the impulse, she could choose how to respond. Perhaps she did need to defend herself in particular situations. But now, she sometimes had the freedom to risk opening to her own need rather than twisting away.

Above all, Bonnie began to experience a sense of aliveness in her body, which she had never even dreamt was possible. She was, as her first yoga retreat had foreshadowed, "finding the missing parts." She was communicating directly with body memory.

BODY MEMORY

We now know that memory resides not somewhere in a "mind" split off from the body, but rather in the cells and neuropathways throughout the body-mind. The skin, the muscles, and the nervous system all record and hold exact memories of how we were touched, held, and soothed—or traumatized and frightened—from the moment of our birth, and even before birth, according to many.

How do somatic memories get laid down in the body? One primary route is through the neuromuscular system. Throughout the course of our lives, our sensorimotor reactions to daily stresses are manifested as contractions in the musculature. Normally, the neuromuscular system "calms down" and muscles relax after a stressful event. However, when groups of muscles are repeatedly contracted as a reaction to an unrelenting stressor, especially traumatic emotional experiences, several things may happen. The stressed group of muscles may over time become shortened and chronically contracted. The body's responses in these muscles do not complete: muscles contract but do not fully release. As a result other muscle groups, which would normally work in opposition to those tensed muscles in order to create balance, become weak and flaccid through underuse. Eventually, we may be unable to voluntarily relax the habitually contracted muscles.

The result is that some degree of hyperalertness persists, as it did with Bonnie. Some tightness in the breathing, in the muscles of the abdomen, or in the shoulders and neck, for example, remain after the traumatic stimulus is gone. In this way, this incompletion "burns" into the hardwiring of the body like a snapshot of the body at the moment of trauma.[13] This leaves us feeling more or less permanently ill at ease. It also leaves us completely split off from insights about why that might be so.

In cases of traumatic emotional stress, or chronic emotional abandonment of the kind Bonnie experienced, contractions may become so deeply involuntary and unconscious that eventually we actually forget how certain muscle groups feel in their relaxed mode.[14] This amounts to a memory loss within the central nervous system. Though we are not aware of it, this memory loss affects us to the very core of our human experience. This "sensory motor amnesia" (as Somatics founder Thomas Hanna calls it) leaves us with a restricted, narrowed experience of our internal self.

CHARACTER ARMOR

A generation ago, Wilhelm Reich, the founder of the science of bioenergetics, coined the term "character armor" to refer to unconsciously held patterns of physical contractions and defenses. It is precisely this complex of bodily defenses that Bonnie penetrated in her first experience of postures. How does body memory function through character armor?

Although most of us tend to assume that muscles make up the greatest percentage of the body's structure, the truth is that connective tissue, or fascia, is the most widely distributed of all the body's tissues.[15] Fascia is the tough but thin elastic connective tissue that forms an uninterrupted three-dimensional network from head to foot, knitting the body together like one huge sweater, and connecting the viscera, the musculature, and the outer layer of the skin.[16]

Subcutaneous fascia, which lies directly below the skin, stores fat and is richly embedded with nerve endings. Our entire body is connected via this web of tissue. What affects one part of this myofascial system will have an impact elsewhere as well. So when I have a trauma in my right hip, contracting and pulling it into a knot, the entire "sweater" is pulled and slightly distorted. It is not surprising that a symptom would begin to show up in my right knee, or my right ankle, or the left hip, which has now begun to compensate for the pulling on the other side.

This accounts for the well-known piece of folk wisdom spoken by Ida Rolf, the founder of the deep bodywork system known as Rolfing. "Where you think it is," she said, "it ain't." A symptom is the body's voice speaking, but we must know the body's language in order to understand its message. Because of the way in which the entire body is connected, through nerve cells and chemicals, and through the myofascial system, both emotional and physical trauma can travel through the body and "land" somewhere, perhaps distant from the original site.

When neuromuscular patterns become chronic and unconscious, they are patterned into the whole myofascial system, and the original reaction becomes locked into the cells as a body memory. Fascia, which is originally highly plastic and malleable, becomes increasingly frozen and rigid as our body-mind becomes chronically set in certain defensive postures. This increases geometrically with age and lack of exercise. The "armor" is complete.

ENERGY CYSTS: *SAMSKARAS*

Sophisticated new studies of psychoneuroanatomy have taught us a good deal about the biochemistry of the body's defensive postures. But from the yogic view there is a deeper level than Western science has yet explored. In the yogic view, the energy of trauma, of contraction, of resistance to life, of holding on—in yogic terms, the energy of the afflictions—is understood to penetrate deeper than the neuromuscular systems. The energy of holding on penetrates into the organs, the fluids, the glands, and the most subtle tissues of the body. Even further, it penetrates into the subtle energy body, the pranamayakosha, where it is finally held.

From the yogic point of view, contraction is the nature of the afflictions (the kleshas). The conditions of asmita, raga, dvesha, and abhinivesha have a physical basis: they function to inhibit the normal pulsatory rhythms of the physical body. The contractions caused by the afflictions are held in "energy whorls," which are tightly condensed balls of energy collapsed in on themselves—you might say the "black holes" of the human body. These unconsciously held energy knots are called *samskaras*. Even though they are reflected in the mirror of the physical body, they are finally held in a deeper place—the subtle energy body.

Not surprisingly, contemporary bodyworkers who are particularly sensitive to energy have begun to intuit this phenomenon, and many have sought ways to express it. For example, John Upledger, an osteopath who teaches craniosacral therapy, believes that what he calls the "energy of injury" can go further into the body than the external location of the original trauma.

> A blow on the foot or ankle might go through the leg all the way to the pelvis. When it reaches its maximum penetration, it stops and forms a localized "ball" of foreign or external energy that doesn't belong there. If the body is unable to disintegrate it for normal healing to occur, the energy is compacted into a smaller and smaller ball in order to minimize the area where tissue function is disrupted. Eventually, it becomes compressed into what [Upledger] calls an "energy cyst."[17]

This is a description that the yogi recognizes. Constrictions that show up in the annamayakosha (the physical body) also have increasingly subtle energy equivalents in each succeeding energy structure or layer. Indeed, the yogic view is that samskaras (or impressions left from emotional or physical trauma) are primarily retained in the subtle bodies and are subsequently reflected through physical symptoms of tension in the gross bodies. Until the energy knots themselves are treated, the structure and function of the tissues will continue to reflect them.

In the yogic view, this picture becomes slightly more complicated— or more interesting—because these energy cysts may be the result of holding patterns acquired not only in this life, but also in past lives.[18]

The patterns may already be in place in our energy body when we're born. Because yogis view infants as "coming in" with their own karmic-samskaric balance, they might view Bonnie's predicament through a slightly different lens from that of the ordinary Westerner. For example, it is possible that Bonnie played a role in her abandonment. This may have arisen in two different ways, karmically speaking. Perhaps Bonnie brought in with her such a deep hunger for holding and soothing, that even a normal, "good enough" mother could not have met her level of need. Perhaps, too, Bonnie, responding to her own samskaras, may have subtly abandoned her mother, turning away from her and not responding to her cues and offerings—thus helping to precipitate her mother's abandonment of her.

While Bonnie went through a period of time when she was experiencing her rage at her mother for the abandonment, eventually she had to acknowledge that whatever her mother's role, her body's patterns belonged to her, and she would have to be instrumental in unwinding them. In fact, this is precisely what she had been doing in unwinding the "twist" in her hip.

CALM ABIDING: CULTIVATING THE EQUANIMITY OF THE BODY

At one point during her summer of intense work, Bonnie had a dream that her house was on fire. In the dream, there was a big, pot-bellied stove in the living room that was overheating. It had been fed with so much fuel that the cast iron had turned bright red and had begun to melt. The house, which was made entirely of wood, was about to ignite into a giant conflagration. Bonnie awoke with a sense of dread and foreboding. She intuited that the fire referred to the fires of transformation raging in her body, or, perhaps, to the fire of rage and grief held in her solar plexus. She was terrified that these fires were about to burn out of control, that she would be consumed. Had she turned the heat up too high?

Her dream pointed her toward an important concern. Deep-body awareness cultivated without an equal amount of physiological equanimity truly does risk leaving us in a burning house. Without the presence of the calmly abiding body, the physiological dimension of self-soothing, we will not be able to bear the "heat" produced by the unwinding of samskaras.

Throughout the course of regular posture practice, the physical and energy bodies go through a profound reorganization. It is, as Trungpa Rinpoche said about meditation, "an operation without anesthesia." Even a beginner's practice, if it's regular, can begin to create this transformation. Without a strong container of calmly abiding self, we cannot bear the disorganization of self that results.

American yogis, practicing in the context of a will-driven and ambitious culture, work very hard at the transformation of awareness. But we chronically give short shrift to relaxation, integration, and rest. In my early years at Kripalu, it was clear that for many students the fires of transformation were literally burning out of control. Many were doing deep practice without giving equal time to integration. As a result, yogis got sick. Chronic fatigue was not uncommon. I didn't get sick, but I did learn a valuable lesson: Real witness consciousness cannot be built in the body without giving equal time to the cultivation of both awareness and equanimity.

During her summer of intense transformation, Bonnie learned that trusting the wisdom of the body also means learning to respond when the body says "no." There are times when it may be abusive to keep practicing postures—times when continued practice may move more energy around the system than we can bear. Over the course of my own long-term practice, I have been through periods when I needed to *not* practice postures. In fact at one point, I needed to make a regular nap be my practice for an entire year. I called it (quoting a former psychotherapy client) "sheet therapy." The posture my body wanted most every day at about two PM was to get between the sheets and go to sleep. At first I resisted. I thought there must be something wrong with napping at my age. But then I began to listen. I discovered that I was deeply tired. I needed to rest. And I needed to do it until my body said that I'd rested enough. It was only through surrendering to the reality of my exhaustion that I was eventually able to go on to the next stage of my practice. As psychologist and poet Tom Yeomans says, "Sometimes, rest is the highest spiritual practice."

And so it was for Bonnie. Particularly during the summer of her deepest work, she needed to rest. She needed to sleep. She needed to "do nothing." Sometimes she needed to sit and stare at the grass. She needed to do deep yogic relaxation, *yoga nidra,* every bit as much as she needed to do postures. Real healing happens in relaxation, and unless we're relaxing, we are not healing.

HEALTH, STRENGTH, AND EQUANIMITY

Relaxation is not the only key to the calmly abiding body. Health and strength can be important components of equanimity, as well. And no one, I think, has understood this better than yogis. Postures build the "hardwiring" of the body—the physical structure capable of containing the reorganization of the psyche. Though Westerners generally have a limited view of yogic practice, we are not wrong in one belief: it is the perfect exercise. Yogic practice intentionally re-creates the physical structure: the musculoskeletal, neurological, digestive, respiratory, circulatory, and immune systems are all literally remade through the regular practice of postures and conscious breathing.

Physiologists say, "Function maintains structure." Or, more simply, "Use it or lose it." If our bones are not regularly used to bear substantial weights and to sustain strong forces, they become soft. If our muscles are not regularly challenged, they become weaker and less responsive. If our brain cells are not systematically involved in a wide variety of voluntary activities, they deteriorate.[19]

"What you practice gets stronger." It's as simple as that. The practice of postures is intentionally meant to create the physiological foundation for the "steadiness and relaxation" of which Patanjali speaks. It does this through enhancing both function and structure. Yoga postures challenge every system of the body to, in effect, practice their function, and to be the best they can be. Consider just this partial list of effects:

~ *Muscles.* Yoga creates a relaxing and massaging effect in the musculature, reducing accumulated tension and stress, relieving conditions that are directly related to muscular tension— headache, backache, muscle spasm. It builds muscle mass and tone, and it aids in the removal of waste materials like lactic acid. It massages and stretches the smooth muscle of the organs. And it helps the development of control of the diaphragm, the only semistriated muscle in the body. When the muscular system is balanced, the skeletal system is brought back into natural alignment, reducing the risk of wear-and-tear conditions like osteoarthritis. Also, when the musculoskeletal system is aligned there is more energy available and energy is used to optimum advantage.

~ *Bones.* We tend to think of bone as a kind of "nonalive" rock-like, mineral structure. Nothing could be further from the truth. Bones are a living community of cells like everything else in the body. They require a steady supply of blood and nutrients and a flow of energy or prana. Postures provide this in an especially effective way. Stimulation of the bones in postures is helpful for bone growth. Also, postures help to stimulate and distribute the flow of synovial fluid, which lubricates the joints between bones.

~ *Circulatory system.* Yoga facilitates the return of deoxygenated blood to the heart. It provides exercise for the heart itself and creates elasticity in the arteries and veins. And it reduces stress, which is the number one enemy of the circulatory system.

~ *Digestive system.* Many postures directly massage and stimulate the abdominal area; they also release muscular stress, which robs blood from the digestive system. Relaxation in the deep abdominal muscles reduces spasm and allows more blood to flow to the tissues of the digestive tract. Both postures and pranayama increase the "fire" of digestion.

~ *Nervous system.* Postures and pranayama bring the two hemispheres of the brain into balance. They increase the flow of blood and nutrients to the nervous system, facilitating the healthy production of brain chemicals and neurons. And they calm the restlessness of the mind, allowing the nervous system and brain to rest.

REINVENTING THE BODY

Peak functioning of the systems of the body is not an end in itself in yogic practice, as it often is in our Western concept of exercise. It is, rather, a way of enhancing the steadiness and relaxation of the calmly abiding self so that the windows of perception can open to the more subtle sheaths of the body.

The maturation of the human being is really an astonishing learning process—developing a repertoire of functions that allow us to interact at remarkably subtle levels with ourselves and with our environment. Unfortunately, in our culture, no sooner do we learn this repertoire than we begin to cease to use it fully, entering into "retirement" and "the long, slow good-bye" of aging. Some have said that life is a race between maturation and senility. Our culture is stuck in a tragically incorrect view of aging, thinking, as Bonnie had, that loss of function and structure is inevitable. It is not.

Bonnie is an inspiring example of this. At fifty-one, eight years into her practice, she is still consciously reinventing her body, creating a new physical self that is strong, steady, relaxed, flexible, and awake, and that contributes to her peace of mind, her sense of steadiness and centeredness in the calmly abiding self. Through the course of her first eight years of practice, Bonnie had made two major changes in her physical structure and function, which contributed enormously to the cultivation of equanimity:

1. Grounding: increasing the strength and steadiness in the legs. There was nothing Bonnie needed more than grounding. Bonnie's awareness of her legs was completely split off. Often she wasn't even aware of them. She couldn't begin to sense her real body until she felt her real feet touching the solid ground beneath her, holding her up. Through her legs she found she could connect with the energy of the earth. She didn't have to count just on herself: she could be supported.

At one point, practicing the standing postures like the warrior or the tree became central in her healing. She learned to hold her ground, to stay with her internal experience of need, however shaky she felt. She learned to feel the strength in feeling real feelings. She didn't fall over. She felt the fundamental strength of coming from her true ground, even if the feelings were scary and primitive. It was only as she developed her grounding that she could begin to access her aggressive, assertive feelings, her natural hostility, and the rage that resulted from her abandonment.

Bonnie's legs had, since toddlerhood, been used in the service of the false self—being responsible, running errands, taking care of others. There was, she discovered later, rage in those legs that terrified her. As she learned to kick and push with her legs, she freed up huge amounts of energy for her life.

2. *Reconnecting with the life force at the center of the body: relaxation of the abdominal muscles.* The false self is habituated to resist the feelings in the belly—out of the ancient, unconscious fear that if I am needy no one will want me. *I will be abandoned. I will be hated and despised. No one wants a baby.* The feelings of need that arise when the musculature releases may initially be experienced as disgusting and degrading, but as they are embraced, they can, for the first time, be truly met.

It was unsettling at first for Bonnie to feel so much energy at the core of her body. It took a long while for her to allow the waves of feelings to move through her belly, pelvis, hips. She literally had to practice letting it happen. This meant experiencing the wave of breath in the belly for the first time in decades. It meant experiencing a new sense of aliveness and energy.

As Bonnie learned to relax her abdominal muscles, she also began to feel her diaphragm free up. Her digestion improved. The wave of breath was less suppressed, and that nagging tightness between the shoulder blades was relieved. She had moments of feeling a soreness in her sternum, just at the heart.

Simultaneously, she felt a release of the tension at the back of her neck and jaw, which had been holding and inhibiting both rage and sadness. Her eyes became clearer, her face relaxed, and she had periods of feeling that it was easier to concentrate. She had fewer headaches.

THE REDISCOVERY OF THE SELF

Bonnie, her brother Michael, her twenty-four-year-old son Danny, and I were sitting in front of a blazing fireplace at her home in Boston, having cocoa.

"Bonnie," I said, "do you realize it's been eight years since your first yoga retreat?"

"Wow, Mom. You've been doing that for eight years? Don't you think you should be, you know, like better by now?"

Bonnie gave Danny a mocking glare. "What? You mean it's possible to get better than I already am?"

"You're just the same old Mom. That New Age stuff hasn't changed

you. I know what changed you. It was Alan moving in that changed
you. You've been different ever since the day you met that guy."

Michael and I looked at each other. "You're the same old Bonnie,"
Michael said, "but there's something different. Way different. It's like,
I don't know—you're the same, but you're more Bonnie than ever.
Personally, I think that's why Alan wanted to move in, in the first
place."

I sat quietly with my own thoughts on the matter. It seemed to me
that Bonnie was very different indeed. In fact, I knew that over the past
eight years, Bonnie's yoga practice, both on and off the mat, had pre-
cipitated a crisis for the whole family. At first, they resented her taking
time for herself, because it eventually meant that she didn't take quite
such scrupulous care of everyone else. The entire extended family
missed her former self-sacrificing qualities. They felt challenged by her
self-care. Bonnie looked better. She felt better. She modeled a way that
they could do the same. Finally, the survival strategies of her entire
lineage were challenged and subtly changed by her own transformation.

The rediscovery of the self, frowned upon as selfish in Bonnie's culture of origin, led, in Bonnie's case, to a great deal of social creativity
and the capacity for true generosity. Through yoga, Bonnie had freed
up the energy to reimagine her life and her caring. And this had made
a difference to a great many people. Yoga had clearly changed the life
of this family. Bonnie could now both contribute more effectively to
others and find happiness for herself.

15

MEDITATION IN MOTION

The stillness in stillness is not the real stillness.
Only when there is stillness in movement can
the spiritual rhythm appear which pervades
heaven and earth.

—Ts'ai-Ken T'an,
in Fritjof Capra, *The Tao of Physics*

"Yo. Steve. You wakin' up or what?"

I pulled my mind reluctantly from a deep fog of dreaming and turned over to see the outline of Tony standing next to my bed. I put the pillow back over my head. "Go away. I'm sleeping." Tony seemed ridiculously perky for 4:30 in the morning.

Tony took the pillow off my head. "No, I don't think so. C'mon. Or we won't get our spot."

I dressed quickly, gathered my blanket and threw it around me. "OK, let's go," I mumbled. As we stumbled toward the main chapel, we passed dozens of ghostly figures in the near-darkness of the hallways, on the way to their own particular "spots" for morning yoga.

The hour just before sunrise is thought, in Hindu culture, to be the most auspicious time of the day for most kinds of spiritual practice. It is called the "hour of Brahma" and it is believed that the quality of prana is particularly pure and strong at that time.[1] It is also believed that the mind is particularly quiet and clear, having just arisen from dreaming and deep sleep, and that the "deep structures" of the mind are especially available for direct observation.

Tony and I found our favorite place at the back corner of the main chapel and spread out our yoga blankets. The candles were already lit on the high altar; the low drone of an Indian raga and the smell of incense softened and warmed the room. We entered silently into our morning yoga routines.

Ordinarily, after I dropped into my own sequence of postures and breathing exercises, I was completely unaware of Tony. But on this morning, I could feel that Tony had entered an unusually deep state of concentration. It was so deep that I was getting a kind of contact high from it. My own concentration deepened. Halfway through the hour-and-a-half session, I became aware that Tony had gone into a bridge pose and had stayed there. He had held it for at least ten minutes. He began to moan and groan. Grunting. Panting. At one point he began to growl like a dog, and I could feel a powerful wave of aggression and anger.

Finally, Tony released the posture and began to flow spontaneously from one deep pose to another, at times flinging himself violently around the back corner of the chapel. He was making strange sounds. Spontaneous pranayamas were occurring. Many of his movements were jerky—rapidly vibrating an arm, a shoulder, or a leg. I stopped my own practice and created a boundaried space for Tony so that he could let go.

The postures, pranayamas, and *mudras* (literally, "gestures," often with the hands) lasted about twenty minutes and ended as spontaneously as they had begun. Tony entered the lotus posture and remained in what appeared to be a state of samadhi for another half an hour. Then, as others were silently gliding out of the chapel toward breakfast, he just lay down in corpse pose and entered into deep relaxation.

I sat down next to Tony and meditated for the next half an hour. Finally, he rolled over and looked at me.

He smiled. "I guess I'm enlightened now."

"Fat chance," I said.

STILLNESS IN MOVEMENT

When the practice of postures is combined with conscious breathing and deep states of concentration and absorption, prana will sometimes spontaneously "take over" the practice. Suddenly, energy itself will begin to direct the flow of postures. In these moments we may have a sense of effortlessness, of complete surrender to a force greater than ourselves. This experience can be surprising, compelling, and blissful. And, it appears to be completely out of our control. We cannot make it happen. We can only let it happen.

When Tony and I talked about his experience that morning, he described it as "being lost in the dance of energy." "There was a deep sense of calm and quiet at the center of the dance," he said, even though the dance itself had been vigorous and at times even violent. He said that he had found himself spontaneously entering postures he had never before been able to execute and some postures he had never even seen before. "The only thing I did," he said, "was to keep allowing it to happen. Other than that it was completely effortless. I was not the doer. I was pure witness. It was like I was pure prana."

In watching Tony's posture flow, I could literally see the manifestation of the wave, what bioenergetic therapists call "the original organismic self-expression." His body pulsed with life, alternating between expansion and contraction. His whole organism appeared to be breathing itself, all aspects of the gross and subtle bodies moving in synchrony like an amoeba under the microscope.

"My mind was so focused that all distractions were tuned out," Tony said. "I wasn't aware of you or anyone else around me." Tony went on to describe a sense of unwinding. "It was kind of like I was one of those wind-up kid's tops, and the whole outpouring of movement was, like, winding me down. Finally, I just got to the end of the wound-up energy, and I was completely still inside. The relaxation afterward was unbelievably deep.

"But here's the most amazing thing. For part of the time I was actually flying. I was on the ceiling. I was over the altar, looking down. I was in Bapuji's alcove, watching the whole scene. I was, in a way, everywhere at once." Tony described this as the discovery of his "astral" body. He was, in his experience, no longer confined to his physical body. "And then this other thing happened. Sometimes my body was huge, filling the whole room. Sometime I was as small as an ant. It was better than acid."

Through the years of my teaching career at Kripalu I have seen many spontaneous posture flows, yogis surrendered to the wave of prana. When it happens, it can be entrancing to onlookers, just as

Tony's was to me that morning. It seems that our own minds are captured by another mind and body that is deeply surrendered to absorption and spontaneous movement.

But what is actually happening? Is the body being taken over by the magical power of prana? By some higher intelligence? Do we have any control over the conditions that create this kind of altered state? And how do we describe Tony's experience of flying?

THE STATE OF FLOW

Tony's posture flow was not magic. Nor was it the result of some secret "transmission" from a powerful guru or enlightened being. Prana is not a kind of alien substance, or "third force," which was taking over Tony's body. The entire experience of his posture flow was a manifestation of one of the central laws of yoga: energy follows awareness. As states of concentration deepen in the body-mind, prana also becomes more concentrated. Deep states of mental and physical absorption gather and focus prana into a powerful stream. When these conditions of absorption are merged with an attitude of surrender and nonreactivity, the spontaneous flow of postures can easily emerge.

Psychologist Mihaly Csikszentmihalyi has done extensive research on what he calls "the state of flow," or "the psychology of optimal experience" in everyday life. These are the states, for example, characteristic of the jazz musician "in the groove," or the athlete "in the zone." He identifies three elements, in particular, that typify these altered states of mind and body:

~ the merging of action and awareness in sustained concentration on the task at hand
~ the focusing of attention in a pure involvement without concern for outcome
~ self-forgetfulness with heightened awareness of the activity[2]

Csikszentmihalyi found what he believed to be the key prerequisite for dropping into the flow state: the mental and physical flexibility to track and adapt to the changing demands and input of the environment on a moment-by-moment basis. In the case of posture flow, this means the capacity to fully attune to and respond to the changing signals of the prana body. In rapid states of movement like the one Tony experienced, the attention must be highly tuned to rapidly changing discrete moments of sensation. This quality of mental one-pointedness has the effect of drawing the mind even more deeply into absorption.

A second requirement is the ability to "forget the self" in action. All self-consciousness is dissolved for short periods of time, as awareness of the activity itself is heightened. The "actor" then has a sense that he is not acting at all. He is not the doer. He abides as the still point around which the movement takes place.

The state of flow can be blissful, because it gives us a compelling taste of action unimpeded by anxiety—that is to say, action completely detached from concern for outcome. The resulting experience results in a sense of bliss, rapture, contentment, and harmony. These states of harmony are characteristic of a heightened stage of yogic concentration known as *dhyana*.

DHYANA

As the mind develops the capacity to remain one-pointed and settled on the object of concentration (sensations and feelings in the body) during the practice of riding the wave and holding the posture, we may penetrate momentarily into a deeper phase of concentration, dhyana. In the *sutra* describing dhyana, Patanjali uses the word *ekatanata*, which means "extending continuously or unbrokenly"—referring to the absence of interruptions from distractions. One commentary on the *Yogasutras* adds: "This continuity may be compared to the continuity of the flow of water in a river or that of oil being poured from one vessel into another."[3]

When we penetrate into the state of dhyana, a sense of easy flow will saturate our experience—a sense of the "streaming" of the mind. In this new phase of concentration there is a marked quality of effortlessness, a sense of receptivity to a natural process, and a miraculous sense of dropping into a state of pure union with the object of our concentration. The mind experiences a visceral, alive connection with the subtle sensations of the energy body and seems capable now of penetrating into its very core. As Patanjali says, the mind "shines with the object."

All of the contemplative traditions recognize that with this maturation of concentration some startlingly new features arise in consciousness. Most traditions have a name for this new level of skillfulness. In Buddhist traditions, for example, it is called "access samadhi," or beginning samadhi. There are two experiences in particular that characterize absorption at this level. First of all, there is the achievement of a whole new quality of steadiness. Once stabilized, the yogi can hold his concentration for long periods of time and can therefore hold postures in a "steady and relaxed" fashion.

Secondly, there is a remarkable change in the yogi's perception of the body. As the yogi's mind becomes more and more one-pointed, the object itself (in this case, the body) seems to become more and more subtle, drawing the mind deeper into itself. In postures, there will then arise a state of absorption in pure physical sensation, without any elaboration, association, judgment, or reactivity by the mind. In one study, psychologist Dan Brown found that yogis experiencing dhyana were primarily attentive to, and occasionally absorbed in, the pure perceptual features of the object of their attention—the texture, color, and movement of subtle sensation.[4]

As Brown describes this experience,

> the yogi has stopped the mind, at least in the sense of its so-called "higher operations": thinking and pattern recognition. The yogi keeps his awareness at the more subtle level of the actual moment of occurrence or immediate impact of a thought or of a sensory stimulus.[5]

This state gives rise to what Buddhists have sometimes called "bare attention." All associations and comments of the mind are completely pared away from consciousness. The practice period

> is experienced as a succession of discrete events: pulses, flashes, vibrations, or movements without specific pattern or form. . . . Though mental and bodily events occur moment-by-moment in uninterrupted succession, attention remains fixed on each discrete moment. Awareness of one event is immediately followed by awareness of another, without break for the duration of the sitting period, or for as long as this level of concentration remains.[6]

When the yogi has reached this point of skillfulness, something astonishing can begin to happen, as it did to Tony that morning. As attention becomes "bare," not only does the subtle energy body dominate the stream of consciousness, but the perception of the body itself also undergoes changes and becomes increasingly unstable. The body seems to lose its solidity, its hard edges.

> The object changes size, shape, location and luminosity. It may become, for example, as large as the ocean or as small as a mustard seed. What once seemed to be a fixed internal representation is now experienced as an image in constant change.[7]

Tony's perceptions had become so refined that he had begun to deconstruct the gross physical anatomy. He experienced this as his astral body. He could fly.

A SPIRITUAL WARRIOR

Tony was the youngest son of a first-generation Italian-American family in which an impulsive and violent father had dominated everyday life. Tony had grown up on the streets of Chicago with three older brothers, one of whom was particularly jealous of Tony's status as "his mother's baby." Early on, Tony learned to defend himself around his father and his older brothers. Later, he learned to fight his way through school. He had been smaller than the other boys in his grade and he had adopted an exterior toughness—a tough-guy stance. As a result of all of this, Tony had a kind of flash-point response to any perceived threat—a real "in your face" attitude.

Underneath the tough-guy exterior, Tony had a huge heart. He'd been drawn to spirituality early, as an altar boy and a choirboy in the Roman Catholic Church, and he still thought of himself as a devout Christian. He had stayed on in the home longer than his brothers, to protect his mother from his father. He was deeply attached to his mother and felt, as he put it, "ready to sacrifice his life for her"—but it wasn't clear that she wanted things any other way than the way they were.

When I first got to know Tony, it was clear to me that he was carrying a lot of baggage. But Tony had never been particularly interested in psychotherapy. Instinctively he took the direct route of the body, of energy, for working with his anger and hurt. He had become interested in martial arts early on and had excelled in them. One of his martial arts instructors had interested him in yoga, and when he got involved with yoga postures, he did them like a warrior.

In his yoga practices, Tony was fearless, total. He regularly got up somewhere in the wee hours of the morning. There were frequent sightings of him in the main chapel at four AM, doing his intensive yoga *sadhana*. The whole program had to be finished by 7:30, so he would be available for his job in the kitchen.

Tony had been practicing deep states of concentration in postures, and though he wouldn't have described it this way, he had refined his attention so that he could easily drop into states of dhyana. This practice gathered and focused enormous amounts of prana, which further supported his practice. So great was his connection with energy that he seemed to need astonishingly little sleep.

Tony had a particular devotion to Bapuji, whom he saw as a kindred soul, a kind of warrior of the spirit. His practice was, indeed, leading him in the direction of Bapuji's practice—the sadhana of effortless surrender to prana.

PRANA SADHANA

For thirty years, Bapuji did his daily practice in a windowless, underground room at the temple of Kayavarohan in Baroda—the ancient temple he rebuilt at the command of his own mysterious guru, Dadaji. Bapuji's sadhana room was underground so it would remain cool in the 125-degree heat of Gujarat summers. His daily session of asana, pranayama, and mudras was a strictly solitary practice that very few other human beings ever witnessed. But those few who did see it attest to the fact that his sadhana was to enter into a deep state of absorption and then to surrender his body completely to the movement of prana. The result, according to one close follower, was an outpouring of movement that was very often spastic in appearance, rude, crude, rapid, and violent, or, at other times, very, very slow. The spontaneous flow of postures, mudras, and sounds could last for hours. Sometimes he was completely motionless for hours on end.[8]

Bapuji explained that prana (or, in his case, a highly concentrated form of prana called *kundalini shakti,* which we will explore shortly) is possessed of all the wisdom of buddhi—enlightened mind. Prana moves automatically to the places in the body-mind where there are blocks to the free flow of energy—the energy cysts, or samskaras, described in the last chapter. When prana encounters blocks to its flow, it creates a kind of swirl of energy, which challenges the block. Spontaneous movements and postures are simply the forms that arise as prana moves into some particular block. Spontaneous gestures are held just long enough to accomplish eroding the samskara.

Bapuji called this phenomenon "a spontaneous *kriya* of chitta and prana"—literally, a purifiying action of mind, or consciousness, and energy. He taught that through the surrender to the flow of supercharged prana, the body-mind is freed from any obstructions and its capacity for channeling prana is thereby increased. There is a deep surrender involved, because the adept is fully absorbed in the experience, but is not guiding it or directing it in any way. As my friend Gitanand describes it: "The image of a posture arises spontaneously in the mind. You wonder if it might happen. Sometimes it does, following your thought; and sometimes it doesn't. It is completely beyond your volition."

Bapuji, it must be remembered, found that he had to lead a monastic lifestyle in order to follow the rigorous demands of prana sadhana. He did ten to twelve hours of practice a day. He lived in almost complete silence for thirty years. He practiced celibacy throughout that time, as well as the strictest of yogic diets. His energy body had been cultivated and matured to the maximum capacity of a human being.

Astonishingly, Bapuji never really studied postures with a yoga teacher. His guru, Dadaji, gave him only one posture, the lotus pose for meditation, and one pranayama, a pattern of alternate-nostril breathing called *anuloma viloma,* familiar to most beginning yoga students. The entire hatha yoga vocabulary of hundreds of postures and pranayamas—postures and pranayamas that he had never seen—were revealed to him spontaneously in his practice.

THE SERPENT AWAKES: KUNDALINI

The Sanskrit word *kundalini* refers to a highly condensed and distilled form of prana thought to lie "coiled and sleeping like a serpent" at the base of the spine. In Tantric philosophy, kundalini was depicted as a snake coiled three and a half times around, awaiting the arousal that comes only through dedicated practice of purification and hatha yoga.

In the Tantric formulation, the ultimate goal of practice is to increase and manipulate the flow of prana through the nadis (the energy channels, see chapter 13) so that its flow is first balanced and finally moved up through the central nadi of the shushumna, or "the most gracious channel." This is the process known vaguely to millions of Westerners as "raising the kundalini." As the kundalini moves up through the shushumna, the energy vortices of the chakras are opened one by one, "as the blooming of a lotus flower," and the major knots in the energy body are pierced through and released. The realized yogi can consciously regulate the flow of prana through the nadis and send it with full force to any aspect of the body-mind.

Kundalini is also identified as the essence of divine goddess energy—the energy of Shakti, who longs to meet her consort, Shiva, pure consciousness, where he resides in the crown chakra, at the other end of the shushumna. The union of Shiva and Shakti is accomplished when shakti moves upward through the shushumna and arrives at the crown. When this is achieved, the goals of hatha yoga have been realized. Yogis believe that at this stage the practitioner will not only have reached the goal of awakening transcendental consciousness but will also have put on "the divine body"—immortal, transcendent, and light filled.

The arousal of kundalini is really very serious business. Bapuji taught that only one yogi every five hundred years will actually bring the kundalini experience to a successful conclusion. Of the few Westerners who dared embark on this path during the heyday of Kripalu's guru years, all, I think, abandoned it after being "fried" in the heat of intense practice to the brink of their endurance—and sometimes beyond. Bapuji himself, who devoted virtually his entire life to the path, did not claim to have achieved "the divine body." He made clear over and over again to his Western students that practice for them would necessarily be about "building the fortress of the self"—creating awareness and equanimity—and not about raising the kundalini.

It is hard to overstate how hot the fires of transformation are in true prana sadhana. When yogis are dedicated to working at this level, the demands are so great that they have to live in a protected environment where their physical needs for food and shelter can be met. As Bapuji said, in this practice "the rope of ego is burned to ash." Kundalini yogis' capacity to take care of the business of ordinary life dissolves to some extent, and they literally cannot function in day-to-day life without support. They forget to eat. They may wander around naked, lost in ecstatic states and trances. Followers of the great nineteenth-century Bengali saint Ramakrishna were full of such stories about their own "God-intoxicated" teacher:

> The Master's mind was so constantly turned towards God that even when he was eating he would often not be conscious of it and someone would have to tell him when he had eaten enough. "Have I taken enough?" he would ask, and if the person said that he had, then at once he would stop.[9]

The "holy fools," like Ramakrishna, who have taken the path of energy all the way can sometimes look a lot like lunatics in our eyes. But those followers who inevitably surround these remarkable beings say that they experience something quite the opposite of lunacy—a mind and body completely absorbed in God, completely sunk in a blissful union with Brahman. They experience a consciousness that fully manifests the fruit of yoga: sat-chit-ananda, being, consciousness, bliss.

Bapuji believed that much of the conventional Western understanding of kundalini is completely inaccurate. Most of what is thought to be kundalini awakening is simply the awakening of a slightly more concentrated form of prana. One of the most knowledgeable Western scholars of the process, Georg Feuerstein, agrees: "Many of the supposed kundalini symptoms brought to the attention of psychotherapists today are caused not by genuine kundalini arousals, but by what are known as 'pranic awakenings.' "[10]

These so-called "pranic awakenings" are wonderful and important experiences in themselves. They are the experiences that many of us who develop hatha yoga practices will actually have. And they require careful preparation.

There are many, many stages to go through before the human body can fully open to the movement of prana. Each of them is necessary before we can experience prana in its most highly condensed form. All of these stages prepare the body for the raging powers of kundalini shakti, an experience most of us will not have in this lifetime. The two most important preparatory stages, according to the yogis of the Kripalu lineage, are first, *pranaprabalya,* the intentional strengthening and purification of the prana body; and second, *pranotthana,* the spontaneous purification of the musculature, organs, and glands through the initial awakening of prana, a spontaneous energy experience that precedes kundalini awakening and prepares the way for it.

STRENGTHENING THE PRANA BODY

In order to be able to tolerate even the initial awakening of prana, and to channel it properly, the "hardwiring" of the nadi system must be extremely strong and resilient. Most of us have nadis that would, metaphorically speaking, only accommodate a 110-volt current. Through the process of pranayama and postures, we can upgrade that so that it will accommodate, say, 220 volts. Without the proper preparation, the experience of pranic awakening would be like opening a 1,000-volt current into a 220-volt wire. The wire would simply melt, and the body would be destroyed. Kundalini energy, of course, would be more like 10,000 volts.

I've taken this "electrical" metaphor from B. K. S. Iyengar, whose description, in *Light on Pranayama,* is worth quoting at length:

> The generation and distribution of prana in the human system may be compared to that of electrical energy. The energy of falling water or rising steam is made to rotate turbines within a magnetic field to generate electricity. The electricity is then stored in accumulators and the power is stepped up or down by transformers which regulate the voltage or current. It is then transmitted along cables to light cities and run machinery. Prana is like the falling water or rising steam. The thoracic area is the magnetic field. The breathing processes of inhalation, exhalation and retention of breath act like the turbines, while the chakras represent the accumulators and transformers. The energy generated by prana is like electricity. It is stepped up or down by the chakras and distributed throughout the system along the nadis, which are the transmission lines. If the power

generated is not properly regulated it will destroy the machinery and the equipment. It is the same with prana.[11]

There are a number of very simple pranayamas—in addition to full yogic breath, or *dirgha pranayama* (already described in chapter 13 as "abdominal-diaphragmatic breath")—that are specifically designed to balance and purify the nadis. *Ujjayi* breath, or "ocean-sounding breath," for example, and *nadi shodhana* (alternate-nostril breathing) are practices that use "circular breathing," breathing without pauses between inhalation and exhalation. These simple, safe practices do not use the more advanced techniques of retention of breath *(kumbhaka)*. But even these basic pranayamas balance the flow of prana, purifying the nadis and opening both sides of the energy body.

AWAKENING THE PRANA BODY

Students often have a fantasy that the awakening of the prana body will be like taking a drug that gives us more energy for our pursuit of the perfect body, the fully realized career, the most fabulous, high-powered lovemaking—whatever ideal is in the mind about how we should be. If this is what we hope for—and who doesn't?—we will be disappointed.

As the nadis are opened, purified, and balanced through pranayama practice, and as our consciousness remains attuned to the energy body, a kind of enriched prana will begin to move through the system. This, however, is not as much fun as we might hope it will be. In fact, prana will move right to the densest areas of our attachments, where we want to feel solid and armored, and begin to erode this sense of solidity. Prana moves methodically through the physical and energy bodies, unwinding blocks, holdings, and karmic "knots." Anywhere there is a blockage to energy, prana will be at work. The symptoms that we may feel—the discomfort, the sometimes bizarre energy experiences—are simply the process of unwinding, the release of the blocked energy. These releases—or kriyas ("purifying actions")—can be short, intense, and dramatic, or they can last for months and be extremely subtle.

Many kriyas come under the heading of what I call "weird energy experiences." Sylvia Boorstein, a well-known Buddhist teacher, author, and former yoga teacher, tells the story of her bizarre three-year energy experience. It began during an intensive retreat in which she awoke to the existence of her energy body. She felt her whole body streaming with what she described as "lines of energy." "I feel like an acupuncture wall chart!" she said to Joseph Goldstein, a senior American teacher of Buddhism. "Those charts are true. We really do have energy bodies!" After her retreat, Sylvia found that the energy experiences continued and were "unpleasant and disturbing." "My limbs would vibrate or spasm in random movements in public places, and sometimes I would awaken in the middle of the night to find my teeth chattering. My actual body temperature stayed normal, while I experienced periods of shivering with cold or imagining that I was radiating heat. . . . I felt sharp pains around my heart."[12]

These unpredictable energy experiences are almost always beyond the capacity of Western medicine to explain or treat. Several years into my most intense practice, for example, my neck went into a kind of death-grip spasm and I couldn't move my head for about a month. It was hard to teach yoga. My head just wouldn't budge. I saw every conceivable form of health practitioner. No one seemed able to treat it. Finally, it just disappeared.

At another point in my practice, I went through almost an entire year of sweating profusely at night, usually soaking through three T-shirts and sometimes having to completely change the bedding in the middle of the night. I've had quite a few yogi friends who have been through that. (Interestingly, one of the foundational medieval texts on hatha yoga mentions several common symptoms and signs of the awakening of the prana body.[13] The first of these is profuse sweating. The next is quivering, trembling, and shaking uncontrollably.) For a while, my whole scalp broke out in a nasty eruption of pimples. "Never seen it before," said the understated dermatologist, who was, by that time, used to me. At another point, whenever I went into a deep state of relaxation, I found my right leg violently kicking and shaking.

Buddhist teacher Jack Kornfield describes his own experience of kriya, and the helpful instruction his teacher gave him about working with it:

> Early in one year-long training retreat, I experienced a period
> of very powerful release where my head began shaking back
> and forth for hours. Some days later my arms started to invol-
> untarily flap like a bird's wings. When I would try to stop them,

I could barely do so. If I relaxed at all, they would flap continuously. When I asked the teacher about it, he inquired whether I
was being fully aware, and I said, "Certainly." Later he said,
"You're not really being aware. Look more carefully and you
will see that you don't like it. You subtly want it to go away."
When I saw he was right, he said, "Simply go back and observe
it," and over the next two days the movement subsided, and I
sat there feeling my arms throb, bringing hours of deep bodily
release.[14]

Kornfield's teacher identified the very instruction that hatha yoga
adepts give to their students: When an energy experience hangs around
long enough to become troublesome, it is usually because we are subtly
resisting it. And what we resist persists. The recommendation is usually
that we bring our awareness to the sensations, without judgment, and
that we open to the experience of the energy, if we can tolerate it. It is
the nature of prana to move. And eventually it will.

With experience, we will learn to trust the movement of prana, so
that we don't need to try to control it, or to stop it. With some practice,
we may find that we're no longer afraid of it. We can just allow the
energy to move, knowing that it will move in exactly the right way to
work through the next samskara that is ready to be released or diminished. Prana moves at just the right pace, in just the right way. And
usually not in a way that we cannot bear.

If we let the prana move, we will eventually end up with a greater
capacity to tolerate "the winds of life." We will feel more alive, more
open to experience. As Sylvia Boorstein said, after her dramatic energy
experiences subsided, "I think the experience left me with an enhanced
sense of vibrancy, a sensual liveliness that I enjoy and that pleases
me."[15]

PUTTING ENERGY EXPERIENCES INTO PERSPECTIVE

In a culture saturated with *The X-Files*, the psychic TV network, and an
inexhaustible fascination with the esoteric, many yoga students will at
some point be drawn to colorful notions of exotic energy states, yogic
alchemy, supernormal yogic powers, and enlightenment. Inevitably,
some will long for the awakening of kundalini shakti and the divine

body. In this context, it is wise to remember Jacob Needleman's triad of essential attitudes toward spiritual phenomena—openness, common sense, and skepticism.

The yogic path, more than any other contemplative discipline, seeks to work directly with energy, and in the process it is guaranteed that we will have a multitude of interesting, sometimes difficult, sometimes pleasurable energy experiences. I have found that, when dealing with energy experiences, many students lose their balance, becoming either too open or too skeptical. It is useful to keep these energy experiences in some perspective. Here are some frequently asked questions:

1. Are the chakras real? The so-called "seven energy centers of the body" seem to be one piece of yogic lore that has particular appeal for the Western imagination. "Have you experienced all your chakras?" new yoga students ask me. "Are you able to 'see' them? How can I develop mine? I saw a white light the other day in my meditation—was that a chakra opening?"

The truth is, though almost all hatha yoga adepts believe in the reality of energy centers in the body, different individual practitioners may have widely varying experiences of them. Indeed, the classical scriptures vary widely in their accounts of these energy centers—some describe seven chakras, others describe thirteen, some describe eleven.

Are they real? The chakras we see diagrammed in books are, indeed, just mental pictures. In that sense, they are not at all real. They are concepts. Usually, they are described with much attendant baggage, including particular sounds, colors, archetypal images, and Sanskrit mantras and sounds that supposedly accompany each chakra. In my experience, it is not at all useful to have preconceived notions about the kinds of energy experiences we will have in yoga.

In fact, many great hatha yoga teachers and scholars—as well as masters from other contemplative disciplines—steer their students away from concern with the chakras. When we have these ideas in our heads of "what is supposed to happen" in our bodies, we very often spend time looking for these experiences and feeling badly or inadequate when we don't have them. In the meantime, we miss what is really happening. The idea of chakras actually distracts us from the real work of yoga—attuning to precisely how it is for us in our bodies right now, and directly and immediately exploring this energetic landscape.

2. *Do energy experiences mean I am closer to enlightenment?* Contemplative practice is notoriously full of colorful energy experiences. But the guidance in both Buddhist and yogic traditions is clear. These supernormal energy powers are a by-product of intense states of concentration. Some people get them and others don't. They should never become the goal of practice. In fact, as the Buddha said, "They should be counted as nothing."

It seems that many Western yogis are attached to the wonderful esoteric ideas of chakras and kundalini. But reaching for these supernormal experiences simply reinforces the kleshas of clinging and craving, and can only serve to remove us from a fresh, direct exploration of our immediate, moment-to-moment, day-to-day experience of the subtle body.

Energy experiences are not the goal of practice. They should not be seen as particularly sacred, or as special signs that we have become enlightened. Some more advanced students have multitudes of colorful energy experiences, while others have absolutely none. There is no evidence that they are, in themselves, barometers of any special spiritual accomplishment. Actually, the less we can stay preoccupied with them, grasping toward them or resisting them and pushing them away, the better.

3. *If I have a "weird energy experience," how should I proceed?* Use awareness: If it is possible, explore the energy state more deeply. Move repeatedly with compassionate and balanced awareness into the sensation. How, exactly, is it? Does it move? What is its texture?

It is wise not to resist the movement of energy, if we can tolerate it. What we resist persists. We should open to the experience and bring our awareness to the sensations, without judgment. If fear arises, or terror, we can simply bring awareness to those. Usually, we will discover that either craving or aversion are the engines that are subtly keeping the energy experience alive.

4. *If the energy experience is difficult to bear, what can I do?* For the most part, energy experiences are the result of prana moving upward in the body from the lower energy centers. There are very concrete steps we can take to bring the energy back down. For myself, I find that it helps if I connect with the ground—gardening, getting my hands dirty, or walking in the woods.

Most of all, in damping down prana, it is important to stop practices that heighten purification in the body and mind, and that encourage the energy to move upward in the energy body. These energy experiences tend to be heightened during periods of sexual celibacy. Having sex can often lower their intensity.

If energy feels intolerable, or dangerous in some way, focus on practices that cultivate equanimity. There are techniques that may help to dampen the flow of prana, and relieve the symptoms of the energy release. (When I need to do this, for example, I go out for some heavy foods—foods referred to as "tamasic" in yogic tradition—which help bring the energy back down to the ground.)

TONY: MEDITATION IN MOTION

What learnings, then, should we be taking away from our energy experiences? It might be useful, here, to revisit Tony's "weird energy experiences," because he is an example of a Western student who has worked particularly effectively with deep states of pranic awakening—both physically and psychologically.

Tony's experience of the relationship between his prana body and his physical body was fairly typical. There were areas where he could feel the movement of very subtle energies, and other areas that just always felt blocked, numb, cut off from the connection to prana. His back was the most obviously split-off area. Paradoxically, his back was (physically speaking) overdeveloped in relationship to the rest of his body—powerfully muscled and seemingly full of energy. And yet, even though his back seemed flexible, Tony rarely had the sense that it was open to the waves of prana that sometimes coursed through other areas of his body. He had the vague sense that he was holding on to something back there—that there were things he was "keeping behind him."

Several months before the posture flow I described at the beginning of this chapter, Tony had had an energetic breakthrough during a long meditation retreat. As he sat in the retreat hour after hour and scanned the sensations in his body, he began to become aware of an intense sensation between his shoulder blades—a kind of death grip, which he could feel tighten the muscles all the way around his chest. It felt to him like an iron barrel stay. This tight band prevented him from breathing deeply and from feeling the pulsation of life in the area of his heart. As Tony continued to sit and explore, and as he breathed into this vortex of energy, it began to soften and open. As if for the first time, he could feel the throb of breath and life in this area. A little door had been opened. It felt like bliss just to have some energy moving there.

When Tony came back from the retreat and started practicing postures again, he found that for the first time he was attracted to deep back-bending poses—the camel, the bow, and the cobra. Whenever he went into either the bow or the camel, he had deep spasms and tremors between his shoulder blades. He found that he really wanted to hold the postures deeply, so that he could feel the throbbing and the movement, and explore it. As Tony began to allow more energy to move into his back, and as he let the energy build, he would have amazing experiences upon releasing the posture: his arms would move and flail spontaneously, and sometimes he would begin to kick—aggressive, angry kicks, coming from his hips and lower back.

Tony found that after holding these back-bending postures, his body was taken over by a wave of energy that just had to express itself in a spontaneous flow of movement. And he learned how to let the resulting energy wave move him, surrendering to the intuitive wisdom of his body. He learned how to move with the wave of prana, rather than against it. And he found himself entering into a dance called forth from within. As he learned to trust the movement, he found that the flow would eventually wind down, leaving him with a peaceful sense of having literally "unwound" the knots in his body-mind. Afterward, he would often collapse into a deep relaxation.

For several months, Tony had the experience of prana working methodically on his back. Sometimes during these posture flows, he would experience an exhilarating openness in his chest. His chest visibly relaxed and expanded, and he felt the wave of breath going into areas of the body and lungs that he had never sensed so deeply before. As he allowed the breath to go deeper into this expanded chest, he felt the beginnings of big heaving sobs that seemed to originate in his belly. When he later put this grief into words, it seemed to be about the loss of himself, the loss of his vitality for so many years. He couldn't feel the prana body now without realizing how long he had lived without it.

Over a period of months, these catharses brought to the surface a mourning process that had been locked in his physical structure. Both the long-denied energy and the rage and aggression toward his father and brothers were available for him to feel in his body for the first time. Eventually, Tony came to understand that he had put all of his aggression and rage behind him, and there it had remained—lodged in his back, right between his shoulder blades.

Tony's front-back split was one of the most deeply unconscious aspects of his physical-energetic structure, precisely because the feelings and experiences it held were some of the most painful he would have to face. Not only had his rage and aggression been inhibited by muscular contractions in the back. His natural reaching out had also been inhibited and blocked in the same part of the body. And something else as well. His back was rigidly holding the false-self posture of self-sacrifice—doing for others out of an overdeveloped sense of responsibility and feeling, unconsciously, as though he were carrying them on his back.

Entering the back side of his body was, for Tony, entering his shadow side. It was dangerous and it was exhilarating. It was the most profound experience of coming home to the split-off aspects of his own self.

As Tony's practice matured he found that long holdings of postures were no longer for the purpose of "getting them right," or perfecting anything, but only for the opportunity to get more deeply absorbed in the subtle sensations in his body. Tony was experiencing a version of Bapuji's "spontaneous kriya of chitta and prana." He discovered that the more frequently he penetrated into these states of absorption—or dhyana—the deeper he was able to go. In this discovery, he confirmed one of the major findings of Csikszentmihalyi's research on flow: Csikszentmihalyi found that being in the state of flow, over time, sharpens the perceptual apparatus and increases the capacity to focus attention in a one-pointed fashion, to concentrate deeply, and to tune out distracting and irrelevant stimuli.

Tony had the sense that his increasingly deep altered states were transforming him in some subtle fashion, that each time he returned from penetrating into states of dhyana, he was slightly changed. Was this so? And if so, what is the mechanism of change?

THE MIND IN SECLUSION

Scientists researching the effects of contemplative techniques have precisely described the mechanisms of change in dhyana. There are several key elements. First of all, as the mind gains this level of one-pointedness and becomes quite free from distraction, the mind goes deeply into seclusion—becoming completely cut off from conflict, from normal experiences of reactivity, attraction, and aversion, restlessness and doubt. The mind is now deeply secluded from the kleshas. As a result of this deep seclusion, two other factors automatically arise—rapture *(piti)* and *sukha,* or happiness (sometimes described as "comfort"), which manifests as a kind of all-pervading sweetness. There can be a deep opening of the heart in this state of bliss, and an unutterable sense of well-being. The defensive structures in the body and mind are relaxed. The agitation of worry is completely eliminated, and anxiety is eased.

Secondly, as the reactivity at the surface of the mind is calmed, the deepest patterns of reactivity are brought to the surface. The process of purification heats up. Even a few seconds of dhyana have a powerful purifying impact on the mind, because they are moments during which the mind has detached from its customary, habitual patterns. Even momentary penetration into states of dhyana begins to create the meltdown of the five afflictions and the four erroneous beliefs. The mind is secluded from clinging and craving. It is beginning to be changed by its direct apprehension of the impermanence and mutability of objects it once took to be permanent and immutable. It is experiencing itself as nonseparate from the whole field of mind and matter. We have direct perceptions that reality is not what we had thought it to be.

As a result of sustained moments of dhyana, the yogi finds himself overwhelmed by a powerful insight. Beneath what we usually think of as "the mind"—discursive, restless, craving, and clinging mind, as well as rational, logical, deliberative mind—there is an intuitive, awake intelligence that sees clearly into the nature of reality. Buddhi, the awake mind, is saturated with a kind of discernment and wisdom that we have never before experienced in such a distilled fashion. Even momentary experiences of this subtle sheath of mind leave us irrevocably altered. Each time we experience dhyana, one small root of avidya is severed. In an instant, we know that we are not who we thought we were. We are not separate from the whole field of mind and matter; we are not our minds, or our personalities, or our bodies; ultimately, we discover that we are not even the seer, but that we are saturated with the clear seeing of the awake mind. We are, in effect, pure seeing—pure witness consciousness.

In the more mature stages of practice, these highly refined aspects of mind become the instrument for penetrating into the essence of things. Clearly, this is a mind that has developed capacities of which we in the West have been almost entirely unaware. It is the mind capable of penetrating the unmanifest realms beyond time and space. It is the mind of pure being—the mind of brahman.

THE DIVINE DANCE

Through his experience with posture flow, Tony had discovered one of the most astonishing truths about the practice of hatha yoga: through teaching us to attune in the most visceral way to the spontaneous wisdom of the body, this ancient path takes us all the way to union with the mind of God. What begins as an experientially grounded practice—one that asks us to take nothing at all on faith, indeed, asks only that we pay attention to the body—brings us finally and inexorably back to God. The physical is revealed to be spiritual. The spiritual is revealed to be physical.

The yoga philosopher might put this truth in a slightly more metaphysical way: The still point of consciousness always shines at the center of the dance of form. The paradox is that the more deeply we penetrate the phenomenal world (the body, the earth) with our attention, the more we discover that the world and its forms are full of God—indeed, are God, or more accurately from the yogic point of view, god and goddess.

There is no escaping this fundamental truth of yoga: as attention becomes highly concentrated in the state of samadhi, life is revealed to be simply a dance that happens between the still point of pure consciousness and the play of pure energy. We have a direct experience of the world being brought into existence moment by moment through the interplay of the two forces of pure being, and pure becoming, shiva and shakti.[16]

Yogis discovered that, under the surface of the mundane world, energy and consciousness are always arcing toward one another—creating what Bapuji called "the ineffable dance of *chitta* (consciousness) and *prana* (energy.)" As Bapuji himself discovered through years of dedicated practice, whatever separates us from God is finally destroyed in this dance. And God, by way of the dance, is always bringing us back to herself. Ramakrishna articulates this view when he says, "The whole world is God alone. The universe is a manifestation of God's power and glory. God has created all these—the sky, stars, moon, sun, mountains, ocean, men, animals. They constitute His Glory. He is within us, in our hearts. Again, He is outside. All of Life is simply the play of God in his mansion of mirth."[17]

Tony was as surprised as anybody when his devotional heart was aroused by his yoga practice—when he discovered God to be right in his own body. Indeed, for Tony this was a somewhat bewildering development, and he and I spent many hours in conversation about its meaning. Eventually, again to his surprise, he began to make tentative forays back to the Catholic Church of his youth. He found himself compelled to revisit this side of his religious nature—searching for an appropriate form for the universal spirit of *bhakti* that yoga had reawakened in him.

"All spiritual journeys have a destination of which the traveller is unaware," said theologian Martin Buber. Most of us who start out on the yoga mat do not realize that, if we dedicate ourselves to practice, it is only a matter of time until the mat becomes an altar.

Part Five

THE ROYAL
ROAD HOME

16

THE ROSE IN THE FIRE

You thought that union was a way you could decide to go.
But the soul follows things rejected and almost forgotten.
Your true guide drinks from an undammed stream.

—Rumi,
Translated by Coleman Barks

It was the final morning of Kripalu's first weeklong conference on psychotherapy and yoga, in 1994. The main chapel was packed with hundreds of psychotherapists and yogis from all around the globe. Gurudev was seated in his armchair, to one side of the main altar, dressed in an elegant gold silk robe, feet tucked in lotus, radiant with the stimulating exchange that had taken place during the preceding five days between himself and the speakers at the conference—all well-known figures in the burgeoning American conversation about psychotherapy and spirituality. We sat in the chapel together, awaiting the arrival of our distinguished guests. Among them: Marion Woodman, one of the greatest living students of Carl Jung; Sylvia Boorstein, psychologist and senior American teacher of Buddhism; Jacquelyn Small, pioneer in the synthesis of spirituality and addictions work; and Tom Yeomans, poet, psychologist, and one of the leaders in the field of spiritual psychotherapy.

As the room came into stillness, the keynote speakers entered quietly to take their seats for the final panel discussion. In deference to the presence of the guru, the room was a sea of white. But as if to balance the overweening whiteness of the crowd, Marion Woodman had dressed herself in shocking red, and had thrown a boldly patterned red and purple silk scarf around her neck.

"Do you know whose colors these are?" she asked, when Gurudev expressed delight with her garb.

"These are the colors of the whore of Babylon." She looked right at him. "Red and purple."

The room erupted wildly in laughter and applause. Through the week, Marion had acted as a "tuning fork" for what was hidden, unspoken, outcast, rejected, forgotten. Calling for the red under that sea of white. Calling for the sexuality underneath the spirituality. Calling for the feminine, the divine Mother, even as she stood on the altar of patriarchy—the old Jesuit chapel under the portrait of Bapuji and the mosaic reredos of Ignatius Loyola, the seventeenth-century founder of the Jesuit order.

I had already come to know Marion as a relentless witness for the feminine archetypes—for Shakti, for the goddess, and for the divine Mother. "The feminine," she would insist, "is full of paradox. Imperfect. Messy. Chaotic. Human. To know the wisdom of the feminine, we have to love the matter of our own bodies. Matter equals *mater* equals Mother!"[1]

On this final morning of the conference, Marion was talking explicitly about balancing the masculine and feminine in our community and beyond: "As long as we try to transcend ourselves, reach for the sky, pull away from ground and into spirit, we are heroes carved in stone. We stand atop the pillar alone, blind to the pigeon's droppings. Don't try to transform yourself. Move into yourself. Move into your human unsuccess. Perfection rapes the soul.

"The entire planet is struggling right now to give birth to the new feminine and the new masculine," Marion went on. "The feminine comes to us in nature. Go outside. Look at the amazing waves of green, of lilacs, of blue mountains. We are in the presence of the manifestation right here. And she's reaching for you." Marion told the story of a client's dream: The dreamer dreamed of a huge wave—a wave so immense, it could be seen from miles away. The goddess was riding atop the wave, and as the wave got closer both the goddess and the dreamer merged into it, becoming a golden drop of water in the sea of life.

"Our work is to bring consciousness and the unconscious into harmony. To bring the new masculine and the new feminine together. Isn't this what yoga has always been about? But what will have to perish in the fire in order for this to take place? That is the question." There was an audible rumble through the room.

That evening, after the conference ended, Jacquie Small and I were having a quiet dinner in Lenox. "When you invoke the shadow, the feminine archetype, messiness, imperfection, the immanence of the soul, death and rebirth, the way we did this week," she said, "watch out. Something is going to happen. Add that together with hundreds of people chanting to Shiva for transformation, and you've added nuclear power to the whole thing. Shiva wants to destroy all of our defenses and pretenses. He wants us to stand in the naked truth."

Throughout the week, there had indeed been the unmistakable scent of death and rebirth in the Kripalu community. Even Gurudev had the sense that this particular event was the outward and visible sign of the birth of something previously hidden and unspoken. On the last day of the conference, he said it: "This is a pregnant moment. Something wants to be born. A new community. It's already birthed, as far as I'm concerned."

Little did we know how pregnant the moment really was. Within less than six months, the community would be turned upside down. We would ask for and receive the resignation of Gurudev. Many of the senior members of the community, some residents for twenty years or more, would leave. There was, even as Marion foreshadowed, a large wave headed right for our shores. And the goddess was certainly riding atop it.

WHEN THE DREAM SHATTERS

The psychotherapy and yoga conference had been the culmination of several turbulent years in Kripalu's history. After twenty years of dedicated practice, many community members had discovered that life was feeling stale, confining. Even in the midst of the "path of reality," the faint odor of unreality and inauthenticity was unmistakable. After the conference, it became unbearable. The traditional guru-disciple relationship was keeping a lid on personal empowerment and on the energy of cocreativity in the community. For some younger members it was inhibiting the very fundamental work of individuation and identity-formation. The yogic sublimation of sexual energy had turned, for some, into a strange kind of sour hatred for the embodied life. A kind of yogic spiritual perfectionism was killing the soul. As Marion had pointed out, the exclusive focus on purification, transcendence, and spirit was keeping at bay the energies of immanence, grace, and soul.

Over the course of the two years preceding the conference, the 350 residents of Kripalu had begun to ask some serious questions. Can the classical forms of yoga really serve the growth and transformation of modern Western students? We subjected the forms of yoga, and the realities of our life together, to the light of many of the most masterful practitioners of the Western healing, psychological, religious, and transformational arts. Community members were brought into dialogue with psychoanalysts, Jungians, Reichians, addiction specialists, family therapists, Buddhists, Sufis, rabbis, priests, and healers of all descriptions. A well-known psychodrama coach from Boston had us acting out the ashram's dramas in intensive three-hour sessions, often with one person role-playing the guru. This proved sometimes to be both hysterically funny and alarmingly real. A bioenergetics therapist had us screaming and grunting and wailing on the floor, adding a whole new emotional and quasi-sexual dimension to "meditation-in-motion."

Through the course of one entire year, Gurudev and the senior members of the community went through a kind of family therapy process with very skilled systems-centered therapists. All of the family's dirty laundry was spilled onto the floor of the resident chapel, as Bapuji and all of the saints of the lineage looked on (perhaps amused) from their perch on the altar. At one point, a senior male member of the community charged across the room, driven by twenty years of suppressed resentment and anger. With his face right in the guru's he unloaded. "You never really respected us. You're a complete phony."

Once the shadow was invoked it was everywhere. Marion's tidal wave from the unconscious had hit landfall. Aspects of community life that had once been idealized were now devalued. There was a longing for a new level of authenticity. "Let's get real" was the code word. A new allergy to "spiritual language" erupted. There was a burgeoning emphasis on egalitarianism and femininism, on cocreation, individuation, sexuality. The search for nirguna Brahman, transcendence, had collided directly with the spirit of American pluralism, democracy, realism, and self-reliance. What would survive?

Amrit was by no means unaware of the powerful forces of idealization and projection that had previously sustained the teacher-student roles. And he knew that they were now dissolving. He seemed to say, in so many ways, that he understood that the old paradigm, especially the guru-disciple model, had to die at Kripalu. In an article published in *Yoga Journal*[2] just after the conference described above, Amrit Desai wrote movingly of the "death of the dream," which, paradoxically, his own teaching—and the qualities of transformational space he had helped to build—had made inevitable:

> Twenty-two years ago, at a time when younger Americans were disenchanted with materialistic society, many spiritual seekers came to live at Kripalu to explore a spiritual lifestyle. Many experienced the feeling of finally "coming home" and the possibility of living in a conscious community with a guru, a spiritual father who would nurture their spirits, love and care for them. Even with its simple lifestyle, austere conditions and demands of spiritual disciplines, ashram life held the promise of personal and spiritual fulfillment. Many believed, "This is it! My life will be whole and complete!"[3]

In this article, Amrit revealed that he had some understanding of the psychological needs that brought students to live with him—the need for merger, the need to be safely held and soothed, the need to find a home. He seemed to understand the peculiarly American relationship between orphans and gurus.

ORPHANS AND GURUS

Among the hundreds of people of all ages, races, and religions who have been residents at Kripalu, I can safely say that almost all came seeking some version of the idealized family. In the guru and in the community at Kripalu, thousands of seekers sought the perfect Dad and Mom. In their fellow community members they sought the perfect brother and sister—and, of course, at one point in the life of the community we even used those words to describe one another.

"Orphans" bring a tremendous amount of idealization and projection into their relationship with teachers. We fall in love with our teachers, and with our communities, and as a result we do not see them at all clearly. Psychologist Jack Engler addressed this phenomenon in a discussion we had with him at the time of Gurudev's resignation. "With our teacher," said Jack, "our longing for love and recognition, for perfect goodness and caring, for perfect fairness and justice, is so deep that we project it and see it whether it is there or not. A spiritual teacher is the greatest receptacle of these projections in any culture, but especially in ours where everyone else seems to have defaulted—parents, teachers, priests, ministers and rabbis, therapists, corporate CEOs, elected officials and the president of the United States. So we often see our teachers as we want them to be, not as they are, in all their humanness."[4]

All the paradoxes of the unconscious that we have discussed throughout this book apply as well in our relationships with teachers and communities. While we may be aware of a wish to awaken and come into transformational relationship, we may be unaware of an equally powerful wish to remain hidden and to withdraw. While we may be aware of the wish for empowerment, we may be unaware of the wish for passivity and dependence. While we may be aware of spiritual longing, we may be denying our unconscious sexual longing. Relationships to spiritual teachers and communities are subject to the law of parallel process—they are equally characterized by love and hate, wish and fear, hope and dread, self-love and self-punitive guilt. Generally, in these relationships, one side of this duality is deeply submerged in shadow.

Many Eastern teachers, not understanding the depth of the Orphan archetype in the West, walk right into situations in which they are highly idealized. If the teacher is not aware of his own unresolved needs to be admired, highly praised, and adored, he or she may begin to believe the idealizations of the students. An air of unreality begins to suffuse the entire situation, as it did at Kripalu. Teacher and student grow further and further from an understanding of their complicated unconscious motivations. It is only a matter of time until the situation collapses of its own weight. The powerful forces of idealization are suddenly transmuted into a bonfire of devaluation, hatred, and rage, usually coming on the heels of some dramatic revelation that the teacher, the hoped for god-man or god-woman, is really all too human.

OPTIMAL DISILLUSIONMENT

As Amrit's article continues, it reveals his insight into the next stages of growth toward which the community was moving:

Many entered into a spiritual lifestyle and discipline to fulfil their dreams. But, in order to keep the dream alive, they suppressed a lot of their feelings. In time, these suppressed feelings were destined to shatter their dreams. We tend to believe that love ends when dreams are demolished. In reality, the shattering of dreams is the opportunity for the emergence of true love. . . . In these situations, what is perceived to be the failure of relationship is, in reality, the failure of the dream. . . . I and those at Kripalu who are committed to spiritual growth are determined to use the failure of the dream as an opportunity to enter into an authentic relationship. . . . This new level of honesty is sometimes uncomfortable for us, but it is making a profound impact on our community life. . . . We are in the process of dismantling the old form, which has served its purpose.[5]

Here, Amrit points to perhaps the central truth about psychospiritual growth with which the community was grappling. If we do, in fact, receive a "good enough" experience of being safely held and soothed, as so many of us undeniably had at Kripalu, we then need help and support with the next important developmental task—separating out of the merger and incorporating those capacities to soothe into ourselves.

If we don't manage this task, then we will remain children. In effect, we will play the Orphan throughout all of our lives. We will look for merger in every relationship and we will have major difficulties in living, because, especially as adults, there are very few persons who will be willing or able to play the role of perfect parent for us. We will be terribly disappointed over and over again, and we will become hungrier and hungrier—unconsciously wanting to eat people up, to incorporate them whole, in order to get their center inside us.

We need our powerful love objects to help us learn to separate from them. There is nothing more difficult. Initially, we can only separate through the process of disillusionment. We begin to see the other more clearly, as other, as not self, as not just exactly like us. Under the best of conditions, our idealization of the other is let down softly and gently, through a process therapists call "optimal disillusionment."

One of Semrad's graduate students, for example, describes his own process of "optimal disillusionment" with his beloved mentor.

My first reaction to Dr. Semrad had been to develop a strong positive transference. He represented the idealized "good, wise, all-knowing, all loving, all accepting father." Only as I had more contact with him did I gradually develop a more realistic sense of Elvin Semrad, the man. I learned that, indeed, he wasn't perfect. I began to notice his obesity, his heavy smoking, his habitual lateness for appointments, his frustrating passivity at times, his long hours of overwork, and what seemed a constant sense of sadness underlying his smile. . . . Though I could see imperfections and began to read apparent inconsistencies within the volume of notes I was accumulating, I realized that the more I knew Dr. Semrad, the more I liked him. In fact, by the end of residency, I felt a strong love for him.[6]

Our self-objects can help us to make the disillusionment "optimal" by allowing us to separate while still reassuring us that we're always held in their hearts and minds. We are deeply sustained, knowing that they hold us continuously at the center of their own being. They also support us with their faith that we can learn to hold, soothe, and support ourselves. And in the process of separating, we will need occasional refueling, going back to being held again, perhaps even physically.

We are now working at the "graduate school" level of transformational space. And, on this level, there is one more difficult lesson. According to Heinz Kohut, we finally need to experience the self-object as a "benignly opposing force who continues to be supportive and responsive while allowing or even encouraging [us] to be in active opposition, thus confirming an at least partial autonomy."[7] We need self-objects who are assertive, adversarial, and confrontive, without losing the self-sustaining responsiveness.

This entire process of merger followed by separation is precisely the way in which the relationship between teacher and student is described in the yogic scriptures. Inevitably, the womb experience gives way to the birth experience. The student's own consciousness is birthed. The very best teachers awaken the inner guru—the sadguru, or the awakened mind and heart—of the student. The best teachers eventually leave the students—as Dadaji left Bapuji—or demand that the students leave them (while still being available for occasional "refueling"), precisely so that the student can discover and rely on his own connection with the source. The teacher's final role is to awaken the lotus of the heart, so that the student's own consciousness is called forth.

STANDING IN THE NAKED TRUTH

The experience of separation from the teacher is always painful, and no matter when it comes, it always feels premature. Bapuji longed for and cried out for his guru throughout his life. But Dadaji, in his wisdom, reappeared very infrequently. How would Amrit handle this final developmental challenge? Would he, and the community, survive it? Judging by the perceptive conclusion of his *Yoga Journal* article, Amrit appeared to be ready:

> We need to figure out how to strike a balance between personal freedom and responsible cocreation and how to live in a nonseparative, nonviolent consciousness while being rigorously honest at the same time. Rigorous honesty doesn't always feel good, but it is the only path that leads to authentic, intimate relationships.[8]

This was truly remarkable language for an unsophisticated "poor boy from Halol." Amrit's apparent flexibility sparked a new version of the dream: the hope that together this community could feel its way into new forms to embody the essence of yoga—forms that would be more appropriate for Western adults at the end of the twentieth century; forms that would create the transformational field in which Westerners could mature to full aliveness; forms that would find a new role for the teacher.

At the conference, Sylvia Boorstein had emphasized the importance of creating a "strong-enough container," a container capable of holding the painful truth of new insights, the painful revelation of hidden and previously unbearable truth. Marion Woodman evoked the classic yogic archetype of the fire: "A life truly lived constantly burns away veils of illusion, burns away what is no longer relevant, gradually reveals our essence, until, at last, we are strong enough to stand in our naked truth.

"The rose," Marion said, explicating a line from T. S. Eliot's *Four Quartets*, "is the Western counterpart of the sacred lotus—the symbol

of consciousness. It must stand in the fire in order to burn away illusion
and delusion." Had the community developed a strong-enough container to withstand the bonfire of the opposites that was about to ignite? Could we really acknowledge, experience, and bear the truth?
Did we have the resources to contain our exploration of areas of unconsciousness in our spiritual community and in our teacher? Could we
stand in the hottest fire of yoga?

SHADOWBROOK BURNS AGAIN

One evening, not long after the conference, as I was walking down the
long corridor toward my little former Jesuit's cell on the third floor of
Shadowbrook, I found myself thinking about how well we were doing
as a community. We had really begun to mature—something that most
American contemplative communities had not managed without the
bonfire of a scandal. Just as I turned the corner toward my room, the
ordinarily quiet hallway was pierced by shouting, screaming, and what
sounded like furniture flying.

"You fucked him. For years. You fucked him! Don't tell me you
didn't!"

The entire building stopped breathing in that instant. "Don't lie to
me anymore, you bitch. Stop the lies!"

The raging couple from whom the epithets had originated moved in
and out of an apartment down the hall from me. More screaming.
Slamming of doors. More obscenity than perhaps these walls had ever
heard. The great silence was broken.

I hardly slept that night, knowing, but not knowing, what was to
come. The next morning, as I sat in my office, there came an urgent
knock.

"Come to my office, immediately," said my friend Rani. "We're in
meltdown." Several of the senior members of the community were
huddling in Rani's office. Some looked stricken. Others giddy. The
sense of panic was palpable.

"What's going on?" I demanded.

"Sit down," said Rani. "You're not going to believe this."

The whole sad story poured out. Gurudev had had an affair with
Krishnapriya—the senior administrative officer of the ashram. For
years. Right under everybody's nose. Right under the nose of Mataji,

Amrit's wife, who was much admired and widely considered to be the real saint in the family. But there was even more. Several longtime community members were stepping forward to say that they, too, had had sexual relationships with the guru.

Events unfolded rapidly. A huge community meeting in the main chapel with Gurudev and his family. Shame. Disbelief. Rage. Betrayal. The board of directors' demand for Amrit's immediate resignation, for a public acknowledgment of his inappropriate actions, for direct amends to the women, for financial remuneration where appropriate, and for immediate psychological treatment. These demands must be met, declared the board, before Kripalu could have any further relationship with its founder.

Within days, the guru and his entire family were gone. Press releases were written, forthrightly declaring the details of the scandal. The therapists with whom we had been working throughout the previous year were called. Group sessions. Individual sessions. Standing in the naked truth was difficult to bear, but we were doing it. There was some sense of exhilaration in how effective we were being through this crisis. We were relentlessly honest with the press. Everyone was interested in integrity. We were standing in the best traditions of yoga. We had learned something. This was good.

But the bonfire did not stop there. There were legal maneuverings. Lawyers' bills mounting into the millions. Challenges from former residents. New allegations of sexual misconduct. We worked with consultants—a center for clergy sexual abuse, a mediation firm. The meltdown continued. As the center for clergy sexual abuse had forecast, there was polarization in the community. The guru's throne was smashed to smithereens in the main chapel. The flames raged on. As it turned out, Shadowbrook would have to burn again, almost to the ground, before it could be raised up. The former multimillion-dollar organization came within a hairbreadth of having to declare bankruptcy and close its doors.

Over the course of the next four years, the community would go through a complete death and rebirth. Many of the senior members would leave, to find their way in the world and to bring into the marketplace what they had learned on the mountaintop. Most did well. The more vulnerable remained deeply wounded from the betrayal and death of the idealized family. The entire organization was restructured, from the board down. We sold much of our property. We would no longer be a largely volunteer organization (in the wake of the betrayal, we struggled repeatedly to define the difference between selfless service—or seva—and giving oneself away) but henceforth would hire employees.

Within several years, signs of rebirth were in the ascendant. But the dream had to die, the guru had to leave, and the idealization had to be irreparably broken. The old forms had to be not just challenged, but immolated in order for the new forms to be born. The wave had to break on our heads. This had not been an optimal disillusionment.

THE ROSE IN THE FIRE

The bonfire of Kripalu was full of paradox. The greatest of these, certainly, is that it was in many ways the teachings of Amrit Desai themselves that made the conflagration inevitable. Just as one cannot chant to Shiva and expect to avoid the fire, so, too, one cannot teach the reality project and expect to avoid the complete revelation of whatever is hidden, rejected, abhorrent, and split off from consciousness. One cannot teach the reality project and expect to avoid the bonfire of opposites.

Curiously, Amrit seemed to intuit this. He often said that he believed that, in teaching this way, he was "raising a snake pit in his backyard." During the conference, he had even compared what happens to a psychotherapist in the heat of transference to what happens to the guru: "First comes the idealization. Later on," he said, "just as the therapist is crucified, so is the guru." He paused, beaming, and then added, "I'm delighted." The paradox, and, perhaps, the tragedy, is that though he gave lip service to this notion, he did not really understand its potential power.

Ironically, though, in retrospect, we might say that Desai should indeed have been delighted: as transformational space goes, what Desai and his community had created was better than most. The best transformational space must always be preparing the ground for its own transformation. And the community at Kripalu had indeed done much of that work. Even so, where the processes of transformation are particularly hot, as they were at Kripalu, it is not always possible to avoid "burning down the building," especially when the forms themselves become reified and sacred. Under these conditions, it sometimes takes the energy of the profane to dislodge them. The fire of real transformational space eventually burns up its own forms.

Many still mistakenly see the second immolation of Shadowbrook as a sign of the failure of the community at Kripalu. Those who do are not appreciating how deeply the twins of success and failure are related. It was not the scandal that forced the death of the old forms of yoga at Kripalu. Quite the opposite: It was the impending death of the old paradigm that required the scandal. It is clear that the fact of Amrit Desai's affairs had been in the unconscious of the community all along. It was not new information. Quite a few individuals held the secret. It was simply information that could not be brought to the light of consciousness until the community was more or less ready for it. In 1994 when the scandal erupted, Gurudev had not suddenly changed. In fact, the sexual misconduct was by that time many years old. Amrit was who he had always been—ambitious, brilliant, sometimes a sincere yogi, sometimes just a smooth performer, too often a teacher who was too charming for his own good. It was the community's own capacity to see and bear the truth that had changed.

The bonfire was just as much a sign of success as of failure. The community had created enough maturity, enough of a calmly abiding center, that it was ready to stand in the naked truth, and to be burned by it if necessary. It was ready to let sexuality and spirituality stand hand in hand. It was ready to accept that the Mother has many aspects—not just the good, nurturing Mother in white, but the dark, irrational Mother of shadow as well. It was ready to see failure and smallness where there had been only a halo of success and magnificence. To acknowledge the lie as well as the truth.

"So what is the rose in the fire?" Marion Woodman had asked. "It is soul suffering in the fire of physical pain and passion. It is spirit languishing as it descends into physical limitation. It is matter ascending towards spirit. It is time in timelessness. It is light in matter.

"We learn to live in paradox," she went on, "in a world where two apparently exclusive views are held at the same time. In this world, rhythms of paradox are circuitous, slow, born of feeling rising from the thinking heart. Many sense such a place exists. Few talk or walk from it." The question for the community was—could we walk in this level of paradox?

In many ways, the bonfire of the opposites was entirely predictable, especially for those who might take seriously the Tantric lineage of the community. It's anybody's guess what caused the first fire at Shadowbrook. (Was it the shadow of the Jesuits, one can't help wondering?) But it is clear to me that the second fire at Shadowbrook was the fire of Tantra. Through this fire, Kripalu came into its heritage, into its place in the true lineage of its Tantric forebears—Lord Lakulish, Dadaji, and Bapuji. For as Hindu scholar Sir John Woodroffe says, "The Tantric sadhak is not interested in conventional survival so much as in the fathoming of life and the discovering of its timeless secret. His goal is to incorporate the excluded forces as well as those accepted generally, and experience by this means the essential nonexistence of the antagonistic polarity—its vanishing away, its nirvana."[9]

In yogic lore, it requires a hero (vira) to confront and assimilate both sides of the truth, to embrace the whole world of the creatrix (Shakti). It is only when the lotus of transcendent consciousness stands in the fire of embodied life that the naked truth is revealed in all her power. The second immolation of Shadowbrook was neither failure nor success, but an initiation into the deeper mysteries of yoga, an initiation that, paradoxically, we had all been sincerely invoking.

THE FIRE AND THE ROSE ARE ONE

"You know, Stephen, trying to be a god or a goddess all week long can flip us into wanting to be an animal on the weekend," said Marion, as she took a sip of wine.

Ross and I howled. It was four years after the conflagration, and Marion, her husband Ross, and I were having dinner in Lenox.

"Do you realize what you unleashed when you stood up in the main chapel and invoked the whore of Babylon?" I said.

"Well, it had absolutely nothing to do with me. The shadow was screaming to be heard. Didn't take Carl Jung to see that.

"In the patriarchy, Stephen, everything is split," Marion went on. "It's the way it is in this culture. It's either or. But the wisdom of the feminine is both and. And it's right there in the yogic tradition, too: Shakti embraces and sustains all of creation. All of it must be seen. Embraced. But first, you must be ravished by the irrational. And in the orderly world of the Father, surrendering to the shadow is not easy to accomplish. Sometimes it's just impossible to avoid the fire."

We talked for a while about the drama of the conference. "You know, your community had created enormous light. I guess just through years of yoga—purification, practice, meditation, reaching for God. When I stood up in front of that sea of white, the light was practically blinding. There had to be a huge shadow there. What did Gurudev say, 'The back is as big as the front'?"

"With the wisdom of time," I explained to Marion and Ross, "it seems to me that in many ways, the sexual scandal, difficult as it was, was a cover for what was really happening. A large group of talented adults had given themselves away to their idealized version of a father, had sacrificed too much in order to be safely held and soothed."

"Well, a guru cannot be a guru unless a group of people want to be disciples," said Ross. He was right: Many in the community wanted to be disciples. Wanted the perfect daddy. Wanted the perfect family.

"It's not as if you just invented this stage of spiritual growth, for God's sake," said Ross. "It's what the entire Reformation was about. Moving beyond the priestly intercessor. In Christianity, remember, the Second Person of the Trinity had to ascend, had to leave, before the Spirit could infuse the whole community. It's a stage you just can't skip. It's an archetype—shows up in fairy tales, in children's stories. Across many different cultures. It's basically the parable of Dorothy in the Wizard of Oz, you know."

Ross explained that at the end of Dorothy's journey to see the Wizard of Oz, Glinda, the Good Witch, tells her that she could have gone home anytime she wanted to. She was never a captive in Oz. When Dorothy asks why she hadn't told her this earlier, she replies that Dorothy simply would not have believed her. And this was so. Dorothy had to make the journey toward her fantasized great and powerful Wizard, the all-knowing and all-powerful idealized object who would save her. It was through the course of the quest to find the Wizard that Dorothy developed the skills and self-confidence to see through the Wizard once she confronted him. Only later would she understand that it was her own clear seeing that had finally killed the Wicked Witch. And it was her own power that would finally get her home—not the magical power of the Wizard.[10]

"Exactly," I said. "In many ways, the community had to raise up the idealized father, then expose him—pull the curtain away, as Dorothy did."

Paradoxically, without the experience of having been safely held and soothed, we cannot grow up enough to make the soother our adversary. And, finally, in order to grow up we need the adversary. We need the worthy opponent. We need to feel the effects of our own power in the world, and to experience our own mastery. To acknowledge, experience, and bear reality—and, finally, to bring it into perspective.

The final initiation was terrible. It required the death of the idealized father. However far he had been raised up, that far would he be thrown down. So, for some of those who had made of Amrit Desai a god, he would now inexorably become a devil (at least for a time).

"But the community's job," Marion said, now looking at me quite intently, "is to take back the projections. To acknowledge both the idealizing and devaluing projections, and to suffer the consequences. And the consequences are two-sided. First, the disappointment, the loss of the dream, the acknowledgment of delusion, the grief of letting go of yet another illusion from childhood. But the other side is empowerment—seeing that it's not out there. It's in here. And always was. Remember, when Dorothy gets back to Kansas, she looks at her glittering red shoes, and says, 'Now I realize that it was all *right here* to begin with.' This is mature spirituality. Reality always brings us to this crossroads.

"Life wants us to be whole. Life wants us to remember ourselves. Everything nudges us in that direction," said Marion. "The real will always triumph."

"Here's the most fascinating paradox of all," I said. "After the conflagration, I started reading the history of our lineage. I discovered that the Pashupat lineage, from which Kripalu springs, was probably one of the earliest and most influential of the Hindu religious sects dedicated to Shiva. It was a classic left-handed path. That is, it was devoted to the shadow and to incorporating all of the things that most people rejected—to finding God in the dung heap, in the lowest of the low, in sexuality. Pashupats would hang from trees and act like monkeys. Walk around naked, making lewd gestures, taking daily baths in ashes."

"And in some deep way, you're marked with that consciousness, Stephen," said Ross. "It's planted like a seed. The shadow was bound to reassert itself."

"This is so much the wisdom of Jung," continued Marion. "If we allow ourselves to be ravished by the irrational, we are compelled to face our own evil. Trust takes on a new dimension. In knowing our own darkness, we know what another's darkness can release. We learn to forgive and to love. Then, we don't know from moment to moment what will happen next. As your Pashupats clearly understood—this is God's country, not ours."

17

THE TRIUMPH OF THE REAL

> After long searches here and there, in temples and
> in churches, in earths and in heavens, at last you
> come back, completing the circle from where you
> started, to your own soul and find that He, for
> whom you have been seeking all over the world,
> for whom you have been weeping and praying in
> churches and temples, on whom you were looking
> as the mystery of all mysteries shrouded in the
> clouds, is nearest of the near, is your own Self, the
> reality of your life, body and soul.
>
> —Swami Vivekenanda

It was a sweltering August weekend in the Berkshires, not unlike the
weekend of my first meditation retreat at Kripalu ten years earlier.
Once again I was sitting in the resident chapel with seventy other silent
meditators, rivulets of sweat rolling down my back. Images of my first
retreat welled up in my mind, and I thought with some satisfaction how
different this retreat would be from that one. Now, I prided myself on
knowing my way around the meditation cushion. Frequently over the
past several years, I had penetrated deep states of concentration either
in meditation or in yoga postures. Just as the ancient texts promised, I
had had experiences of dissolving my physical body into light, had
watched discrete mind-moments move one by one past the still point of
my consciousness, and had observed thoughts and sensations, like individual frames in a movie, arise and pass away. I had had momentary
flashes of insight—of seeing through the erroneous beliefs, knowing

the root of suffering to be ignorance. I had experienced transcendent moments of well-being in various states of samadhi.

On this particular weekend, I longed to go there again. I had spent months looking forward to this retreat, to the sweetness of deeply concentrated mind, still body, bare attention. But during the morning session on the second day, I realized that I couldn't hold my attention steady at all. Everything annoyed me: the little catch in the overhead fan that made a ticking noise every time it circled; the noise of the dumbwaiter below. These annoyances had begun as the faintest sounds, almost imperceptible, and they now seemed unbearably loud. Water torture! I felt enormous aversion to sitting, an aversion I watched build into a cataract with the ferocity of Niagara Falls. Nothing was satisfactory. I was having what Buddhist teacher Sylvia Boorstein calls a "multiple hindrance attack"—attacked on all sides by the kleshas, by doubt, aversion, clinging, craving, restlessness.

Nonetheless, I persevered. "Bring the awareness back to the breath. Observe sensation. Let yourself feel the aversion. Where is it in your body?" After two days of sitting through the assaults of the dark forces of Mara, of delusion, I found myself exhausted. Clearly I was trying too hard. Too much effort. Too much clinging. Too much craving. Too much disappointment. I couldn't seem to let go of my hopes for how this weekend would be. Finally, I was at my wits' end. I wanted to go outside and howl like a wolf.

Yet with all the voices of aversion screaming their loudest, there was a small voice that kept saying something like, "Give up. Just give up." For a while I swatted it away. Spiritual warriors do not give up. I'm going to tame this wild mind. "Give up." Finally, from someplace deep inside, the white flag was raised. The final holdout cell had given the order: Surrender!

Then, as if from afar, I watched myself do something radical: I got up, left the meditation hall, and walked outside. My body seemed to know that in this particular case, giving up required a physical act of surrender. The air was sultry, and the sweet smell of freshly mowed grass wafted up from the lawns. The August day was full of the ripeness of mature summer—lush greens and a high blue sky. I walked up the hill and through the orchard to a path that led through a stand of woods to a small, clear, green pond.

I sat on a bench just at the edge of the pond, surrounded by utter quiet. What a relief to drop all that effort and straining. As I settled into my perch, I realized I was not alone. Just at my feet was a row of twenty or twenty-five frogs sunning themselves on rocks and logs. I watched the frogs for a while. These frogs knew how to meditate, I thought—talk about "just sitting, just breathing." I exhaled a huge, pent-up sigh. Somehow, their mud-covered primeval presence spoke to my cells. They certainly had "nowhere to go and nothing to do"— except to catch the occasional fly.

I sat with the frogs for hours that day. I let them teach me nondoing. Because I was calmed down enough, and quiet enough just to sit with them, to breathe with them, I had epiphanies of insight. Just sitting there in the sunlight, I had insight into impermanence, into no-self, into suffering—the so-called three marks of existence. This is what I had been trying for in the meditation hall, but here it was, right here with the frogs.

The great Theravadan monk Ajahn Chah used to teach that the whole world is teaching the dharma (the truth) to us all the time. "All times and all places become occasions for us to hear the dharma," he said.[1] The lesson is right here, but where are we? In order to hear the teaching, we must slow down, cultivate awareness, and tune in. Most of all, we have to drop our hopes and dreams and preconceived notions of how it should be. We must look at how it is. We must look with a mind that lets go. Then we will see.

In the entire path of yoga, there is really only one lesson. It is the one lesson we have to learn over and over again. And each time, it arrives as an epiphany, as it did, again, to me that day with the frogs: Whenever we relinquish our craving, clinging, and grasping, whenever we stop the war with reality, whenever we are totally present and undivided, we are immediately in union with our true nature.

In every such moment of presence, we come back to the still forest pool—the quiet mind that reflects the real with utter clarity. Whether samadhi happens on the mountaintop or in the marketplace, it is the same still forest pool to which we return, over and over again.

"Try to do everything with a mind that lets go," says Ajahn Chah. "Do not expect any praise or reward. If you let go a little, you will have a little peace. If you let go a lot, you will have a lot of peace. If you let go completely, you will know complete peace and freedom. Your struggles with the world will have come to an end."[2]

Such a simple lesson. Such a difficult lesson. It doesn't matter what we call it: Yoga. Buddhism. Christianity. Relaxation. Consciousness. As

Ajahn Chah says, "Teach the essence of freedom from grasping and call it what you like."[3] When we relinquish the identification with the poles of opposites, when we stop choosing for and against experience, we are established in the witness, and in the state of yoga. But that state is here right now. There is no distance to travel, nothing to do. Every moment in which we simply watch the arising and passing away of thoughts, of craving, of aversion, is a moment of enlightenment. Every moment of witnessing, rather than attempting to divide or separate pleasure from pain, choosing one over the other—that moment is a moment of being awake.

In these moments, we know that it's alright to be happy, to do nothing, to enjoy ourselves—to have a full life in our body. In these moments we know that we don't have to pay for whatever we enjoy. We naturally feel our interconnectedness with other beings. In these precious moments, we awake from the dream of separation and striving in which we usually live, and we experience the hidden depths of life, which are right here for us to see. We experience the essence of all spirituality: generosity, gratitude, and love. And in these moments of transparency we feel more real than ever.

As I sat with the frogs that afternoon, I mused upon how many years it had been since my experience of samadhi on the ladder at Coach's house. And how many "footsteps" I had taken on the path. And yet, had I really discovered anyplace new? Was the so-called developed consciousness of this spiritual seeker any match for the grace of the ladder moments? And that grace had been with me all along—before yoga, before meditation. It had been there always.

In the practice of yoga, the end is in the beginning, and the beginning is in the end. Ramakrishna says this so clearly: "Only the Divine can worship the Divine." It is only because we are already divine that we recognize our own divinity. It is our awake mind and heart that recognizes itself in the mirrors of the phenomenal world. Consciousness is born from consciousness. Indeed, as Ramakrishna says, "How can a maple tree grow from an acorn?"

WHO SEEKS NIRVANA?

I stayed all afternoon at the pond. As the sun began to drop beneath the high oaks and maples, I sauntered back down the hill to Shadowbrook, taking my place once again in the meditation room for the evening dharma talk. The teacher was a bright, young American man— Ivy League educated, and trained in meditation by a very well reputed Theravadan Buddhist monk. He told colorful stories of his time in India and Burma and of his relationship with his fabled teacher.

"Every other afternoon," he said, "I had to walk down the path to my teacher's little mud-and-tile house for an interview and instruction session. As I entered, my teacher would sit completely still and watch my every move. After a while, he would examine me about my practice, often asking some of the classic teaching questions that help to ferret out wrong practice. But the most amazing thing," he continued, "was that I was sure every afternoon when I walked through that door, that my teacher knew every detail of my practice, before I even said a word."

A little buzz of energy was palpable in the room. I could feel all seventy or so students in the room lean a little closer. "His mind was so refined and so subtle that he could penetrate me like a laser beam. He knew me better than I knew myself. I'm convinced that he could see directly into my mind, into my practice." Students in the class nodded knowingly. Suddenly the room was filled with magic.

I recognized the buzz all too well. My belly knotted up and I heaved an audible sigh. So predictable, I thought. We always go for the magic powers, the secret knowledge. We so desperately want to idealize our teachers. We want them to be all-knowing and all-seeing, to have supernormal powers, *siddhis;* we want them to be able to levitate and see directly through us. We desperately want to believe that somebody knows—finally, completely, fully. We want to believe that we will eventually find a "way" that is incontrovertible. A teacher who is incontrovertible.

The funny thing was, I'd been around the world of yoga and meditation long enough to believe that this young American teacher may well have been right. His teacher may indeed have had supernormal powers of intuition. And yet, I'd been far enough down the path of magic with Amrit Desai to know incontrovertibly that there was no pot of gold at the end of that rainbow. As soon as we begin idealizing our teachers, craving their powers, wishing to participate in the glow of their siddhis, it won't be too many months or years until we begin to devalue them. If we make them into gods, we will eventually see them as devils. The back is, after all, as big as the front. And the worst part is that at the same time that we're leaning in toward the magic powers, we will miss the real, more subtle, ordinary magic of transformation in our lives.

As I sat with myself for the rest of the hour, I could feel how much greed and grasping there is in our practice. Our longing for God, for freedom, for being awake is as filled with craving and aversion as any other longing. And because this is so, any active, willful practice that we do to "achieve" God, enlightenment, or samadhi is likely to be simply reinforcing "me," "mine," and "I." My enlightenment. My spiritual progress and perfection. My special powers. My freedom.

Anyone who's been in a spiritual community for even a few weeks, has seen that this is so. Clinging, craving, greed, and hatred are just as prevalent here as anywhere else. There is perfectionism, self-domination, self-rejection, clinging to life, and fear of death. Only the objects are changed. Now, instead of a new Porsche, we're going for a new and higher experience of samadhi, or for perfection in "right speech." Now, we crave some really psychedelic experience of dissolution of the physical body while holding a long, intense yoga posture. Now, instead of our addiction to sex, drugs, or rock 'n' roll, we're addicted to the light. Addicted to the dark side, addicted to the light— what's the difference?

As I left the meditation hall that evening, I felt disillusioned, sad, and a little angry. But mostly, I felt tired. I felt a great wave of skepticism about the entire project of spiritual practice. My afternoon with the frogs had awakened a thought: this is all probably much simpler than we make it. Why does it have to be such a big deal, taking up so much room in my life?

I realized that I was tired of spending all my vacations on retreats, meditating, doing yoga, eating "clean." I wanted to have more fun. To turn back to the world. Hadn't I been a true spiritual warrior, going for enlightenment? Yes, and I was tired. Worn out from it. It was clear that I still had enough greed, hatred, and delusion for many lifetimes. I still had the kleshas, and the erroneous beliefs. Apparently, I was not going to be transformed into a saint in this lifetime. Whatever transformation was happening was surely going to be by grace, not effort. Through letting go, rather than hot pursuit.

Spiritual practice had brought me to a new stage of disillusionment. At that moment, I did not realize that my exhaustion and depression had wisdom in them. It was the wisdom of the Hindu *tantrikas,* who, having tried the way of transcendence, finally declared, "What is gained by *moksha* (liberation)? Who seeks nirvana? After all, water mingles with water."[4]

When all is said and done, most of the stages of spiritual practice are stages of grief work. We have to let go of our deeply cherished dreams and illusions. And there's no way we're going to let them go until we have pretty much worn ourselves out trying to make them work. As Trungpa Rinpoche said, "The shoe of ego is only worn out by walking on it." The moment of raising the white flag, then, is a precious one, one that usually comes only as the fruit of exhaustion. Finally, we step deeper and deeper into the reality project not because we should or because we want to, but because we have to. The shoe is worn out.

THE DISCOVERY OF THE INNER ROOM

"Excuse me, everybody," said Paula over the buzz of conversation, "but can I just have your attention for one minute?"

The conversations stilled. Tom and Geoff, Nina, Paula, and I had stretched out on the patchwork of blankets we'd spread on the mansion lawn for our Sunday afternoon picnic. The late August sun was just beginning to set over Lake Mahkeenac, and Geoff had already lit the big citronella candles to defend us from the onslaught of mosquitoes.

"Drinks in your glasses everybody," demanded Paula. "We're going to raise a toast to the completion of Steve's yearlong sabbatical that in the actual physical realm of space and time just happened to take almost exactly, ahhhh, well, ten years."

Everyone cheered and stood up with glasses raised. Tom picked up his harmonica and played a fanfare. "Speech, speech," yelled Geoff. And as we all sat back down, I felt the challenge and the opportunity of this moment. It was clear that it was time to say something meaningful about my "sabbatical" to this group of friends.

Earlier in the afternoon, as we swam and lay in the sun by Lake Mahkeenac, Paula had reminded me that at the dinner the night before my departure, ten years earlier, I had been full of urgency. I had left as the hunter, with a deep air of purpose. Even, perhaps, an air of desperation. And we remembered how her life, too, at that time, had seemed up for grabs.

In the moment, all of that seemed like a dream. Here we were again, remarkably the same as before. Happier, perhaps. More comfortable with ourselves. And certainly ten years older. Tom had bought and renovated a new home, and he continued to pursue his private practice. Nina had finished her psychoanalytic training and, in addition to her private practice, had now gone about the business of child rearing. Geoff's legal career had, indeed, prospered—and he'd managed to stay out of politics. Paula's company had failed, and she'd found herself very happily teaching yoga and meditation. Only Mark was missing. He had died of AIDS, almost exactly seven years earlier.

As for me—what was my accounting to be?

"Gather round," I said. "Get a little of Tom's outrageous rhubarb pie to keep you company." I topped off everybody's drink from a large thermos of lemonade.

"I'm going to tell you one of the great parables of yoga, a tale shared around campfires and in sacred circles like this one for thousands of years. This is the story about the quest for the true self. Because yogis see this as what our lives are really about. Lifetime after lifetime we're hunting, looking, sniffing out our true self."

I launched into the story of Viveka—how he'd gone to live in exile; how he'd forgotten who he really was; how his mother had come to him in a dream; and how he'd set off on his pilgrimage home. I told the story of his encounter with the seer and his later rescue by the Mother—and the lessons he had learned from each. And I shared how I had followed in Viveka's footsteps for the past ten years—of the seers and Mothers in my life.

"But in the tale," I continued, "Viveka has a final essential lesson— one that I haven't even had a glimpse of until recently. It's the one Viveka must put in place in order to fully recognize his inner kingship." I paused. "The palace in the story represents the Self. And Viveka must find his way to the symbolic center of the Self, the kingship—just as, in Teresa of Avila's masterpiece *The Interior Castle*, the pilgrim must eventually find her way into the mystical 'inner room' of the castle.

"In the final approach to the center, Viveka must enter into an entirely new dimension of practice: he must let go of the longing for enlightenment itself. This is his final—and most difficult—letting go. Paradoxically, in order for his quest to bring him to his final destination, he must call off the search altogether. As Ramakrishna said of this mysterious stage, 'The key to this door truly turns in the opposite direction.' " (With regard to this stage of practice, Viveka's tale carries an important warning for the practitioner. Timing is all-important.

The search must not be called off prematurely, out of aversion, but only when the self has been fully prepared through its efforts.)

I described to my friends my own disillusionment with spiritual practice, and my discovery that craving and greed infect the spiritual life just as they do every other aspect of life. "What I thought I was leaving behind," I said, "I found right here—the kleshas, the erroneous beliefs, creating new spiritual knots." I explained that all spiritual traditions based on direct experience of awake mind have had to deal with this great obstacle: how do we actually practice our true nature without falling into another bind of attachment?

"I'm just beginning to see that for me, the next phase of my journey has got something to do with completely letting go of all my grand schemes for the quest. And, somehow, living into the mantra 'Everything is already OK.' I'm already free. The secret is that I don't have to get to the inner room of the castle. The castle is already in me. I'm already the king."

In order to stand in his true nobility as a fully alive person, as a jivan mukti, Viveka must return to the palace and embrace his dharma—his vocation, his sacred duty in the world. Having discovered who he really is, he must turn back toward the world, which he now understands as God. He must dedicate his life to the world—to the awakening of all beings. Through his renunciation of the life of bliss in the unmanifest realms, the practitioner at this stage makes it clear that the task of moksha—liberation from the vicissitudes of time—was not the highest good. Samsara (this ever-changing, finite, and temporal world) is finally revealed to be the same as nirvana.

At this crossroads, the seeker's profound disillusionment turns to quiet joy. He is at home in the world at last. As Walter Neveel says in his study of Ramakrishna at this stage in his quest,

> he was now able to enjoy the normal conscious state of man.
> For he came to see the Mother not only in the ecstatic trance,
> but all around him in the affairs of man and nature. The frenzy
> of separation abated and we find a man at ease with the world.[5]

THE MATURATION OF THE REALITY PROJECT

All summer I had been wrestling deeply with the final chapter of the Viveka tale. Was it time, now, for me to leave the ashram and find my way again in the world? Gitanand—who was himself preparing to leave—had directed me back to the *Bhagavad Gita:* "You can't really understand this stage of the yogic path," he had said in one of our evening talks, "without understanding this pivotal scripture." I remembered then that Amrit had alluded to this in one of my interviews with him so many years earlier. But only now was I truly ready. The *Bhagavad Gita* had become my latest transitional object. I carried my little paperback copy with me everywhere.

On this particular afternoon, it was tucked into the inside pocket of the now stained and weathered leather-bound journal Mark had given me at my departure dinner. His last photo and a copy of his obituary from *The New York Times* were pasted into the inside cover.

"If you guys are willing, I'd love to tell you just the broad outlines of this story of the *Bhagavad Gita.* I wish Mark were here, because this story is putting together for me something he was trying to teach Paula and me in one of our final talks before he died."

Heads nodded all around the circle.

I briefly recounted the story of Arjuna and Krishna as Desai had told it to me so many years ago (see chapter 5). I told them about Arjuna's impossible choice—acting on his sacred duty as a warrior and facing the karmic consequences of fratricide, or retreating from his duty into inaction and facing the sin of "dereliction of dharma." I spoke of Arjuna's "fit of dejection" as he throws down his arms and declares, "I will not fight this enemy." Of Krishna's teaching that Arjuna "is not who he thinks he is," and his revelation to Arjuna of the secrets of the soul. And finally, of Krishna's revelation of "the divine body."

"OK, so he's 'born divine,'" interjected Tom. "So what? He's still faced with the same difficult choice, isn't he?"

"Exactly. And now we're coming to the central point of the teaching," I went on. "Krishna finally shows Arjuna that there *is* a way out of his dilemma. Arjuna, he says, cannot avoid acting out his dharma. As a warrior, it is his sacred duty to fight in a just war—which this clearly is. This duty, this dharma, came to him from God, and he cannot renounce it without creating further suffering. We cannot escape our true nature."

Finally, however, teaches Krishna, there is no need to renounce action in the world. Rather, what we must renounce is our attachment to the fruits of that action. "Do your duty," says Krishna, "dedicate it to me (meaning both to him personally and to him as a representative of God) and let go of the outcome." Action that is done "desiring the welfare of the world," in alignment with duty and without "attachments to the fruits," is action that leaves no residue of karma, no bondage, no stain of any kind.

Ascetic withdrawal from the life of the world and from the life of the senses had previously been held as the pinnacle of the mature yogic life and ultimately the only way to avoid the accumulation of new karma. Krishna now helps Arjuna to envision a path beyond this earlier ideal, a path that frees the spiritually inclined being to live in the world and to remain free nonetheless from the stain of karma. It allows the devotee to live a full life in the world in any capacity that is "true dharma."

"There is one more essential component to Krishna's teaching," I continued. "In the process of their interaction *in extremis* on the battlefield of Kurukshetra, Arjuna falls in love with Krishna. Krishna encourages Arjuna to take refuge in him, and to act out his duty as an expression of his love for Krishna—and for the One and the many, the God in whom all beings live, and the God who causes all things to be."

This is the most revolutionary aspect of Krishna's teaching, as I explained to my friends. Love is at the core of all true dharma. The enactment of our vocation in the world stands in the stream of love that flows from the divine Self to the individual soul. The *Gita*'s prescription is filled with heart and is colored by an emotionally poignant connection between the god and the man, between the divine and the human. Through love, Krishna teaches, we rise above the field of opposites, of action and inaction, of nature and spirit, of passion and dispassion, to find a synthesis of them all.

At the end of the story, Arjuna has awakened to his true self: "Destroyed is my delusion. Memory has been regained. By Thy grace, O Unfallen One, my doubts are gone. Thy bidding will I do."[6] Arjuna is now established in reality. At the last, the story of the dialogue between Arjuna and Krishna on the battlefield of Kurukshetra is revealed to have been a dialogue between the soul and its eternal source, through which the soul "remembers herself"—knowing her true nature directly once again. Established in the real, Arjuna is free to be fully himself, to live a full life in the world, and to transcend the bondage of karma.

INACTION IN ACTION

As I finished telling the tale, I could feel a kind of exquisite grief welling up inside. The moon had risen higher on Lake Mahkeenac and shimmered in the distance. The coolness of the evening had begun to descend, and Paula and Geoff had pulled a blanket over themselves, their heads just peering out. Everyone seemed lost in thought.

"It's a beautiful story, Steve," said Paula. "But tell us why it means so much to you. I'm not sure that I totally get it."

"OK," I said, understanding that of course my friends had not really felt it the way I had. After all, I'd been living in this story for the past few months as I considered what form my own turn back to the world would take. "Let me back up a bit. I'll tell you why it's so compelling for me right now."

I explained, first of all, that in the yogic view, the great problem of life is desire—clinging, craving, greed, holding on. The afflictions and the four erroneous beliefs are all driven by desire or by its opposite, aversion. Our desire for life to be the way we want it to be, rather than the way it is, is finally what chains us to the great wheel of karma, the wheel of suffering, that goes round and round through endless eons.

This is the great dilemma with which Indian spirituality has wrestled for thousands of years, I explained. And for a good part of that time, the best solution was thought to be a life of renunciation. If action in the world is driven by desire and is therefore binding, then let's not act in the world. Renouncing the phenomenal world seemed to many like the only answer to the conundrum. Spiritual practitioners in the West pretty much came to the same conclusion: monasticism became the featured way of life for the spiritually serious.

But then, as spiritual practice matured on the subcontinent of India, there arose a radical new understanding of the paradox of action and inaction. This was the doctrine of inaction in action (*naishkarmya-karman*), which eventually gave birth to a synthesis so profound that it forever transformed the human conversation about this paradox. This teaching, laid out most eloquently in the *Bhagavad Gita,* had particular meaning for me just now, because I had come to see that a life of renunciation was no longer what I was being called to. Having had a remarkable monastic experience of yoga, I could begin to see the broad outlines of the next phase of my journey. I wanted to be in the world again—knocked about by it, perhaps. I wanted to stop trying to transcend desire in any way, and the pain that it might bring. "Act in the world," teaches Krishna, "in alignment with your true vocation, your true self, and turn over the fruits—and you can rest assured that, then, you are not the Doer of the action."

"The *Gita* added one more critical piece," I continued. "Krishna counseled that devotion is the key to the doctrine of inaction in action. Arjuna must be devoted to seeing God in all beings. He must dedicate his action to the benefit of the One and the many. He must turn over his actions to God and let God hold their fruits. This leaves him beyond the field of opposites—beyond praise and blame, fame and ill-repute, gain and loss, wish and fear, hope and dread, dark and light."

"I see," said Tom. "You dedicate your passion, your energy, your gifts, to something bigger than yourself, and then you just live it fully— and the outcome is none of your business."

"You're right, Steve," said Paula. "This is what Mark was trying to teach us."

I remembered well. The last time Paula and Mark and I had had lunch in New York, he was looking very pale and weak. He was in a philosophical mood. As we sat in a deli munching on oversized tuna sandwiches, Mark had been telling us some of the lessons of his life. "Don't wake up at the end of your life," he said, "and find that you've had yourself at the center of it all along." He went on: "You have to find some one, some thing, some purpose greater than yourself to which you're devoted, and cultivate that devotion. Really give yourself over to it, whether it's teaching, music, family, the law, children, meditation, yoga, gardening. Whatever."

"It's not an idea that belongs exclusively to yoga or Hinduism," I said. "It's an idea that belongs to mature spirituality in many traditions. For example, St. Teresa makes it clear that service in the world is the final outcome of the journey to the center of her 'interior castle.' As she says, 'The spiritual marriage engenders forgetfulness of self. The soul does not worry about honor, heaven, or life. She literally trusts that God will look after her, if she looks after what is His.' "[7]

As it turned out, the entire Kripalu community was struggling with an attempt to integrate the philosophy I was trying to communicate to my friends that afternoon. Many of my peers, and, indeed, my seniors, had left to explore this next stage of their own quest: vocation in the world. But those of us who stayed were determined to transform the organization, rewriting the by-laws in order to make the transition from an explicitly religious organization to a nonprofit educational center—declaring ourselves to be a global community dedicated to creating a compassionate world by helping people create a relationship to spirit.

By the end of my tenth year, I had once again resolved the question I had already faced so many times: to leave or to stay. I knew that my own personal, developmental challenges and those of the community were enough alike that I could probably continue to thrive in the community. And so, once again, I decided to cast my lot with this group of seekers on the mountain in western Massachusetts.

AT HOME IN THE ETERNAL NOW

I was only just beginning to understand, myself, this next phase of the Quest. The final freedom is not freedom from the world. It's freedom in the world. Being "in the state of flow" doesn't mean that we spend all of our time in bliss in the nondual realms. Flow means allowing ourselves to be surrendered to life, to the way it is, and to forget ourselves in pure involvement in our work, our task at hand, our love—without worry over the outcome. As Robert Frost said, "Freedom means moving comfortably in harness."

As yoga matures within us, the intellectual idea that we are born divine becomes transformed into a way of life. We move ineluctably toward trust in the basic OKness of things and in the remarkable intelligence of life itself. We let our dharma—the plan life has for us—find us. And when we surrender to life's plan for us, we discover that we are not the doer. God is the doer.

Paradoxically, in spite of all that has ensued, I still go back again and again to Amrit Desai's credo; set forth in his sixtieth birthday book:

I have no plan for my life.
I accept the plan life has for me.
I follow that plan and what it provides me moment to moment.
I am not the roles I play in following the plan.

I am the witness of all that I interact with in my life.
I was a child, an adult, and will soon be an old man.
I was a son, a brother, a husband, a father, and a grandfather.
I was an artist, a businessman, a yogi, a guru, a friend.
I have been healthy, sick, successful, a failure, awake, and asleep.
Behind all those changing experiences, I am the changeless consciousness
*   that is constantly present.*
I am that I am, in spite of the changes that "I am" experiences.
I am That.
My present is pregnant with all my past.
My future unfolds from the way I live my present.
My being manifests in the present.
I am present.
I am at home in the eternal now, living the plan life has for me.[8]

THE STILL POINT OF THE TURNING WORLD

The moon was at its highest point now, lighting Lake Mahkeenac and the surrounding Stockbridge Bowl with a shimmering blue haze. We huddled together in silence, old friends looking out together on the silent mountainscape. Out of the quiet haze the ghosts of this place arose in my mind's eye: Jesuits, Andrew Carnegie, Bapuji, nineteenth-century picnickers in broad-brimmed straw hats, Mahicans gathered around great ceremonial fires.

I sat with them all, as if at the still point of the turning world. In my mind, I saw the waxing and waning of forms: the gilded houses of the past, the philosophies of East and West, communities, families, relationships, empires, rising and falling. And nothing had really changed.

On the mansion lawn, in the cool of that August evening, my friends had joined me at the still forest pool. For several sublime moments, the boundaries that separated us, our complicated personalities, our struggles, our tragedies, all receded into the stillness of Lake Mahkeenac. We were together on the ladder, in the meditation hall, on the mountaintop. We were young. We were old. We were successful. We were failures. We were at the end of our lives. We were at the beginning of our lives. And everything was absolutely OK. In that ineffable moment, we were joined with the only reality that will remain when all else is washed away by time. The Self is the knower and the seer, and its knowingness and seeingness are immutable. As Krishna says to Arjuna about the Self, "Never is He born or dies. He did not come into being, nor shall He ever come to be. This primeval Self is unborn, eternal, everlasting. It is not slain when the body is slain."[9]

In the shimmering stillness, the world of space and time became transparent, revealing a hidden world in which we were all parts of one another. The many again became the One. We were joined by Mark and Grandma, Grandpa and Bapuji, Vivekananda and Ramakrishna, Semrad and Freud, and all the rest. We were joined by Whitman, who, as if from this same moment, at this same still forest pool, had written:

> *The last scud of day holds back for me,*
> *It flings my likeness after the rest and true as any on the shadow'd*
> *   wilds,*
> *It coaxes me to the vapor and the dusk.*
>
> *I depart as air, I shake my white locks at the runaway sun,*
> *I effuse my flesh in eddies, and drift it in lacy jags.*
>
> *I bequeath myself to the dirt to grow from the grass I love,*
> *If you want me again look for me under your boot-soles.*
>
> *You will hardly know who I am or what I mean,*
> *But I shall be good health to you nevertheless,*
> *And filter and fibre your blood.*
>
> *Failing to fetch me at first keep encouraged,*
> *Missing me one place search another,*
> *I stop somewhere waiting for you.*[10]

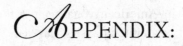PPENDIX:

YOGA METAPHYSICS WITH

A LIGHT TOUCH

When, in 1958, Mircea Eliade first published in this country his majestic study of yoga—*Yoga: Immortality and Freedom*—its publication was the occasion of a delightfully supercilious and all-too-accurate comment on the then-current state of dialogue in this country about yoga.[1] Said the reviewer from *The New Yorker*, "It is altogether free from the intolerable wooliness of thought and the crankiness in which a couple of generations of addlepated theosophist enthusiasts have enveloped the subject; and although it is not light reading it states with clarity and precision what the beliefs and practices of yoga are, and how they originated from the primeval Indic religions."[2]

Addlepated theosophists, indeed. But has the quality of our dialogue improved that much? It's no secret that there's a strong streak of anti-intellectualism in the world of yoga. Amrit Desai often declared, with apparent glee, that he had never read a book straight through. How many times have I heard it?—"yoga is about getting out of your head and into your body." In a culture that perhaps overly values intellect, yoga has often been seen as creating a useful balance.

This is, in my opinion, a misreading and a convenient distortion of yogic tradition. In fact, many yogic paths intentionally work to cultivate not only the powers of the body, but the powers of the mind as well, honing the capacities of intellect so that the more subtle and intuitive capacities of the mind are revealed. The mind is highly valued in yoga, not for itself, but as an essential vehicle to the hidden parts of our nature.

The relentless bias in American yoga against the systematic study and understanding of yoga metaphysics has led to the "intolerable wooliness of thought" to which the reviewer referred, and which most of us involved in the world of yoga know all too well. It has created an enormous amount of confusion about what the practice of yoga really is, complicating the already complicated process of transmission of an Eastern path into a Western culture.

During my first several years at Kripalu I noticed that there was widespread confusion about what the path of Kripalu yoga really was. The confusion was completely understandable. There were elements present of quite a few different yoga traditions—some of them completely contradictory to one another. On one hand, for example, Amrit Desai's descriptions of the path were often saturated with the kind of nondualism characteristic of Vedantic thinking—the individual soul and the cosmic soul were essentially one: God is in every part of us, body, mind, and spirit. But at the same time much of the practice was organized around the rigorously dualistic metaphysic of Patanjali's *Yoga-sutras*, in which spirit *(purusha)* is understood to be completely other than nature *(prakriti)*, and it's only through dissociating from the body that we can identify with our true home in spirit. Indeed, I very often came out of Amrit Desai's yoga talks feeling the way I had in the Calvinist-saturated ethos of my boyhood Presbyterian church: "Gotta try harder. Gotta practice more." This never seemed to fit with the gentle words of the Vedantic *Upanishads:* we are already divine.

This was unfortunately only the beginning of the confusion. On top of this already complicated metaphysic, there was melded a lineage that traced its origins to the Pashupat sect in Gujarat province in India, which worshiped a reincarnation of Shiva—Lord Lakulish. This was a notoriously Tantric path, the primary icon of which is a huge obsidian lingam with the image of Lord Lakulish superimposed with an erect penis, and holding symbols of male and female sexuality. Hello? How exactly does this fit with, say, Patanjali's ashtanga yoga—or with yogic Presbyterianism? To make matters even more interesting, this tradition, in turn, had been joined with an intense form of hatha yoga based on cultivating the free flow of kundalini energy—culminating in the "divine body." Now, add into the mix a large pinch of bhakti yoga (the way of devotion), a very strong dose of karma yoga (the way of service), and . . . aaaarrrrggghh!

"Do I contradict myself? I contradict myself! I contain infinities," said Walt Whitman. What I discovered after a while was that the Indian mind seemed to have vast amounts of room for paradox and for intellectual playfulness—a kind of practiced spaciousness that the Western mind (mine, and most of my peers, at least) did not have. Most of us wrestled with what appeared to be deep logical contradictions between all the various "threads" of yoga with which we'd been confronted. Eventually, many of us gave up. It was a great joke around the community that we were practicing "the pathless path"—because we could never quite put things together in a way that made a complete picture puzzle. The pieces were all there (and then some), but how did they fit together? As a good Episcopalian, I longed for the clarity of *The Articles of Faith:* I could go into any church, pick up the *Prayer Book,* and read exactly what it is I was supposed to believe. And it's all beautifully consistent and linear. Ah, the orderly—and linear—English mind.

But there is a human genius for orderliness in yogic spiritual culture that is just possibly much deeper than the linear mind. Part of the magic of Indian religious culture is that it never throws anything out. It has a genius for preserving the ancient, but adding whatever comes anew, ending up with a vast, tasty stew. One of the great by-products of this is that by and large, it's a culture with an enormous amount of spiritual diversity. Sometimes the tastes blend together and enhance each other. Sometimes they don't. But let's try it, by all means. As Hindu scholar Douglas Brooks has it, "Ideas can be tried on, they can be adopted, they can be assimilated. The Indian philosopher is the intellectual Borg of *Star Trek* lore. He assimilates relentlessly and ruthlessly whatever is good for him."[3]

If you scratch the surface of any of the major yoga lineages that have been influential in the West, you will find a stew similar to the one with which Kripalu students were confronted—slightly different ingredients, perhaps, different tastes, different emphases, but a stew all the same. In my own coming to terms with yoga, I have found it extremely useful to separate out the ingredients of this stew—to look carefully at each of the different aspects of yoga metaphysics, history, and culture that have contributed to the final product.

I have discovered in my career as a yoga teacher, however, that some students are really not so interested in the metaphysical background and historical details of yoga—believing these to be somehow less important than "practice." In fact, mental effort and intellectual rigor are very much considered practice in the yogic traditions. Yogis, as we shall see, do not consider being intellectual different from being physical: in classical yoga, anything that belongs to the realm of the phenomenal world—which the mind manifestly does—is seen as a physical activity. For those readers who wish to extend their understanding of practice—bringing together the metaphysical and the practical—I have added this appendix, which looks a little more closely at important metaphysical questions. The appendix is organized as follows:

I. The term "yoga"
II. The major historical and theological periods in the development of yoga
>   The Vedic period
>   Vedanta
>   The sramanic stream
>   Classical yoga
>   Tantra and hatha yoga
III. The four temperaments
>   Bhakti
>   Karma
>   Jnana
>   Raja
IV. The Kripalu synthesis

I. YOGA: THE TERM

There is certainly no word more subject to "intolerable wooliness of thought" than the word "yoga" itself. Indeed, within the Kripalu community "yoga" seemed to have become one of those words that referred to everything, and consequently to nothing. It became "the yoga of eating," the "yoga of sleeping," "the yoga of consciousness." Part of the root of the confusion is the fact that "yoga" has at least four quite distinct meanings.[4]

1. Any technique of mystic union. The word "yoga" is derived from the Sanskrit root *yuj,* which means to unite, join, harness, contact, or connect. In popular usage, the word yoga can mean any method by which an individual human being is brought into union with God, with reality, with the ground of being, or with source. In this broadest sense, yoga refers to any psychospiritual technology that creates a "reunion with the truth"—in any spiritual tradition. As such, it has at one time or another been used to describe the spiritual disciplines of all of the Eastern contemplative traditions—Hinduism, Buddhism, Sufism, Jainism, and so on. Indeed, it would not be inaccurate to apply yoga in this broadest sense even to the practices of Christianity or Judaism.

One who practices yoga in this sense of the word is a "yogi" or a "yogin." So it's just as appropriate, in this broad sense of the word, to refer to Teresa of Avila or Ignatius Loyola as a yogi as it is to refer to the Hindu god Shiva as a yogi—because they were each practicing a spiritual discipline whose goal was to unite them with ultimate reality.

2. A broad term for Indian spiritual discipline. The second meaning of yoga is somewhat more specific. Yoga refers, here, to a peculiarly Indian psychospiritual technology that began its development as early as 1800 BCE, in the burgeoning culture of the Indus River Valley at Harrapa and Mohenjo-Daro. Archeologists have now uncovered records there depicting human and animal forms and revealing anthropomorphic figures seated in a cross-legged position that most of us, even in the West, associate with this meaning of yoga. This practical spirituality was highly experimental and experiential and usually promoted a kind of radical renunciation and intense spiritual discipline that was discovered to lead to eternal freedom within the yogi's own lifetime. In the post–Indus Valley period, yoga in this sense thrived in what is often referred to as the *sramanic* stream of Indian spirituality. It evolved into countless diverse forms and practices—including the physical practices we know as hatha yoga, as well as the meditation practices designed to lead to samadhi, which laid the groundwork for the later elaborations of Buddhism, and an enormous body of purificatory practices, ethical practices, and so forth.

In this second sense of the term, again, it would be just as appropriate to say that Gandhi was practicing yoga as it would be to say that the great medieval philosopher Shankara or the author of the *Bhagavad Gita,* or Ramana Maharshi, or B. K. S. Iyengar were practicing yoga (or are practicing yoga, in the case of Mr. Iyengar).

3. *Particular forms of yoga.* The next meaning of yoga, thankfully, narrows the field even more. In the context of Indian spiritual practice there arose a number of styles of spiritual discipline, each of which was found to lead to liberation (for different reasons) and each of which was understood to be a particular form of yoga, appealing to human beings of a particular temperament. Here I refer to five styles in particular: bhakti yoga, karma yoga, jnana yoga, hatha yoga, and raja yoga. (I use these terms with the important note that these classifications of yogic styles are quite recent and, though increasingly accepted in the West, they are, as Douglas Brooks asserts, "largely arbitrary"—having meant very different things to different people across the millennia of Indian history.[5]) These peculiarly Indian styles—whatever they may have been called—have waxed and waned over the course of the past several millennia. Each has developed schools, philosophers, brilliant teachers and adherents, adepts, saints, and its own cultural-mythological ethos. For our purposes in this book, bhakti yoga refers to the style of yoga that emphasizes devotion to God, karma yoga to the practice of selfless service, jnana yoga to the path of intellectual discrimination, hatha yoga to the path of the divine body, and raja yoga to the path of meditation.

Within the context of American yoga, most people practice under one of these organizing principles. Most Americans understand yoga to be exclusively hatha yoga. Followers of Yogananda, however, will most likely mean bhakti yoga, students of Ram Dass may mean karma yoga, devotees of Vivekananda may mean raja yoga. In the Kripalu community, I soon discovered that when you ask someone if she practices yoga, she may say yes, but may mean something completely different from your chosen form.

4. *Classical yoga.* In its most specific meaning, the word yoga refers to the most widely accepted codification of the practices of yoga, the path laid out by the sage Patanjali in his concise *Yogasutras,* most likely in about the second century BCE. So brilliant and convincing was this articulation of the yogic path of experiential knowledge that yoga was for the first time accepted as one of the major *darsanas* (doctrine, view, or system of philosophy) of Indian metaphysics, and stood on an equal basis with the other five accepted schools—Nyaya, Vaisheshika, Sankya, Purva Mimansa, and Vedanta.

Even today, many people, when using the word yoga, are referring to this particular school of yogic practice—a school that, as we'll see, is in many ways radically different in its metaphysic from the mainstream of Indian spiritual thought and practice.

II. THE MAJOR HISTORICAL AND THEOLOGICAL PERIODS OF YOGA

Yoga has an astonishingly complicated and nuanced history, spanning at least four thousand years. It is impossible to really come to grips with the views and practices of yoga without understanding at least the broad theological and historical outlines of this remarkable saga.

The Vedic period. This era was the cradle of the fantastic Indian spiritual experiment, and it gave birth to aspects of spirituality that still saturate certain schools of yoga.

The Vedas are four different collections of texts that contain mystical hymns, prayers, and mantras. They were the spiritual texts of the Indo-European sacrificial cult that thrived on the Indian subcontinent in the second millennium BCE. The oldest portions of the four Vedic *samhitas* (or verse-portion texts) date from about 1500 BCE and reached a fixed, but not a written, form about 1100 BCE.

In the Vedic period, "seers"—or holy men and women—were occupied with exploring the human being's relationship with the divine and with the powers of the cosmos. These seers, the earliest yogis, were described as highly disciplined ascetics with long streaming hair who through arduous physical disciplines overcame the limitations of the body. They acquired enormous magical powers, such as the ability to travel through the air and know the thoughts of others. Most important, they were capable of seeing into reality—peering into the unmanifest realms beyond space and time. These Vedic seers expressed what they had seen through sacred poetry. The *Rig Veda,* one of the compilations of this mystic literature, is a treasure trove of these visions, compiled in ten books of verses consisting of 1,028 hymns.

The poems, the collective sacred wisdom of the culture, were originally transmitted orally. They were memorized and handed down from father to son. The poems had to be spoken during ritual sacrifices, and it was essential that they be repeated in an absolutely correct fashion in order to make the sacrifice beneficial. Because of the ritual importance and sacredness of the poetry, an entire new social organization grew up around them. The holders of this sacred wisdom became the ritual, or priestly, class *(varna)* known as Brahmans.

What did the seers discover in their trips into the unmanifest realms? Life was understood to be a battle between the forces of chaos and the forces of order, between the forces of the gods (devas) who propped up and maintained the universe of space and time, and the "antigod" forces *(asuras)* who were seeking a different form of order. Nearly every cosmological hymn talks of creating order, or harmony, in a system that is always on the verge of falling apart. Interestingly, in this view, order is not intrinsic to the universe. It requires cooperation and relationship.

The seers believed that fire was the mouth of God, and that the only way human beings could feed the unseen gods was through offering sacrifices into the fire—into the mouth of God. It was believed that in return for being fed substances they needed, the gods of order would both continue to prop up the universe and feed the sacrificer in return. A request was often made with a sacrifice: "Please bring me a child." There was a give and take relationship with the gods—a sense of inter-dependence between gods and humans.

Vedanta. Literally "Veda's end," "Vedanta" refers to the philosophical traditions that arose on the Indian subcontinent at the end of the Vedic period. There have been a number of different subsets of this tradition, beginning as early as 1500 BCE (though not becoming a real school of thought until the philosopher Gaudapada in the fourth century BCE), and weaving through Indian spiritual history even to the present day. Many of the so-called Vedantist schools (certainly the earliest Vedanta of the important teachers Gaudapada and Shankara, and the later teachings of Ramanuja) hold one fundamental view in common: reality is nondual. All individual souls (atman or Self) are one with the ground of being, the Absolute (brahman). Because we are One with the great river of being, we are all just a single soul—"One without a second." Our true nature is the nature of brahman: *satyam jnanam anantam brahma,* truth-knowledge-infinite is brahman, according to the early *Taittiriya Upanishad;* sat-chit-ananda, or being-consciousness-bliss, according to later *Upanishads.*

The metaphysics of Vedanta were laid out in the astonishing esoteric, gnostic scriptures of the *Upanishads*—perhaps the Indian literature most familiar to Westerners. There are over two hundred *Upanishads*, composed in both poetry and prose, some of them written as recently as our own century. This body of mystical writings includes some of the most inspired and sophisticated scripture in human history. The core writings of Vedanta are the so-called *tritustaya sadhana*, or "threefold resources," the *Upanishads*, the *Vedanta Sutras* of Badarayana, and, most well known to Westerners, the *Bhagavad Gita*. Many of us in the world of American yoga are at least vaguely familiar with the three great maxims of the Upanishadic sages: "Thou art That" *(tat tvam asi)*; "I am the Absolute" *(aham brahma asmi)*; and "All this is the Absolute" *(sarvam brahma asti)*.

The Upanishadic sages taught that the idea of sacrifice, made outward and visible in the elaborate rituals of the Vedic period, must be internalized through the inward act of surrendering attachment and desire. They moved Indian religion away from its highly refined ritualistic roots toward a simplicity that made Upanishadic mysticism a powerful alternative vision. They taught a new kind of metaphysical idealism, focusing upon ecstatic self-transcendance. The "yoga," or spiritual discipline, practiced and taught by Vedantists was the yoga of meditation, a form of inward practice meant to help us separate the real from the unreal—the (capital S) Self from the (small s) self.

The Vedantic teaching provided the metaphysical soil for the growth of yoga in all its forms, because it was fundamentally a path of experiential knowledge (gnosis). The supreme reality (brahman) cannot be reduced to descriptions. Finally, it must not only be described, but it must be realized. Out of this metaphysic arose a view of life that framed the whole of human existence as a movement toward Self-realization. Even with all its metaphysical idealism, Vedanta has always, in practice, retained some coloring of the primitive, archaic flavor of the Vedic period, especially the emphasis on purification, asceticism, heroism, and magical powers still associated with almost all aspects of yoga.

Within the cultural context of Vedanta arose a number of fascinating forms and beliefs that supported the idea of life as a great pilgrimage toward reunion with the true Self. These include views about the continual rebirth of time and space, the existence of unmanifest realms of reality, the existence of countless beings in realms above and below the human realm, the rebirth and transmigration of souls, the belief in the hidden reality of the subtle sheaths of the body (koshas), the four aims of life (arthas), and the four stages of life (ashramas)—and many more.

The two greatest teachers of Vedanta were certainly Shankara (c. 788–820 CE) and Ramanuja (1017–1137 CE). As yoga scholar Georg Feuerstein puts it in his essay on Vedanta:

> [Shankara] succeeded in constructing a coherent philosophical system out of the Upanishadic teachings, and has done more for the survival of Hinduism and the displacement of Buddhism from India than any other single individual. Ramanuja, on the other hand, came to the rescue of *advaita vedanta* tradition when it was threatened with losing itself in dry scholasticism. His notion of the Divine as entailing rather than transcending all qualities encouraged the popular thrust toward a more devotional expression within Hindu spirituality.[6]

The fruit of the spiritual path in Vedanta was jivan mukti—the ideal of "living liberation." Vedantic yogis discovered that through a path of renunciation, meditation, and asceticism they could realize the reality of "truth-knowledge-infinite-brahman," even while living in the human body. Self-realization was a possibility—though it was understood to require a long pilgrimage of the soul through countless lifetimes and incarnations in all realms—god realms, animal realms, unmanifest realms, as well as the human realm. This was a great leap forward for Indian spiritual consciousness, which had theretofore considered freedom and immortality to be available only after death in the land of the spirits and gods. Nonetheless, jivan mukti still required a high degree of transcendence of the human condition. Though nondual, and in some cases radically nondual (advaita vedanta), most Vedantic scriptures describe a path and goal quite saturated with transcendence, rather than the immanence that would come with the later development of Tantrism.

The sramanic stream of yoga. In the midst of traditional Hindu societies that were steeped in some combination of Vedic ritualism and the sophisticated Upanishadic philosophies, there thrived another, more independent stream of yogic practice. This colorful tradition included radical renunciates who thrived at the edge of established religions in India and often existed outside any official sponsorship of powerful hierarchies. They eschewed the traditional paths, insisting that freedom and immortality could be accomplished in "this very lifetime." Their investigations were characterized by a kind of experimental, practical, and almost scientific approach to spirituality known as sramanism (not to be confused with shamanism).

Historically, in India, this kind of yoga was practiced by wandering holy men and women, and it existed in a kaleidoscopic diversity of forms. Yogis of this type rejected the spiritual authority of the Vedic legacy as the ultimate source of truth. The sramanic hierarchy did not share Vedic values, which discriminated on the basis of birth in caste, gender, and even levels of scholastic learning. Yogis in the sramanic stream believed that the only true authority is the soul itself. They believed that the soul could only be known directly, and not through the intervention of powerful priests or bureaucracies. Only through direct realization will the Self be experienced as "infinite, eternal, utterly real and free, as well as immeasurably blissful."[7]

It was this stream of sramanic spiritual thought and practice that young Prince Siddhartha (the bodhisattva who would become the Buddha) joined when he left his palace. He became a wandering mendicant beggar, practicing with and learning from the most accomplished yogis of his day, and adopting the pragmatic, experiential, and experimental framework of yoga. Indeed, it is said that in his six years of practice as a wandering yogi, he had mastered all of the yogic knowledge then available in the sramanic stream (in addition to the knowledge he'd gained in his studies with brahmans), and this knowledge became the foundation of his fresh insight into the nature of reality. In style and practice, the Buddha remained a yogi throughout his life. In his first and most famous utterance, after attaining enlightenment, he referred to a long line of teachers or rishis (seers) who had gone before, and whose line of teaching and practice he was continuing, even as he added revolutionary new insights about practice:

> To you devout monks gathered here I say that I have seen an old path, an old road, traversed by the supremely enlightened ones that have gone before. Along that road I have already gone. Along it I have fully known old age and death. I have also known the path leading to the end of old age and death.[8]

The Buddha was in every way a sramanic yogi, though he ultimately became his own authority, eschewing not only the Vedic legacy as authoritative but transcending even sramanic forms.

Classical yoga: Patanjali's codification of the path. Throughout the millennia of the practice and development of yoga in the sramanic stream, there were many attempts to codify and systematize the practice. Most of these attempts to organize yogic knowledge were foiled by the constant tendency of yogic experiential knowledge to overflow any banks created for it. Yogic knowledge is, by its nature, alive, constantly growing and evolving. At some point quite late in its development, however, a systematic statement emerged that was so inspired, so compelling, that it became widely acknowledged as the authoritative statement of the doctrinal and technical traditions of yoga. (In Sanskrit this is referred to as a darsana.) Patanjali's brilliant codification, called the *Yogasutras,* allowed yoga to stand as a darsana, on an equal footing with the other five major schools of Indian metaphysics.

Paradoxically, the life of the inspired author of this darsana is shrouded in mystery. We know that his name was Patanjali. Most sources suggest that he lived and wrote in the second century CE. We know from his work that he must have been a unique combination of brilliant scholar and very advanced practitioner of yoga—that he knew the path fully and that he happily joined to this experiential knowledge the perspective of a systematizer and compiler of knowledge.

Patanjali sorted through centuries of philosophy and technique, distilling the essential, the time-tested, and the proven into his final formulation. Like the Buddha, whom he succeeded by at least five hundred years, he was scientific and methodical in his pragmatism. He believed that all metaphysical thinking had practical consequences. The path that he describes is not only a *philosophy* but a path of *practical mysticism.*

Classical yoga, as Patanjali's formulation has come to be known, is radically dualist in its description of reality. Rather than one Self (Brahman), the real nature of each soul, says Patanjali, is an individual transcendental self (purusha) that is pure spirit and eternally unchanging. These individual purushas have, through ignorance (avidya) of their true nature, become deeply ensnared in the material world (nature, or prakriti). The material world (prakriti) is quite the opposite of purusha.

Prakriti is eternally changing and absolutely nonspirit. Purusha and prakriti are radically separate. They do not touch at any point. In Patanjali's view, it is impossible to find the true self in the body, or the mind, or anywhere in a human life, because the real self is pure spirit. Our fundamental dilemma is, then, that we are entangled in a realm in which our true nature can never be realized. In the view of classical yoga, freedom (or *kaivalya*) from this ensnarement can be had only by completely disentangling spirit from matter. Kaivalya means "only-ness": one experiences the freedom of pure spirit only apart from and untainted by matter. Self-realization in this system is not about union with the One, but about awakening to the authentic Self, which abides beyond the orbit of Nature.[9]

Patanjali's view, however fantastic it may seem to us, was not just philosophical speculation. It was based on the direct experience of thousands of advanced yoga adepts. Their experience was that this goal of kaivalya can be achieved, even in this very lifetime, but only through the rigorous disciplines of yoga. Patanjali distills the accumulated wisdom and practice of his teachers and their yogic forebears into an astonishing step-by-step path of liberation. The path he describes is based on two wings: *abhyasa,* constant inner practice that leads to the methodical purification of the body, mind, and spirit; and *vairagya,* nonattachment, nondoing, and spiritual surrender.

Patanjali's path was primarily for serious and advanced practitioners of yoga. It required a supernormal degree of renunciation and asceticism—literally requiring the adept to, as Mircea Eliade said, "transcend the human condition entirely." The yogi must transcend the conditions of prakriti—in other words, must transcend conditionality itself. This feat could only be accomplished by "polishing" the human mind and body to such a high degree that, like a mirror or a highly reflective gem, they would reflect the true spiritual nature of purusha. As avidya and all of the other obstacles were attenuated primarily through asceticism (tapas), self-study *(svadhyaya),* and devotion to the Lord *(ishvara-pranidhana),* this reflection would simply call the soul to its true home in pure spirit. The body would be left behind.

The *Yogasutras* are clearly influenced by the archaic spirituality of the Vedas, primarily in their focus on asceticism (tapas) and purification. Also, they are saturated with a description of magical (or supernormal) powers (siddhis) gained through practice. Indeed, over 30 percent of the text of the *Yogasutras* include descriptions of the super-normal capacities that are the fruit of advanced yogic practice. Here, too, we see the influence of more archaic Indian spirituality.

Patanjali wrote in the style of Indian philosophical writings, using pithy, evocative, and very precise half-sentences or aphorisms *(sutras)*, in which every word is rich with meaning. *Sutra* means literally "thread" in Sanskrit, each word being a mnemonic device to connect the mind like a thread to a whole world of associations and meanings. The result is spare, but powerful and poetic. Not only is each word important, as in poetry, but each word's relationship to other words is rich with meaning.

The *Yogasutras,* 195 sutras in all, were meant to be memorized by adepts, held in the mind, repeated, savored, and digested. Medieval yogis came to believe that the very reverberation of the words and the architecture of the sutras in the mind itself had the power to transform consciousness. Consistent with the relentlessly holistic point of view of yoga, words themselves—their sounds, their vibrations, their impact on the physical structure—came to be seen (by Tantric practitioners) as having the capacity to transform the architecture of the mind.

The text of the 195 sutras is divided into four sections—the first section is called the *Samadhipada,* and is the section on ecstasy; the second section, the *Sadhanapada,* is on practice; the third section is the *Vibhutipada,* the chapter on the supernormal powers (siddhis); and the fourth section is the *Kaivalyapada,* the chapter on liberation.

The teachings around which Patanjali organizes his second chapter, the *Sadhanapada* (sadhana meaning "practice" in Sanskrit), are per-haps the most accessible to the beginning student. Included in the *Sadhanapada* is a precise description of the causes of man's enslave-ment to conditioned ways of being—the kleshas, or afflictions, and the four erroneous beliefs. After his description of the ways in which the individual soul becomes ensnared in nature comes a step-by-step tech-nique that unwinds these conditioned "knots" in perception, or sam-skaras. This is the eight-limbed path for which the *Yogasutras* are most well known in the West. This eight-limbed path (or ashtanga yoga) has become deeply identified with the classical form of yoga. The eight limbs are:

1. *Yama:* the restraints, or ethical practices
2. *Niyama:* the observances, or daily practices

3. *Asana:* the physical postures
4. *Pranayama:* breath control
5. *Pratyahara:* withdrawal from external sensory input
6. *Dharana:* the first stage of concentration
7. *Dhyana:* meditation
8. *Samadhi:* ecstasy, or the dissolution of separation between subject and object

The tradition of ashtanga yoga is careful not to use the word "stages" for the eight aspects of practice. The use of the word "limbs" suggests the image of a tree. Though clearly there is a successive nature to these practices (the practitioner must master one before he can move on to the next), they are not true stages because as one moves to the more "advanced" practices the earlier practices are not abandoned. Each of the major limbs continues in play, with its own direct connection to the central life-giving core, the trunk (or spirit). In this sense, each limb of the path is a hologram containing the whole path. Open any door in this remarkable practice, and it opens out onto all of the rest.

Yama and niyama. Bapuji called the practices of the yamas and niyamas "eternal religion," because they represent the core practices of most religious systems. They are also called, in some contemplative paths, the preliminary practices, because they are prerequisites for the more advanced practices of meditation and contemplation. In some texts, the yamas and the niyamas are referred to as the "external instrument" because they begin the process of purification with the most outward and visible aspects of our lives.

The ethical practices (yamas) purify and develop behavior, character, and the capacity for relationship in such a way that the external social container of life is strong, resilient, and clear, and so that the most gross, external obstacles to liberation are worked through.

In the classical system of Patanjali, the yamas are:

1. *Ahimsa:* nonharming
2. *Satya:* nonlying
3. *Asteya:* nonstealing
4. *Brahmacharya:* abstaining from sensual indulgence
5. *Aparigraha:* nonpossessiveness

Through the "daily practices" (niyama), we lay the foundations of awareness and equanimity. We refine the character structure, and learn to organize, focus, and direct energy through it. Through the practice of "witness consciousness" in daily life the mind becomes less reactive and more equanimous. I ✓

The classical niyamas are:

1. *Sauca:* purity
2. *Santosh:* contentment
3. *Tapas:* austerity
4. *Svadhyaya:* self-study
5. *Ishvara-pranidhana:* surrender to the Lord

Through practice of the yamas and niyamas we begin to attenuate the power of the five afflictions (kleshas), and to unwind some of the more gross samskaras. ✓

Asana and pranayama. After the yamas and niyamas, the system of ashtanga yoga proceeds to systematically purify and refine our awareness of and identification with each of the sheaths (koshas) in succession, working from the external to the internal. The physical sheath is developed, known, and purified through asana practice (the postures of yoga); the energy body is refined through pranayama (the breathing practices). Because ashtanga yoga places meditative and contemplative practice at the center of its psychospiritual technique, the purification of the physical and energy bodies is done in the service of cultivating awareness and equanimity, and not for the sake of the supernormal physical powers that inevitably result from these practices. Through asana and pranayama, we begin to learn the rudiments of concentration—the powerful capacity to focus attention in a steady stream, which is the sine qua non of the next four stages of practice.

Pratyahara. The first four limbs of practice are meant to prepare the self for a direct encounter with the more subtle mental sheaths, which are often described as having the energy of a great river or flood.

In pratyahara, the practitioner shifts from the exploration and purification of the so-called external instruments (the physical body and the prana body) to the exploration and purification of the internal instruments—the mental body (manomayakosha); the body of intuitive, awake mind (vijnanamayakosha); and finally, the bliss body (anandamayakosha). Yogis call this natural movement of the mind absorption. The entire practice of ashtanga yoga must finally lead us through this doorway.

Dharana, dhyana, and samadhi. The final three stages of the path are separate, but linked, phases of one project—the development of deep states of meditation: first concentration (dharana), then meditation (dhyana), and finally ecstasy (samadhi). The fruit of these last three stages is the emergence of a buddha, a fully awake being. The buddha lives in a state of jivan mukti—enlightened in a human body. In jivan mukti, transcendent insight into reality becomes a trait of consciousness rather than a momentary altered state. The *jivan mukta* lives in the eternal present, a state of pure witness consciousness. All samskaras have been burned away.

Introversion and extroversion: the architecture of the path. The fundamental goal of yoga practice is introversion, which requires the retracing of those steps that led spirit to become entangled in the material world in the first place. Through the process of extroversion, the purusha gradually became ensnared in the afflictions (kleshas). Through the successive practice of the eight limbs of yoga, the kleshas are systematically attenuated, disentangling the self from its fateful misidentification. (This process is outlined in the chart on page 324.)

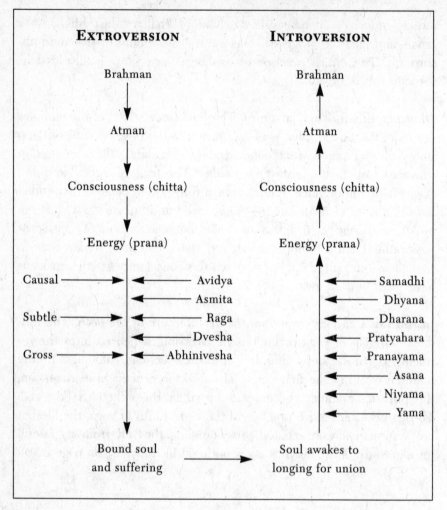

The architecture of the eight-limbed path has been almost universally attributed to Patanjali. Contemporary scholarship, however, is just beginning to reveal that the section on the eight limbs in his *Yogasutras* was most likely a quotation (or possibly even a later interpolation) from a considerably more ancient source. Indeed, we now know that it is most likely that the core of Patanjali's own system was actually not the eight-limbed path, but rather the three stages of kriya yoga—asceticism (tapas), self-study (svadhyaya), and devotion to God (ishvara-pranidhana).

In fact, the eight-limbed path is an ancient system that had been around in some form since the early Upanishadic period. Various versions of the eight-limbed path had been organizing practice in the yogic world since well before the time of the Buddha in the sixth century BCE. Indeed, the Buddha's own eight-fold path, also organized around the practice of meditation, is almost identical in its fundamental architecture to that of ashtanga yoga. Both paths prescribe identical ethical codes, focus on the breath, the purification of the body, and, most important, the same trajectory of meditation and contemplation. It is important to note, however, that while in practical terms the structures of the two paths were quite similar, they differed significantly in metaphysics. Buddhism denied the existence of any ongoing form such as soul or Self, while yoga claimed the existence of individual souls—purushas—which are, of their true nature, pure spirit.

Tantra and hatha yoga. Throughout this essay, I have been describing the Upanishadic-Vedantic tradition of yoga as primarily nondual, and Patanjali's metaphysical framework as dualist. While this is broadly the case, it is nevertheless clear that there is still a quality of dualism in the former. For while Vedanta was a major step for human spiritual culture toward the integration of self and Self, of ego and spirit, of atman and brahman, nonetheless, Vedanta left important questions hanging. Georg Feuerstein has articulated these questions succinctly:

> If there is only the one Self, why should such a struggle be involved in realizing it? Why do we have to think of the world, and thus the body-mind, as an enemy that has to be overcome? To put it more concretely: Why do we have to abandon pleasure in order to realize bliss?[10]

In other words, if our true nature is already awake, enlightened, and free, and if we realize this awake nature when we're not striving, grasping, or clinging, then why do we need spiritual practice?

Eventually, the sophisticated world of Indian spirituality would have to deal with this question. The answer arose with the advent of the movement known as Tantrism, a philosophy that gained ascendancy at least two centuries after Patanjali formulated his *Yogasutras*, and that saturated not just the world of Hinduism, but the Buddhist world as well, thriving across the Indian subcontinent until at least the middle of the second millennium CE.

Tantrism represents a magnificent "great leap forward" for Indian spirituality with regard both to philosophy and practice. Many of the most mature spiritual practices of the human race seek to recognize the identity of spirit and matter, subject and object.[11] They are radically nondual in the sense that they seek to integrate the Self (the Absolute, ultimate reality) and the self (ego, conditioned reality). The Tantric traditions on the Indian subcontinent represented some of the most sophisticated, radically nondualist psychospiritual technologies known to humankind. In the language of Vedanta, the tantrikas (as Tantric practitioners were called) discovered being-consciousness-bliss (and truth-knowledge-infinite) to be right here, right now, always available. In the sophisticated Tantric view, there is no separation between heaven and hell, between ignorance and bliss. In the words of the great Tantric formula, "samsara equals nirvana."

Tantra is truly the path of "nowhere to go and nothing to do." Spirit and the phenomenal world are brought together in its teachings. "The whole world," said Ramakrishna—stating a fundamental Tantric tenet—"is God alone." The Tantric movement is seen by some scholars as an inevitable reaction to the intense dualism of classical yoga—which saw spirit and matter as irrevocably separate. But Tantrism is much more than just a predictable reaction driven by an impulse to balance an extreme view. It represents a quantum leap in spiritual practice, and a much more sophisticated understanding of psychology, philosophy, and practice.

In Tantra, the world is seen as the outward manifestation (the "shining forth") of what exists as pure potential in the godhead. The emanation and embodiment of this potential takes place through a process of condensation from subtle to gross (or a "devolution," or unraveling of subtle into gross), through a series of stages, or cosmic categories, the tattvas—usually numbering thirty-six.

Though in the view of many Tantric practitioners the ultimate transcends all duality, it is conceived as having two poles, or aspects—the masculine and the feminine. The feminine principle, or shakti, is active, and the masculine principle, shiva (or brahman) is pure consciousness. Life is understood to be simply a play of these opposites (lila), and liberation is gained not through renunciation, but through realization of the plenitude of the world, and entering into the dance of energy and consciousness. Feminine entities (goddesses) are especially numerous in this system, which sees the entire cosmic process of world creation as the work of the feminine principle (shakti).

Hatha yoga, the yoga most well known in the West, is the offspring of the Tantric movement, and is in every way philosophically rooted in the Tantras. Indeed, it was the Tantric literature that first comprehensively described the hidden realities hatha yoga sought to explore—the awakening of the so-called kundalini shakti (the coiled serpent energy at the base of the spine), the esoteric physiology of the subtle body (the chakras and nadis), the pathways of prana in the subtle body, and the purification of all the sheaths of the physical, energy, and mental bodies.

Hatha yoga, or "the yoga of force," sought to harness the most subtle energies of the body, initiating a purification of the physical structure that resulted in what was called "the divine body," or "the adamantine body"—the diamond body. Hatha yoga is rooted in a Tantric metaphysic that takes the goals of self-realization one step further than ever before in Indian spirituality: not only can one realize brahman, one can become brahman—one can achieve immortality in the body. The psychospiritual technology of hatha yoga was refined between the seventh and fourteenth centuries CE, primarily by two social groups of northern India: the Nathas and the Siddhas. Its most influential scripture, the *Hathayogapradipika*, was not written until the fourteenth century.

III. THE FOUR TEMPERAMENTS: BHAKTI, KARMA, JNANA, AND RAJA

We have looked very briefly at some of the major streams of Indian metaphysics around which yogic practice has grown. To complete the picture in even the most rudimentary fashion, it is important to understand another major organizing principle of Indian spirituality, which, beginning with the Vedic period, flows in a kind of horizontal way through the evolution of all of these overarching views.

Each of the "views" we have explored in this essay seeks in a general way to do two things—first of all to provide a description of ultimate reality, and secondly to provide the aspirant with a path through which she may realize that reality, whether reality is seen as brahman or purusha. This final organizing principle relates to the second of these two goals—the practice of "the Real."

From earliest times, the cultures of the Indian subcontinent have

been spiritually curious and inventive. In their relentless quest for freedom and immortality, they discovered that there are different human
temperaments, which require different kinds of paths to God. Classi-
cally, Indian spirituality has found it necessary to create parallel paths
for four different kinds of temperaments: bhakti, jnana, karma, and
raja. These four are not paths, or schools, or metaphysics, as has sometimes been suggested. They are, rather, styles of practice, styles that
are found in some combination in all of the overarching systems—
Vedic, Vedantic, classical, and Tantric.

Bhakti. The bhakti temperament wants more than anything to develop
a direct, intense, personal relationship with the divine (or simply with
life—bhakti does not necessarily require the presence of "God"). Such
a person is by nature intensely devotional and is drawn to ritual worship, prayer, mantra, and surrender to some particular image of the
divine, or symbol of the life force. Some religious views lend themselves more to this kind of personality than others. Obviously, Tantric
god-worship (especially focused on Krishna and Rama) might attract
mostly bhakti temperaments, while the classical yoga of the *Yogasutras*
might not. Even so, there is room for bhakti even in classical yoga.
Patanjali makes frequent mention of "devotion." Sometimes, at the end
of a long list of other kinds of practice, for example, he will simply say,
"or by devotion."

Karma. The karma yogi is by temperament action oriented and is
drawn into the world of human affairs. She can transform her action in
the world into a spiritual path through dedicating her action to God
and letting go of the fruits of her actions. Karma yoga is the path of
selfless service (seva)—a way perhaps best described in the *Upanishads*, and particularly in the *Bhagavad Gita*. Sri Krishna teaches the
path of karma yoga to Arjuna on the battlefield of Kurukshetra.

Jnana. The jnana yogi is most drawn by the path of discriminative
intellect. As Swami Prabhavananda puts it, "The jnana yogi rejects all
that is transient and apparent and superficial, saying 'not this, not this'
[neti, neti], and so comes at length to brahman by the process of elimi-
nation."[12] The jnana yogi is drawn to the study of scripture, to reason,
to argument, and to debate, and to systematically separating the unreal
from the real. Some of the most remarkable saints in all of the Indian

pantheon—Shankara and Ramanuja, for example—have been jnana yogis.

Raja. Raja yoga as a category has sometimes been used interchangeably with the yoga of Patanjali's sutras, or the so-called "royal road" of the eight-limbed path. It is this, indeed, but it is much more as well. It might be fair to say that the raja yogi is the psychologist of yoga. The raja yogi is drawn to the methodical, scientific development of the psychospiritual capacities of the human being, for the purpose of "waking up" to the true nature of the real. The raja yogi is by temperament curious, scientific, and drawn not to an intellectual experience, but to a direct experience of the real, often through a systematic combination of bhakti, karma, and jnana practices. The practice of raja yoga inexorably culminates in the most sophisticated and scientific meditative practices of the final four stages of Patanjali's eight-limbed path, or the "internal way"—pratyahara, dharana, dhyana, and samadhi.

IV. THE KRIPALU SYNTHESIS: AWAKE IN THIS VERY MOMENT

This has been the briefest overview of the "stew" of Indian spirituality that we presently have on our plate. By any accounting, it is a remarkable melange—the archaic, magical thinking of the primitive religious imagination is tossed together with the world's most sophisticated metaphysics; animism is intertwined with unitive consciousness; fundamentally nondualist propositions are, in practice, deeply mixed with fundamentally dualist cosmologies.

And yet, each yogic lineage manages to cobble together some lively working synthesis of this four-thousand-year history. In describing the Kripalu synthesis, it is helpful to keep in mind that the contemplative traditions often describe themselves in terms of two categories: view (metaphysics) and practice. In this regard, the approach described in this book might be said to have **a view** saturated with elements of the nondualism of both Vedanta and Tantra, and **a practice** organized principally around the eight-limbed path, with an idiosyncratic hatha yoga technique practiced in the greater context of the meditative goals of raja yoga.

The fundamental tenets of this approach are:

Born divine: First of all, this approach is in every way nondualist, with deep roots in the Upanishadic nondualism of Vedanta. At the center of our true nature is atman, and atman is one with brahman. We are born divine.

Nonseparate: The "whole world," as Bapuji used to say, "is one family." We are all part of a unified field of mind, matter, and soul. In the most literal sense we are all part of one another, just as we are all part of the One.

Already awake: Awakening involves only the process of exposing and relinquishing the false view of the self, and choosing a direct experience of the Self. The experience of our true, awake, enlightened nature is available in every moment when we choose it. There is no distance to travel and nothing to "earn" or prove. Enlightenment is a done deal. It is already our true nature. Because of our deeply conditioned misidentification, however, we may need to use elements of the eight-limbed path to find our way back to reidentification with our true nature.

The body as the temple of the divine: This approach seeks to bring spiritual practice down to earth, and holds with the Tantric view that God is everywhere. Our true nature must be realized in the body, in this embodied lifetime. Realizing our divinity does not in any way require transcending the body or the human condition. The emphasis is on immanence rather than transcendence. In this context, hatha yoga is practiced as an intimate trip to the core of our true nature, as discovered in the physical body and in the energy body.

Life is transformation: This approach focuses on learning to trust the basic wisdom and intelligence of life, to trust energy, and to transform the materials of everyday living into transformational space. How we breathe, eat, sleep, dream, move, speak, and love all contribute to the daily expression and re-creation of our true divine nature. The eight-limbed path may help us to organize life as transformational space, but there is no need to leave life in the world. Life itself is the path. In this way, Kripalu yoga is deeply Tantric, with its roots in trusting the spontaneous wisdom of prana (energy), and in the great Tantric dictum that *samsara* equals nirvana. It's all right here, right now.

The sacredness of the moment: "There is absolutely nothing wrong with this moment." This very moment, however it is showing up, allows us entry into our true nature. Our very humanness is the doorway to our spiritual connection. The vicissitudes of the embodied life are themselves a bridge to the Self. There is no need to escape to some wished-for transcendent realm. As we turn to embrace the world, and our own lives, we will discover that our suffering, conflicts, misfortunes, and neuroses are windows into the real, the divine, the true nature of our mind and heart.

Even this very sketchy and incomplete overview of yogic theology and history reveals the richness of the forms of yoga. And yet, at the risk of confusing the reader, it must be said that change, flux, impermanence, and evolution are at the very heart of yoga itself.

One of the central views that connects our postmodern culture with the ancient cultures of yoga is the understanding that all knowledge is situated in experience. It does not exist apart from the observer, or the participant. All living knowledge is constructed, not discovered. It is inevitably rooted in a particular historical and cultural setting. In the final analysis, it is wise to remember that in our vision of yoga, as in our vision of all things, we see the world not as it is, but as we are.

The living truth of yoga exists only in the tension between its multifarious forms and the realities of immediate practice in the life of real human beings. As the *Upanishads* have it, "Knowledge comes alive only through practice."

NOTES

Introduction

1. In 1994, *Yoga Journal* commissioned a Roper poll, which found six million Americans doing yoga on a regular basis. Current analysis of the growth of yoga, benchmarked to that study, suggests the figure of eleven million by the end of 1999.

Prologue

1. See, for example, Barbara Stoller Miller's discussion in her *Yoga: Discipline of Freedom* (Berkeley: University of California Press, 1996), p. 22.

Chapter 1: Waking Up Is Hard to Do

1. Carl Jung, *Collected Works*. Translated by R. F. C. Hull. Edited by Sir Herbert Read, et al. 20 vols. Bollingen Series XX (Princeton: Princeton University Press, 1953–1979), vol. XI, p. 509.
2. Ibid., vol. VIII, p. 784.
3. Carol Pearson, *The Hero Within: Six Archetypes We Live By* (San Francisco: Harper & Row, 1989), p. 51.

Chapter 2: To the Mountaintop

1. See Mark Epstein on "Transitional Space," in *Thoughts Without a Thinker* (New York: HarperCollins, Basic Books, 1995), p. 122.
2. From, "When Is Religion Transformative?" (a conversation with Wilber, Needleman, and Anthony) in Dick Anthony, Bruce Ecker, and Ken Wilber,

eds., *Spiritual Choices: The Problem of Recognizing Authentic Paths to Inner Transformation* (New York: Paragon House Publishers, 1987), p. 340.

Chapter 3: Brahman: Ecstatic Union with the One

1. Reported by Daniel Goleman, in "Truth and Transformation in Psychological and Spiritual Paths," an edited transcript of a workshop presented September 21, 1985, at the New York Open Center in New York City, copyright 1985, Transpersonal Institute. Published in *The Journal of Transpersonal Psychology,* vol. 17, no. 2, 1985, p. 188.

2. The word *samadhi* is used in subtly different ways within the vast array of distinct yoga traditions. While it always refers to deep states of concentration (union) in which subject/object boundaries dissolve, in some traditions—particularly the classical traditions as codified in about the second century CE—it is seen as the final and most advanced stage of a highly esoteric path of awakening. In this context, my experience on the ladder would be understood not as samadhi itself, but as one of the early, preliminary stages of samadhi— *dharana*, or *dhyana.* See the appendix for an examination of the classical understanding of samadhi.

For simplicity, in the opening chapters of this book, I have used samadhi in its most generic sense, "a deep state of concentration." Later on, especially in chapter 15, where I undertake a detailed description of the state of dhyana, I will explore a more nuanced understanding of samadhi.

3. The *Yogasutras* of Patanjali, III. 3; translation by Georg Feuerstein in *The Philosophy of Classical Yoga* (Rochester, VT: Inner Traditions, 1996), p. 86.

4. A paraphrase of Ramakrishna's words, in Lex Hixon's *Great Swan: Meetings With Ramakrishna* (Boston: Shambhala, 1992), p. 270.

5. Edmund Colledge and Bernard McGinn, trans., *Meister Eckhart* (New York: Paulist Press, 1981), p. 203.

6. Shankara, *Crest Jewel of Discrimination* (Hollywood, CA: Vedanta Press, 1975), p. 115.

7. John Welch, *Spiritual Pilgrims: Carl Jung and Teresa of Avila* (New York: Paulist Press, 1982), p. 105.

8. Hixon, *Great Swan,* p. 270.

9. Teresa of Avila, *The Interior Castle,* Kiernan Kavanaugh and Otilio Rodriguez, trans. (New York: Paulist Press, 1979), quoted in John Welch, *Spiritual Pilgrims,* op. cit., p. 139.

Chapter 4: Shakti: The Play of the Divine Mother

Epigraph is quoted in Hixon, *Great Swan,* p. 16.

1. Hixon puts a charming version of this tale into the mouth of Ramakrishna.

Hixon, *Great Swan,* pp. 173–174. My version is a paraphrase of his retelling. Quotes in the following two paragraphs indicate I'm using Hixon's words. The *Puranas* ("old narrative and ancient lore") is an ancient Indian collection of legends, myths, and customary observances—encyclopedic in breadth and scope.

2. Kali is one of the chief of the fecund, life-giving goddesses. Her insatiable hunger for life must be constantly replenished by blood sacrifices, and she is often represented as black, naked, and adorned with parts of human bodies.

3. Strictly speaking, Brahman and Shiva cannot be identical—as Brahman is formless (*nirguna,* "without form") and Shiva has form (*saguna,* "with form"). Nonetheless, many Shiva traditions say Shiva is Brahman, just as many traditions that honor Krishna say that Krishna is Brahman. In some Tantric lineages, however, such as those of Kashmir Saivism, the story is different, says Hindu scholar Douglas Brooks, "because they are true theists insofar as the absolute is the consciousness who is Shiva and Shiva becomes the world in the form of his Shakti. We might also say that the conceptual scheme of shiva and shakti is simply an *upaya,* a skillful way to articulate the experience of the absolute as both nirguna and saguna. This allows us to have it both ways, since nirguna- and saguna-style talk is not much in the *Tantras* which prefer *saskala* and *niskala,* with and without aspectual nature." (From review notes prepared by Dr. Brooks for this book.)

4. Hixon, *Great Swan,* p. 283.

5. Heinrich Zimmer, *Philosophies of India* (Princeton: Princeton University Press, 1951), p. 576.

Chapter 5: You Are Not Who You Appear to Be

1. Hinduism is a complex body of social, cultural, and religious beliefs that evolved over the course of 4,000 years on the Indian subcontinent. Yoga—a particular discipline by which the individual prepares himself for union with the universal spirit—is only one system of beliefs and practices that evolved in the context of Hinduism.

2. Barbara Stoler Miller, *Yoga: Discipline of Freedom* (Berkeley: University of California Press, 1996), p. 46.

3. Swami Rajarshi Muni, *Awakening the Life Force: The Philosophy and Psychology of Spontaneous Yoga* (St. Paul, MN: Llewellyn Publications, 1994), p. 79.

4. Alain Danielou, *Virtue, Success, Pleasure and Liberation: The Four Aims of Life in the Tradition of Ancient India* (Rochester, VT: Inner Traditions, 1992), p. 3.

Chapter 6: A House on Fire: The Identity Project

1. Quoted in Georg Feuerstein, *Yoga: The Technology of Ecstasy* (New York: Jeremy Tarcher, 1989), p. 81.

2. See the excellent discussion of this in Michael Washburn, *The Ego and the Dynamic Ground: A Transpersonal Theory of Human Development* (Albany: State University of New York Press, 1995), chapter 4.

3. Ibid., p. 99.

4. Ibid., pp. 104–107.

5. Ibid., p. 100.

6. Ibid., p. 105.

7. Albert Camus, *The First Man* (New York: Knopf, 1995), p. 26.

Chapter 7: The Suffering of the False Self

1. Epstein, *Thoughts Without a Thinker*, p. 44.

2. See the excellent discussion of this in Stephen A. Mitchell, *Hope and Dread in Psychoanalysis* (New York: HarperCollins, Basic Books, 1993), p. 132.

3. Ibid., p. 132.

4. David Remnick, *The New Yorker*, March 10, 1997, vol. 73, no. 3, p. 56.

5. Stephen Johnson, *Humanizing the Narcissistic Style* (New York: W. W. Norton, 1987), p. 54.

6. Ibid., p. 54.

7. Bhagwan S. Rajneesh, *Yoga: The Science of the Soul* (Rajneeshpuram, OR: Rajneesh Foundation International, 1976), pp. 6–7.

Chapter 8: From the Unreal to the Real

1. Though I heard Desai declare these views many times, they are also concisely stated in his sixtieth birthday celebration book, Christine Deslauriers, ed., *In the Presence of a Master: Gurudev, Yogi Amrit Desai* (Lenox, MA: Kripalu Publications, 1992), pp. 12, 203.

2. Quoted in Mitchell, *Hope and Dread*, p. 133.

3. Quoted in Prabhavananda and Isherwood, *How to Know*, p. 15.

4. Feuerstein, *Yoga: Technology*, p. 123.

5. This section relies heavily on Johnson, *Humanizing*, pp. 159–161.

6. Ibid., p. 121.

7. Ibid., p. 160. Here, Johnson writes about taking "a personal stand opposing the longstanding sacrifice of self in pursuit of compensatory objectives."

8. This, too, is an idea taken from Johnson, ibid., p. 160.

9. Ibid., p. 145.

10. Ibid., p. 143.

11. John Patrick Shanley (screenwriter), *Moonstruck* (Los Angeles: MGM, 1988).

12. Ken Wilber, *Transformations of Consciousness: Conventional and Contemplative Perspectives on Development* (Boston: Shambhala, 1986), p. 72.

13. Ibid., p. 72.

14. Deslauriers, *In the Presence,* p. 27.

15. Ibid., p. 27.

16. Prabhavananda and Isherwood, *How to Know,* p. 94.

Chapter 9: The Twin Pillars of the Reality Project

1. *Bhagavad Gita,* II. 48, as quoted in Feuerstein, *Yoga: Technology,* p. 16.

2. Susan Rako and Harvey Mazer, eds., *Semrad: The Heart of a Therapist* (Montvale, NJ: Jason Aronson, 1988), p. 17.

3. Ibid., p. 16.

4. Ibid., p. 86.

5. Ibid., p. 106.

6. This particular list is drawn from the work of Daniel Buie, M.D., presented to a Harvard Medical School training course, "Personality Disorders: Treating Deficits in Self-Maintenance Functions," Nantucket Island, August 12–16, 1996.

Chapter 10: Equanimity: On Holding and Being Held

1. For many of the ideas in this chapter, including the phrase "safely held and soothed," and the importance of the concepts of "evocative memory" and "aloneness," I am heavily indebted to the work of Daniel Buie, who develops this material in the context of his unpublished work on the "five psychological self-maintenance functions" of the adult.

2. Quoted in Feuerstein, *Yoga: Technology,* p. 20.

3. Ibid., p. 20.

4. Quoted in Walter G. Neveel, Jr., "The Transformation of Sri Ramakrishna," in Bardwell L. Smith, ed., *Hinduism, New Essays in the History of Religions* (Leiden: E. J. Brill, 1976), p. 73.

5. Ibid., p. 73.

6. Buie suggests the use of Ma Joad as an archetype of the Mother.

7. John Steinbeck, *The Grapes of Wrath,* ed. Peter Lisca (New York: Penguin Viking, 1997), pp. 423–424.

8. Rako and Mazer, *Semrad,* p. 16.

9. Steinbeck, *Grapes of Wrath,* p. 419.

Chapter 11: Awareness: On Seeing and Being Seen

1. Margery Williams, *The Velveteen Rabbit* (New York: Alfred Knopf, 1984).

2. This material is quoted from a talk given by Jack Engler at Kripalu in May of 1995.

3. The material on the Used Child draws heavily on Stephen Johnson's work with this clinical syndrome, in both *Humanizing the Narcissistic Style* and *Characterological Transformation: The Hard Work Miracle* (New York: W. W. Norton, 1985).

4. Johnson suggests Doris Finsecker as an archetype of the Used Child.

5. Samuel Beckett, *Waiting for Godot,* in Louis Kronenberger, ed., *The Best Plays of 1955–56* (New York: Dodd, Mead and Co., 1968), p. 308.

6. Buie uses *Godot* in his exploration of seeing and being seen.

7. Georg Feuerstein, *The Shambhala Guide to Yoga* (Boston: Shambhala, 1996), p. 23.

8. Ibid., p. 23.

9. Engler talk at Kripalu, May 1995.

10. Quoted in Feuerstein, *Shambhala Guide,* p. 31.

11. Johnson, *Humanizing,* p. 172.

12. Mitchell, *Hope and Dread,* p. 35.

13. Johnson, *Humanizing,* p. 156.

14. Williams, *Velveteen Rabbit* (no pagination).

Chapter 12: Awakening the Witness

1. By the time I got to Kripalu, this ice-cream story had achieved the status of an oft-told tale of the early years. Though it is assumed to be true, I was never able to identify the original actors in the drama. Therefore, I offer it in the form in which it came to me: more as legend than as fact.

2. Zimmer, *Philosophies of India,* p. 51.

3. Epstein, *Thoughts,* p. 165.

4. Matthew Arnold, "The Buried Life," in *The Poetical Works of Matthew Arnold,* ed. C. B. Tinker and H. F. Lowry (Oxford: Oxford University Press, 1950), pp. 245–247.

5. Daniel P. Brown and Jack Engler, "The Stages of Mindfulness Meditation: A Validation Study," in Wilber, *Transformations of Consciousness,* p. 211.

6. Coleman Barks, trans., *The Essential Rumi* (New York: HarperCollins, 1995), p. 36.

Chapter 13: Riding the Wave of Breath

1. The psychodynamic material in this chapter regarding the experience of the Hated Child is drawn heavily from Johnson, *Characterological Transformation*, pp. 55–163.

2. Ibid., pp. 55–163.

3. See Swami Rama, Rudolph Ballentine, and Alan Hymes, *Science of Breath: A Practical Guide* (Honesdale, PA: Himalayan Institute, 1979), p. 100.

4. Swami Rama, Rudolph Ballentine, and Swami Ajaya, *Yoga and Psychotherapy: The Evolution of Consciousness* (Honesdale, PA: Himalayan Institute, 1976), p. 54.

5. The "Riding the Wave" technique is now taught nationally by one of its major creators—longtime Kripalu teacher Sandra Scherer (Dayashakti).

6. Quoted in Donna Farhi, *The Breathing Book* (New York: Henry Holt, 1996), p. 110.

Chapter 14: Listening to the Voice of the Body

1. The psychodynamic theory in this chapter relating to the Abandoned Child draws heavily on ideas from Johnson, *Characterological Transformation*, pp. 164–242.

2. For more detail, see Johnson, *Characterological Transformation*, pp. 25–27.

3. This section draws on Thomas Hanna, *Somatics: Reawakening the Mind's Control of Movement, Flexibility and Health* (Reading, MA: Addison-Wesley, 1988), p. 33.

4. Johnson, *Characterological Transformation*, pp. 25–27.

5. Hanna, *Somatics*, p. 27.

6. Ibid., p. 27.

7. Ibid., pp. 95–97.

8. Ibid., p. 97.

9. Ibid., p. 97.

10. See Rama, *Yoga and Psychotherapy*, pp. 14–22.

11. Ibid., pp. 25–28.

12. Farhi, *Breathing Book*, p. 100.

13. Mirka Knaster, *Discovering the Body's Wisdom* (New York: Bantam, 1996), p. 127.

14. Hanna, *Somatics*, p. xiii.

15. Knaster, *Discovering*, p. 144.

16. Ibid., p. 144.

17. Ibid., p. 127.

18. Almost all yoga traditions include a belief in *karma*—the law of cause and effect. The view is, simply stated, that every life situation that we face

(whether difficult or happy) is an *effect* of a previous *cause*—some action that we took either in this lifetime, or in a previous incarnation. Yogis believe that every volitional action plants a seed whose fruit we must harvest—for good or for ill. *Samskaras* are, in effect, the outward and visible energy manifestations of these "seeds." Reincarnation is the vehicle through which the seeds bear fruit. Liberation from samskaras means, in effect, the end of suffering from the "effects" of karmic seeds, and the end of the rounds of death and rebirth.

Interestingly enough, Western psychological theorizing in the late twentieth century has begun to generate some intriguingly similar notions, particularly the observation that we "come in" with certain genetic traits and "inborn temperament"—first "causes" that will inexorably germinate into "effects." The laws of karma are fascinating, and at times complicated and esoteric, and I have chosen not to explore them in this book, partly for reasons of space, and partly because they are not essential to a beginning understanding of yogic practice.

19. Hanna, *Somatics*, p. 39.

Chapter 15: Meditation in Motion

1. Feuerstein, *Shambhala Guide,* p. 93.

2. This is Daniel Goleman's rendering of Csikszentmihalyi, in Daniel Goleman, *The Meditative Mind: The Varieties of Meditative Experience* (New York: Jeremy Tarcher, 1988), p. 181.

3. I. K. Taimni, *The Science of Yoga* (Wheaton, IL: Quest, 1992), p. 280.

4. Daniel Brown, "The Stages of Meditation in Cross Cultural Perspective," in Wilber, Engler, and Brown, eds., *Transformations of Consciousness*, p. 198.

5. Ibid., p. 198.

6. Ibid., p. 199.

7. Ibid., p. 202.

8. Personal conversation with Gray Ward, Gitanand.

9. Swami Chetananda, ed., *Ramakrishna: As We Saw Him* (St. Louis, MO: Vedanta Society of St. Louis, 1990), p. 155.

10. Feuerstein, *Shambhala Guide,* p. 119.

11. B. K. S. Iyengar, *Light on Pranayama* (New York: Crossroads Press, 1987), p. 38.

12. Sylvia Boorstein, *That's Funny, You Don't Look Buddhist* (San Francisco: HarperSanFrancisco, 1997), p. 45.

13. From the *Hathayogapradipika*, II. 2.

14. Jack Kornfield, *A Path with Heart* (New York: Bantam, 1993), p. 123.

15. Boorstein, *That's Funny*, p. 46.

16. *Shiva* is the still point in movement, the absolute subject, the One, the nondual reality. He is the formless *brahman—nirguna brahman—*pure spirit

and without attributes. *Shakti* is the primordial power that is ever at play—creating, preserving, destroying. She is *Kali*. She is matter. She is the phenomenal world. She is the dance. There is no object or event that does not disclose her power. And *shiva* and *shakti* are full of each other. The introvert *shakti* herself is *shiva*, the extrovert *shiva* himself is *shakti*. As Ramakrishna put it in one of his most famous utterances, one cannot think of the absolute without the relative, or the relative without the absolute: "If you accept one, you must accept the other. It is like fire and its power to burn. If you see the fire, you must recognize its power to burn also."

17. See Neveel, "Transformation of Ramakrishna," p. 73.

Chapter 16: The Rose in the Fire

1. Here, and several other places in this chapter, I have interpolated some of Marion Woodman's words from her book (with Jill Mellick), *Coming Home to Myself: Daily Reflections for a Woman's Body and Soul* (Berkeley: Conari Press, 1998). I do this with her permission.

2. From Anne Cushman, "Shrinking the Guru," in *Yoga Journal,* November/December 1994, p. 80.

3. Ibid., p. 80.

4. Engler talk at Kripalu, May 1995.

5. Cushman, "Shrinking," p. 81.

6. Rako and Mazer, *Semrad*, p. 14.

7. From Ernest S. Wolf, *Treating the Self: Elements of Clinical Self-Psychology* (New York: Guilford Press, 1988), p. 55.

8. Cushman, "Shrinking," p. 80.

9. Sir John Woodroffe, quoted in Zimmer, *Philosophies of India*, p. 579.

10. Pearson, *The Hero Within*, p. 41.

Chapter 17: The Triumph of the Real

1. Ajahn Chah, *Bodhinyana: A Collection of Dharma Talks by the Venerable Ajahn Chah* (The Sangha, Bung Wai, Thailand: Bung Wai Forest Monastery, 1982), p. 30.

2. Jack Kornfield and Paul Breiter, eds., *A Still Forest Pool: The Insight Meditation of Achaan Chah* (Wheaton, IL: Quest, 1987), p. 73.

3. Ibid., p. 73.

4. Zimmer, *Philosophies of India*, p. 51.

5. Neveel, "Transformation of Ramakrishna," p. 78.

6. *Bhagavad Gita*, XVIII, 73.

7. Welch, *Spiritual Pilgrims*, p. 182.

8. Deslauriers, *In the Presence*, p. 1.

9. *Bhagavad Gita*, XII, 20.

10. Walt Whitman, "Song of Myself," *Leaves of Grass*.

Appendix: Yoga Metaphysics with a Light Touch

1. Mircea Eliade, *Yoga: Immortality and Freedom* (Princeton: Princeton University Press, 1958).

2. *The New Yorker*, 34:67, December 27, 1958, 160W.

3. Douglas Brooks, Ph.D., Professor of Comparative Religion, University of Rochester, personal conversation.

4. See Feuerstein, *Yoga: Technology*, pp. 15–16.

5. From Douglas Brooks, review notes for this book.

6. Feuerstein, *Yoga: Technology*, p. 82.

7. Ibid., p. 118.

8. From *The Sermon of the Turning of the Wheel of Dharma*. See Vivian Worthington, *A History of Yoga* (New York: Penguin Arkana, 1989), p. 3.

9. Feuerstein, *Yoga: Technology*, p. 200.

10. Ibid., p. 251.

11. Ibid., p. 252.

12. Prabhavananda and Isherwood, *How to Know*, p. 156.

ACKNOWLEDGMENTS

The writing of this book has been a collaborative process in every way.

I am grateful to the Board of Trustees and the President of Kripalu Center for Yoga and Health for their enthusiastic support of this project. Without the kind of institutional support they have offered me, few writers could undertake a project of this scope. In particular, I wish to acknowledge Richard and Danna Faulds, Carolyn Lundeen, Terri Schatz, Greg Zelonka, Nan Futoronsky, and Deborah Orth.

I am grateful to my friends who listened, argued, read, criticized, and tolerated the social withdrawal that I at times found necessary in order to complete the work. Particularly to Adam Mastoon, best friend and fellow author, to Paula O'Hara, tireless partisan of the truth, and to Sandra Cope Stieglitz, my twin sister, champion of the intelligent reader.

I am grateful to my tribe of friends in the worldwide Kripalu Community, for helping to create with their lives the fascinating story of yoga in America that I endeavor to tell. Especially Bruce Cornwell, Michael Keane, Kate Feldman, Grey Ward (Gitanand), Jonathan Foust, Christopher Baxter, John Willey, Michael Carroll (Yoganand), David Sands.

I am grateful to my tribe of friends in the worldwide network of dharma teachers, for inspiration, challenge, and ongoing reality testing about the dharma of books. Especially to Sylvia Boorstein, Anne Cushman, Marion and Ross Woodman, Jacquelyn Small, Lilias Folan, Donna Farhi, Erich Schiffman, Douglas Brooks, Georg Feuerstein, and Richard Miller.

I am grateful for my new colleagues in the world of publishing, for their guidance, and expertise. Especially to Amy Weintraub for helping to build this book from the ground up, to Joan McElroy and Lorraine Nelson for expert editorial assistance with early drafts of the manuscript, and to Ryan Stellabotte, Assistant Editor at Bantam, for his steady hand with details.

I am most grateful to Ned Leavitt, an exceptional agent who believes whole-heartedly in the spiritual life.

Finally, and most important, I wish to acknowledge my editor, Toni Burbank, at Bantam Books. She inspired me, supported me, relentlessly confronted me with the truth when necessary, and enabled me to hold to the highest standards for this work.

PERMISSIONS

INDEX

abandoned child
  and false self, 222–226
  psychology of, 222–223
abhinivesha (fear of death), 64
abhyasa (constant inner practice), 319
Absolute (brahman), 40–44, 52, 54–55,
  115, 314, 315
  union with, 42–45
  see also samadhi; supreme reality
acceptance of self, 189
accountability, avoidance of, 158
action and inaction, 301–302
ahimsa (nonharming), 321
allowing (in yoga practice), 210, 211,
  215
aloneness, feeling of, 146
anatta (no-self), 80–82
  and identity project, 82–84
annamayakosha (reality with body), 105–
  106
  see also reality project
aparigraha (nonpossessiveness), 321
arati (ceremony of light), 99, 100
Arjuna (Bhagavad Gita), 62–63, 66–67,
  299–301
arthas (four aims of life), 316
asana (yoga postures), xiv, 6–7, 23, 52–
  53, 67, 202, 321, 322
  and breathing, 208–209, 248
  and calm abiding, 240–245
  and concentration, 248

and developing proprioception (body
  awareness), 229–230
and flow of postures, see flow of
  postures
ascetic withdrawal, 300
ashram (yoga community), 22
  see also Kripalu Center for Yoga and
  Health
ashramas (four stages of life), 316
ashtanga yoga (eight-limbed yoga)
  architecture of, 324
  and Buddhism, 325
  dharana (first stage of concentration),
  321, 323
  history of, 324–325
  niyama (observances, daily practices),
  320, 321–322
  pranayama (breath control), xiv, 67,
  259, 321, 322
  pratyahara (withdrawal from external
  sensory input), 321, 322–323
  samadhi (ecstasy), 39–41, 43, 44, 67,
  321, 323
  yama (restraints, ethical practices),
  320, 321–322
  see also asana (yoga postures); dhyana
  (meditation)
asmita (I-ness), 64, 76, 295
  see also kleshas (five afflictions); self-
  estrangement
asteya (nonstealing), 321
astral body, 249

ABOUT THE AUTHOR

STEPHEN COPE is a psychotherapist who writes and teaches about the relationship between contemporary psychology and the Eastern contemplative traditions. He holds degrees from Amherst College and Boston College. He is currently Scholar-in-Residence at the Kripalu Center for Yoga and Health, in Lenox, Massachusetts, the largest residential yoga center in the world. He is also author of *The Wisdom of Yoga* and *The Great Work of Your Life*.

ABOUT KRIPALU CENTER

Kripalu Center for Yoga and Health in Lenox, Massachusetts, is one of the largest and most successful yoga-based retreat centers in the world. For more than twenty years, Kripalu Center has influenced the growth of contemporary American yoga. Today, the world's top teachers in yoga, self discovery, and complementary medicine offer workshops and training programs, ranging from single classes and weekend retreats to weeklong programs and longer spiritual lifestyle residencies.

The Center is owned and operated by Kripalu Yoga Fellowship, a nonprofit, charitable and educational organization dedicated to teaching a yogic lifestyle. All programs at Kripalu combine time-tested yogic practices with contemporary wisdom about holistic health, teaching practical, grounded ways to take the practice of yoga off the yoga mat and into daily life. Along the way, students experience the body/mind/spirit integration that leads to healthier and more holistic living.

Two award-winning videos, *Kripalu Yoga Dynamic* with author Stephen Cope and *Kripalu Yoga Gentle* with popular senior teacher Sudha Carolyn Lundeen, are available by calling: 1-888-399-1332.

For a free program guide, call: 1-800-741-7353. Visit Kripalu Center on the web at: www.kripalu.org